MCQs in
ENT

MCQs in
ENT

GC Sahoo MBBS MS FIMSA
Professor and Head, Department of ENT
Rajah Muthiah Medical College and Hospital
Annamalai University
Tamil Nadu
India

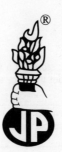

JAYPEE BROTHERS MEDICAL PUBLISHERS (P) LTD

New Delhi • Ahmedabad • Bengaluru • Chennai • Hyderabad • Kochi • Kolkata • Lucknow • Mumbai • Nagpur

Published by

Jitendar P Vij

Jaypee Brothers Medical Publishers (P) Ltd

B-3 EMCA House, 23/23B Ansari Road, Daryaganj, **New Delhi** 110 002, India

Phones: +91-11-23272143, +91-11-23272703, +91-11-23282021

+91-11-23245672, Rel: +91-11-32558559, Fax: +91-11-23276490, +91-11-23245683

e-mail: jaypee@jaypeebrothers.com, Visit our website: www.jaypeebrothers.com

Branches

❑ 2/B, Akruti Society, Jodhpur Gam Road Satellite
   Ahmedabad 380 015, Phones: +91-79-26926233, Rel: +91-79-32988717
   Fax: +91-79-26927094, e-mail: ahmedabad@jaypeebrothers.com

❑ 202 Batavia Chambers, 8 Kumara Krupa Road, Kumara Park East
   Bengaluru 560 001, Phones: +91-80-22285971, +91-80-22382956
   91-80-22372664, Rel: +91-80-32714073, Fax: +91-80-22281761
   e-mail: bangalore@jaypeebrothers.com

❑ 282 IIIrd Floor, Khaleel Shirazi Estate, Fountain Plaza, Pantheon Road
   Chennai 600 008, Phones: +91-44-28193265, +91-44-28194897
   Rel: +91-44-32972089, Fax: +91-44-28193231,
   e-mail: chennai@jaypeebrothers.com

❑ 4-2-1067/1-3, 1st Floor, Balaji Building, Ramkote Cross Road,
   Hyderabad 500 095, Phones: +91-40-66610020, +91-40-24758498
   Rel:+91-40-32940929Fax:+91-40-24758499
   e-mail: hyderabad@jaypeebrothers.com

❑ No. 41/3098, B & B1, Kuruvi Building, St. Vincent Road
   Kochi 682 018, Kerala, Phones: +91-484-4036109, +91-484-2395739
   +91-484-2395740 e-mail: kochi@jaypeebrothers.com

❑ 1-A Indian Mirror Street, Wellington Square
   Kolkata 700 013, Phones: +91-33-22651926, +91-33-22276404
   +91-33-22276415, Rel: +91-33-32901926, Fax: +91-33-22656075
   e-mail: kolkata@jaypeebrothers.com

❑ Lekhraj Market III, B-2, Sector-4, Faizabad Road, Indira Nagar
   Lucknow 226 016 Phones: +91-522-3040553, +91-522-3040554
   e-mail: lucknow@jaypeebrothers.com

❑ 106 Amit Industrial Estate, 61 Dr SS Rao Road, Near MGM Hospital, Parel
   Mumbai 400 012, Phones: +91-22-24124863, +91-22-24104532,
   Rel: +91-22-32926896, Fax: +91-22-24160828
   e-mail: mumbai@jaypeebrothers.com

❑ "KAMALPUSHPA" 38, Reshimbag, Opp. Mohota Science College, Umred Road
   Nagpur 440 009 (MS), Phone: Rel: +91-712-3245220, Fax: +91-712-2704275
   e-mail: nagpur@jaypeebrothers.com

MCQs in ENT

This book has been published in good faith that the material provided by author is original. Every effort is made to ensure accuracy of material, but the publisher, printer and author will not be held responsible for any inadvertent error(s). In case of any dispute, all legal matters are to be settled under Delhi jurisdiction only.

First Edition: **2008**

ISBN 978-81-8448-255-3

Typeset at JPBMP typesetting unit

Printed at Rajkamal Electric Press, B-35/9, G.T.Karnal Road, Delhi-33

In loving memory of my beloved
mother and father
late Smt Ketaki Sahoo and Sri Jadumani Sahoo
to whom I am deeply indebted

CONTRIBUTORS

Adaikappan DMRD Dip NB
Reader, Dept. of Radiology
RMMC and H
Annamalai University

Arulmoli R MD
Prof and Head, Dept. of Anatomy
RMMC and H
Annamalai University

Gandhibabu R MD
Reader-Dept. of Psychiatry
RMMC and H
Annamalai University

Jacinth Cornelius
Prof and Head, Dept. of ENT
Stanley Medical College, Chennai

Jothiramalingam SV MBBS MCh (Neurosurgery)
Prof and Head, Neurosurgery Dept.
RMMC and H
Annamalai University

Lakshmana Rao L BSc MD
Prof and Head, Dept. of Pathology
RMMC and H
Annamalai University

Mishra P MS FRF
Prof of Ophthalmology
RMMC and H
Annamalai University

Mishra SN MS MCh Dip NB
Prof and Head, Dept. of Plastic Surgery
RMMC and H
Annamalai University

Mohan Kameswaran MS FRCS FICS MAMS DLO
Madras ENT Research Foundation, Chennai

Muralidhar P BSc MD
Prof and Head, Dept. of Pharmacology
RMMC and H
Annamalai University

Prabhakar K MSc PhD
Prof of Microbiology
RMMC and H
Annamalai University

Prakash CS MD
Prof of Anaesthesiology
RMMC and H
Annamalai University

Raveenthran V MS MCh
Reader, Dept. of Paediatric Surgery
RMMC and H
Annamalai University

Ruta Shanmugam MS
Prof of ENT
RMMC and H
Annamalai University

Sahoo GC MS FIMSA
Prof and Head, ENT Dept.
RMMC and H
Annamalai University

Sahoo RK MD
Asst Prof of Medicine
JIPMER, Pondicherry

Sampath R MD DMRT
Prof and Head, Dept. of Radiotherapy
RMMC and H
Annamalai University

Sethupathy S MD PhD
Prof and Head, Dept. of Biochemistry
RMMC and H
Annamalai University

Thangavelu A MDS
Prof and Head, OMFS
RMDCH
Annamalai University

Toora BD MD
Reader, Dept. of Biochemistry
APV Medical College
Pondicherry

Tripathy PC MD
Prof of Physiology
RMMC and H
Annamalai University

(Lt Col) Warier MAS
Prof of Surgery
RMMC and H
Annamalai University

PREFACE

In the changing pattern of evaluation system in the otorhinolaryngology and head and neck surgery, especially at the postgraduate level, there is hardly any book on MCQs, available in India at present, keeping in mind the requirements of the students both for MBBS and PG (MS and DLO) Examinations in theory, clinical and practical including viva. The Medical Council of India has also recommended in its regulation for postgraduate medical education in 2000 for a full paper of MCQs to be implemented in five years time. Over and above, most of state and central government recruitment agencies like UPSC also prefer MCQs paper in the selection of various specialist and teachers posts advertised from time to time. It is equally true also in foreign countries like USA, Canada, UK, Australia, New Zealand and even some Gulf countries where Multiple Choice Questions (MCQs) are used in the examination. It is a fact that though basic sciences and allied subjects related to ENT is a full paper at PG level but not much importance is given to that portion. One of the unique features of this book is to integrate all these subjects both horizontally and vertically by contribution from very experienced teachers of these fields to make it a comprehensive book for student-friendly use. It is a humble attempt by a medical teacher in otorhinolaryngology to bring out this book for the academic benefit of the whole ENT fraternity in general and student community in particular. Last but not least, I welcome any positive comment and constructive criticism regarding any omission and errors for improvement in future edition.

GC Sahoo

ACKNOWLEDGEMENTS

I acknowledge with deep appreciation and greatest gratitude from the bottom of my heart for the kind permission given by the authorities of Annamalai University to write this book. I am also grateful for the unstinted support given by my colleagues, especially the contributing authors and the ENT Postgraduates for their meticulous effort to prepare the type script. My sincere thanks to M/s Jaypee Brothers Medical Publishers (P) Ltd, who had done an excellent editorial job to bring out the first edition of this book. I am much indebted to my Professor Dr SK Mahindra, MS, DLO former HOD of ENT Lady Hardinge Medical College, New Delhi for her encouragement and inspiration to do this work. Finally, I would like to thank my son Amit Kumar Sahoo for the computer word processing and all the contributors.

I specially thank, Dr LB Venkatrangan MA, Mphil, PhD, Vice-Chancellor, Annamalai University; Dr M Rathinasabapathi MSc, PhD, MIE, Registrar, Annamalai University; Dr S Vembar MBBS, MSc. Adviser to Vice-chancellor (Faculty of Medicine); Dr PV Hayavadana Rao MS, MCh, Co-ordinator, Distance Education (Medicine); Dr M Ramanathan MS, Dean-Faculty of Medicine; Dr N Chidambaram MD, Medical Superintendent, RMMC and H; Dr S Viswanathan, MD, DMS, Prof and HOD, RMMC and H; Dr VU Shanmugam, MS, Dip NB, AMS, RMMC and H; Dr Ruta Shanmugam, MS, Prof of ENT, RMMC and H; Dr S Balaji, MS, Lecturer in ENT, RMMC and H, Dr R Venkata Ramanan, Dr Prasan Norman, Dr P Mani Maran, Dr N Aravindhan, Dr T Ananda Chockalingam, Dr G Sholai Selvan, Dr D Sridhara Narayanan, Dr NM Arun, Dr Prakash Cherian, Dr R Kanan, Dr R Ramya, Mrs Laxmi Sampath and my wife Mrs Puspanjalee Sahoo and son Anil Kumar Sahoo.

AUTHOR'S NOTE ON TIPS FOR ANSWERING MCQs

It is of utmost importance, the way of approaches to MCQs and the technique of answering the same. Candidates very often leave an MCQs examination without any surety about the performance. The students may unexpectedly fail in the written examination in spite of extensive and intensive preparation, not because of lack of knowledge but simply due to improper examination technique. MCQs often form a substantial component of written (final) examination in most British Medical Schools. Medical Council of India (MCI) should also follow similar pattern of assessment in the PG medical examinations. Prize examinations at regional and National levels are also regularly conducted by the Association of Otolaryngologists of India (AOI) as Quiz competition in MCQs pattern.

The preparation required for an MCQs paper is very different to that for a conventional essay paper. Unlike essay paper where some important and recurring questions can be predicted but in MCQs paper, it is not so because of large volume of questions and a broader range of syllabus. So the best way of preparing of MCQs is to read as widely as possible on a subject with less concentration of memorizing mere facts or data but more on understanding basic principles and concepts. The candidate should follow "Basic Principles for Answering MCQs" as a guideline given in this book.

BASIC PRINCIPLES FOR ANSWERING MCQs

1. Always calculate the time available for each question and stick to the allotted time strictly.
2. Do not spent much time thinking about one particular question.
3. Answer the question using your first impression.
4. Leave the most difficult questions towards the end without much brooding over.
5. Return to these after the first attempt is over.
6. If there is negative marking then don't make wild guess in answering 100% of the questions.
7. It is always beneficial to make an intelligent guess.
8. An understanding of key words and phrases commonly occurring in MCQs is vital for maximum score.
9. Questions which include key words like "Never", "Exclusive" or "Always" are usually false.
10. Questions which include "may", "possible" or "could" are more often true than false.

Even though MCQs are usually perceived as being more difficult than the essay pattern paper but it is more objective and with planned approach to preparation with general overview of the syllabus and careful attention, most of the questions can be answered correctly alongwith educated guesses to score a high percentage of mark.

CONTENTS

Section 1 : Basic Sciences

Section 2 : Otorhinolaryngology (ENT) and Head and Neck Surgery

Section 3 : Allied Subjects

Section 1
Basic Sciences

Anatomy

1. **The following are true about paranasal air sinuses** *except:*
   A. Develop from pharyngeal arches
   B. Develop as diverticula of the lateral nasal wall
   C. Reach their maximum size during puberty
   D. Contribute to the definitive shape of the face

2. **Auditory tube opens into the:**
   A. Lateral wall of oropharynx
   B. Lateral wall of nasopharynx
   C. Lateral wall of laryngopharynx
   D. None of the above

3. **Lateral cricoarytenoid muscle:**
   A. Abducts the vocal cord
   B. Adducts the vocal cord
   C. Tenses the vocal cord
   D. Relaxes the vocal cord

4. **Frontal air sinus opens into:**
   A. Sphenoethmoidal recess
   B. Superior meatus
   C. Middle meatus
   D. Inferior meatus

5. **Vocal folds are abducted by:**
   A. Posterior cricoarytenoid
   B. Lateral cricoarytenoid
   C. Thyroarytenoids
   D. Inter arytenoids

6. **The ear cough is due to the irritation of:**
   A. Internal laryngeal nerve
   B. Great auricular nerve
   C. Arnold's nerve (auricular branch of vagus)
   D. Recurrent laryngeal nerve

7. **Nerve supply to stapedius muscle:**
   A. Glossopharyngeal nerve
   B. Vestibulocochlear nerve
   C. Facial nerve
   D. Mandibular nerve

8. **The nerve piercing the thyrohyoid membrane is:**
   A. Superior laryngeal
   B. Internal laryngeal
   C. External laryngeal
   D. Recurrent laryngeal

9. **Isthmus of the thyroid gland is related to the tracheal rings:**
   A. 2,3
   B. 1,2,3
   C. 2,3,4
   D. 3,4

10. **The nerve involved in temporary huskiness of voice is:**
    A. External laryngeal
    B. Internal laryngeal
    C. Recurrent laryngeal
    D. Phrenic

11. **The central prominent part of tympanic membrane is called:**
    A. Umbo
    B. Tegmen tympani
    C. Fovea centralis
    D. Uncus

12. **Sensory innervation of pinna is by all nerves** *except:*
    A. Greater auricular nerve
    B. Lesser occipital nerve
    C. Auriculotemporal nerve
    D. Posterior auricular nerve

13. **Tonsillar node is:**
    A. Jugulo omohyoid lymph node
    B. Jugulo digastric lymph node
    C. Submandibular lymph node
    D. Submental lymph node

14. **Nose is developed from the following *except*:**
    A. Frontal prominence
    B. Medial nasal prominence
    C. Mandibular prominence
    D. Lateral nasal prominence

15. **Little's area (Kiesselbach's area) is:**
    A. Anterior inferior of quadrant of lateral wall of nose
    B. Posterior inferior of quadrant of lateral wall of nose
    C. Anterior inferior quadrant of nasal septum
    D. Anterior superior quadrant of nasal septum

16. **Suprameatal triangle overlies:**
    A. Mastoid air cells
    B. Maxillary air sinus
    C. Frontal sinus
    D. Sigmoid sinus

17. **The mucous membrane of the larynx below the vocal cord is supplied by:**
    A. External laryngeal nerve
    B. Recurrent laryngeal nerve
    C. Internal laryngeal nerve
    D. Glossopharyngeal nerve

18. **The muscle which relaxes the vocal cord is:**
    A. Criothyroid
    B. Thyroarytenoid
    C. Transverse arytenoids
    D. Oblique arytenoids

19. **The muscle which opens the auditory tube is:**
    A. Tensor palati
    B. Tensor tymphani
    C. Palatoglossus
    D. Palatopharyngeus

20. **Tympanic membrane develops from:**
    A. Ectoderm
    B. Endoderm
    C. Mesoderm
    D. All of the above

21. **Following are correct about auditory tube *except*:**
    A. It is about 35 mm long
    B. It is developed from tubotympanic recess
    C. It gives attachment to levator palatini
    D. It is lined by stratified squamous epithelium

22. **Nerve related to piriform recess is:**
    A. Internal laryngeal nerve
    B. Glossopharyngeal nerve
    C. Greater palatine nerve
    D. External laryngeal nerve

23. **Nasal septum is formed of the following *except*:**
    A. Vomer
    B. Perpendicular plate of ethmoid
    C. Perpendicular plate of palatine bone
    D. Septal cartilage

24. **Of the following one is not an extrinsic muscle of larynx:**
    A. Sternohyoid
    B. Sternothyroid
    C. Cricothyroid
    D. Thyrohyoid

25. **Sixth pharyngeal arch mesoderm gives rise to:**
    A. Hyoid bone
    B. Thyroid cartilage
    C. Epiglottis
    D. Cricoid cartilage

26. **Mastoid antrum:**
    A. Poorly developed in fetus
    B. Anterior extension of the tympanic cavity
    C. Lined by non-ciliated columnar epithelium
    D. Capacity is 5 ml

27. **The cartilage of the second pharyngeal arch forms the following *except*:**
    A. Stapes
    B. Styloid process
    C. Greater cornu of hyoid
    D. Lesser cornua of hyoid bone

28. **Laryngeal cartilage which is immediately above the glottis is:**
    A. Arytenoids cartilage
    B. Thyroid cartilage
    C. Cricoid cartilage
    D. Epiglottis

29. **The following are true about olfactory nerves _except:_**
    A. Are not ' true' cranial nerves
    B. Arise from the neuroepithelium in the roof of the nose
    C. Synapse in the olfactory bulb
    D. Converge on the thalamus before reaching the cortex

30. **The uncinate process of ethmoid bone articulates with:**
    A. Superior turbinate
    B. Middle turbinate
    C. Inferior turbinate
    D. All of the above

31. **True vocal folds are lined by:**
    A. Simple squamous epithelium
    B. Stratified squamous nonkeratinized epithelium
    C. Simple columnar epithelium
    D. Pseudostratified ciliated columnar epithelium

32. **The vestibulocochlear nerve:**
    A. Arises from the nuclei in the midbrain
    B. Is tested prior to diagnosing brain death
    C. Leaves the skull through the jugular foramen
    D. Has a branch which is motor to stapedius

33. **The external ear:**
    A. Receives sensory innervation via great auricular nerve
    B. Receives its blood supply mainly from facial artery
    C. Has muscles which are supplied by facial nerve
    D. None of the above

34. **Which words can not be spoken by a patient with a tracheostomy?**
    A. Nouns
    B. Adjectives
    C. Verbs
    D. Can not speak at all

35. **The nasal cavity is lined by the following _except:_**
    A. Skin
    B. Transitional epithelium
    C. Olfactory epithelium
    D. Respiratory epithelium

36. **The superior laryngeal nerve:**
    A. Is the nerve of the 3rd pharyngeal arch
    B. Is purely a sensory nerve
    C. Divides into external and recurrent laryngeal nerves
    D. Affects the pitch of the voice when affected

37. **The roof of the nasal cavity is formed by the following _except:_**
    A. Nasal spine of frontal bone
    B. Lateral processes of septal cartilages
    C. Anterior surface of sphenoid bone
    D. Horizontal plate of the palatine bone

38. **Choanae are:**
    A. Openings between nasal cavity and nasopharynx
    B. Openings between nasal cavity and oropharynx
    C. Openings between oral cavity and nasopharynx
    D. None of the above

39. **The following arteries supply the nasal cavity _except:_**
    A. Sphenopalatine artery
    B. Greater palatine artery
    C. Anterior ethmoidal artery
    D. Nasopalatine artery

40. **The external acoustic meatus:**
    A. Its lateral 1/3 is cartilaginous and medial 2/3 is bony tunnel
    B. Has sebaceous glands which produce cerumen (ear wax)
    C. It follows a straight course
    D. Only cartiginous part is covered with skin

41. **The cochlea contains the following _except:_**
    A. Scala vestibuli
    B. Scala tympani
    C. Spiral organ of corti
    D. Saccule and utricle

42. **The endolymph is present in the:**
    A. Cochlear duct
    B. Scala vestibuli
    C. Scala tympani
    D. All of the above

43. **The anterior wall of the middle ear contains the following except:**
    A. Pharyngo tympanic tube
    B. Pyramidal eminence
    C. Tensor tympani muscle
    D. Branch from internal carotid plexus

44. **The membranous labyrinth of the inner ear:**
    A. Receives its blood supply via branches of internal carotid artery
    B. Contains the saccule and utricle within the vestibuli
    C. Contains the duct of cochlea which is connected to the middle ear by oval window
    D. Contains the medial, lateral and posterior semicircular canals

45. **The following are sensory receptors of equilibrium except:**
    A. Spiral organ of corti
    B. Macula of saccule
    C. Macula of utricle
    D. Cristae of semicircular canals

ANSWERS

1 A	2 B	3 B	4 C	5 A	6 C	7 C	8 B
9 D	10 A	11 A	12 D	13 B	14 C	15 C	16 A
17 B	18 B	19 A	20 D	21 D	22 A	23 C	24 A
25 D	26 C	27 C	28 D	29 D	30 C	31 B	32 B
33 C	34 D	35 B	36 D	37 D	38 A	39 D	40 A
41 D	42 A	43 B	44 B	45 A			

Physiology

1. **Impulses generated by olfactory receptors in the nasal mucous membrane:**
   A. Pass through the internal capsule
   B. Pass through the thalamus
   C. Are relayed to the sensory cortex via the hypothalamus
   D. Pass to the mitral cells and from there directly to the olfactory cortex

2. **All of the following cells are present in olfactory bulb *except*:**
   A. Tufted cells
   B. Purkinje cells
   C. Granule cells
   D. Periglomerular cells

3. **All of the following are true of olfactory neurons *except*:**
   A. They have short and thick dendrites
   B. There are 10-20 cilia per olfactory neuron
   C. They are constantly replaced with a half life of 24 hours
   D. Bone morphogenic protein exerts an inhibiting effect on renewal of factory neurons

4. **Which of the following is *not true* of vomeronasal organ?**
   A. It is concerned with perception of odors that act as pheromones
   B. Its receptors project to the olfactory bulb and from there primarily to entorhinal cortex
   C. It is concerned with reproduction and ingestive behavior
   D. It has about 30 serpentine odorant receptors

5. **Which of the following substances has lowest olfactory threshold?**
   A. Methyl mercaptan
   B. Propyl mercaptan
   C. Oil of peppermint
   D. Chloroform

6. **All of the following are true of olfactory pathyways *except*:**
   A. There is no relay in the thalamus
   B. The signals do not reach the somatosensory cortex Brodmann's areas 3,1,2
   C. The receptors undergo degeneration periodically but not replaced by new cells
   D. The impulses reach the limbic sytem and are concerned with sexual behavior.

7. **Mechanism of excitation of the olfactory cells include all the following *except*:**
   A. Odorant substance activates the G-protein complex
   B. Increased formation of cyclic AMP
   C. Opening of K^+ channels and depolarization of olfactory neuron
   D. Activation of adenyl cyclase inside olfactory cell membrane

8. **Deficiency of which of the following substances causes the combination of diminished sense of smell and hypogonadism?**
   A. An adhesion molecule
   B. A transcription factor
   C. Nerve growth factor
   D. Gonadotropin releasing hormone

9. **Which of the following does not increase the ability to discriminate many different odours?**
   A. High beta – arrestin content in olfactory neurons
   B. Many different receptors
   C. Pattern of olfactory receptors activated by a given odorant
   D. Projection of different mitral cell axons to different parts of the brain

10. **During deglutition, all of the following take place *except*:**
    A. Contraction of upper constrictors of pharynx
    B. Contraction of cricopharyngeal muscle
    C. Contraction of middle constrictors of pharynx
    D. Contraction of lower constrictors of pharynx

11. **During deglutition reflex, afferent impulses travel in all of the following cranial nerves *except*:**
    A. 5th cranial nerve   B. 7th cranial nerve
    C. 9th cranial nerve   D. 10th cranial nerve

12. **Which of the following is *not true* of Reissner's membrane?**
    A. Stria vascularis is located on its surface
    B. It separates scala media from scala vestibuli
    C. It does not obstruct the passage of sound vibrations through the fluid from scala vestibuli to scala media
    D. It maintains a special fluid in the scala media

13. **Which of the following is *not true* of organ of Corti?**
    A. It contains 20,000 outer hair cells and 3,500 inner hair cells
    B. It extends from the apex to the base of the cochlea
    C. 95% of afferent neurons innervates the inner hair cells
    D. Tips of the hairs of the inner hair cells are embedded in the tectorial membrane

14. **Which of the following statements is true?**
    A. Low frequency sounds cause maximum activation of basilar membrane near the base of the cochlea
    B. High frequency sounds cause maximum activation of basilar membrane near the apex of the cochlea
    C. High frequency sounds cause maximum activation of mid portion of basilar membrane
    D. Specific brain neurons are activated by specific sound frequencies

15. **Which of the following is true of endocochlear potential?**
    A. Endolymph is 80 millivolts positive with respect to perilymph
    B. Endolymph is 180 millivolts positive with respect to perilymph
    C. Endolymph is 80 millivolts negative with respect to perilymph
    D. Endolymph is 180 millivolts negative with respect to perilymph

16. **Crossing over between two auditory pathways takes place in all for the following *except*:**
    A. Trapezoid body
    B. Commissure of Probst
    C. Inferior collicular commissure
    D. Medial geniculate body

17. **All of the following are features of auditory pathways *except*:**
    A. Some impulses are always transmitted to the auditory cortex even in the absence of sound
    B. When basilar membranes moves towards scala vestibuli impulse traffic increases
    C. When basilar membrane moves towards scala tympani impulse traffic increases
    D. When basilar membrane moves towards scala tympani impulse traffic decreases

18. **During tympanic reflex, when tensor tympani contracts:**
    A. The manubrium of malleus is pulled inward
    B. The manubrium of malleus is pulled outward
    C. The manubrium of malleus is pulled upward
    D. The manubrium of malleus is pulled downward

19. **During tympanic reflex, when stapedius contracts:**
    A. Footplate of stapes is pulled inward
    B. Footplate of stapes is pulled outward
    C. Footplate of stapes is pulled upward
    D. Footplate of stapes is pulled downward

20. **In endolymph:**
    A. Concentration of Na^+ is more than perilymph
    B. Concentration of K^+ is less than perilymph
    C. Concentration of K^+ is more than perilymph
    D. Concentration of Cl^- is less than perilymph

21. In perilymph:

A. Concentration of Na^+ is more than endolymph
B. Concentration of Na^+ is less than endolymph
C. Concentration of K^+ is more than endolymph
D. Concentration of Cl^- is more than endolymph

22. Auditory impulses pass through all of the following except:

A. Superior olive
B. Trapezoid body
C. Superior colliculus
D. Medial geniculate body

23. All of the following produce nerve deafness except:

A. Prolonged administration of gentamicin
B. Tumors of vestibulocochlear nerve
C. Tumors of cerebellopontine angle
D. Otosclerosis

24. The human planum temporale is:

A. Larger in the right than in the left cerebral hemisphere particularly in right handed individuals
B. Concerned with detection of rotational acceleration
C. Concerned with frequency determination
D. Generally larger in musicians with perfect pitch, than in musicians without perfect pitch

25. In humans, primary auditory cortex is located in:

A. Posterior part of the occipital lobe
B. Posterior part of the parietal lobe
C. Superior part of the temporal lobe
D. Inferior part of the temporal lobe

26. Determination of the direction from which a sound emanates in the horizontal plane depends upon all of the following except:

A. Detecting the difference in time between the arrival of the sound waves in two ears
B. Detecting the difference in phase of the sound waves in two ears
C. Detecting the difference in the frequency of the sound waves in both ears
D. Detecting the difference in loudness of the sound waves in both ears

27. Mutations in the following nonmuscle myosins cause deafness except:

A. Myosin VIIa   B. Myosin VIII
C. Myosin Ib   D. Myosin VI

28. All of the following features are associated with violinists except:

A. Increase in the size of basal ganglia
B. Increase in the size of auditory area activated by musical tones
C. Increases in the size of cerebellum
D. Altered somatosensory representation of the area to which the fingers they use in playing their instruments project

29. All of the following are associated with the outer hair cells in the organ of corti except:

A. They generate action potentials in the auditory nerve
B. Depolarization makes them shorten
C. Hyperpolarization makes them lengthen
D. They receive adrenergic innervations via an efferent component of the auditory nerve

30. What is the minimum intensity at which sounds are heard as well as felt?

A. 120 decibel   B. 130 decibel
C. 140 decibel   D. 150 decibel

31. Which of the following is *not true* of olivocochlear bundle?

A. It is a prominent bundle of efferent fibers in each auditory nerve
B. It arises from both the ipsilateral and the contralateral superior olivary complex
C. It ends primarily around the bases of inner hair cells
D. It ends primarily around the bases of outer hair cells

32. Which of the following is *not true* of basilar membrane?

A. It is impermeable to perilymph in the scala tympani
B. It is not under tension
C. Its width tapers gradually from 0.50 mm near the helicotrema to 0.04 mm near the round window
D. High frequency sound waves produces maximum displacement at its basal region.

33. **Cochlear microphonic potential has all of the following characteristics *except*:**
   A. It is a receptor potential produced by Na^+ influx at the apical region of the hair cells
   B. It is produced at the apex by low frequency sound
   C. It does not have latency
   D. Its response increases with an increase in intensity of the sound and can be summated

34. **All of the following discriminates loudness of a sound *except*:**
   A. As the loudness increases, there is increase in the number of action potentials from the hair cells
   B. More number of hair cells are activated, as the loudness increases
   C. Certain hair cells respond only when the sound is loud
   D. When the sound is loud, signals from auditory cortex augments the discharge of hair cells

35. **In the auditory cortex, low frequency sound waves are represented:**
   A. Posteromedially
   B. Anterolaterally
   C. Superomedially
   D. Inferolaterally

36. **Destruction of which of the following results in anomic aphasia?**
   A. Angular gyrus in representational hemisphere
   B. Angular gyrus in categorical hemisphere
   C. Wernicke's area in representational hemisphere
   D. Auditory association area in categorical hemisphere

37. **Which of the following areas is more concerned with melody, pitch and sound intensity?**
   A. Brodmann's area 22 on the right side
   B. Brodmann's area 22 on the left side
   C. Left planum temporale
   D. Right planum temporale

38. **Destruction of primary auditory cortex on one side leads to:**
   A. Deafness in the same side ear
   B. Deafness in the opposite ear
   C. Inability to interpret the meaning of the sound
   D. Inability to localize the source of the sound

39. **The sensory area of the categorical hemisphere for interpretation of language is:**
   A. Primary auditory area
   B. Angular gyrus
   C. Wernickes area
   D. Brodmann's area 3,1, 2

40. **Almost all cases of motor aphasias result from damage to:**
   A. Broca's speech area in the left hemisphere
   B. Broca's speech area in the right hemisphere
   C. Wernicke's area in the left hemisphere
   D. Angular gyrus in the right hemisphere

41. **A patient is found to have deafness, elevated plasma renin, hyperkalemia, alkalosis and normal blood pressure. This is due to mutation of which of the following genes?**
   A. The gene for Na^+ channel
   B. The gene for renin
   C. The gene for barttin
   D. The gene for tyrosine hydroxylase

42. **Postrotatory nystagmus is caused by continued movement of:**
   A. Aqueous humor over the ciliary body in the eye
   B. Endolymph toward the helicotrema
   C. Endolymph in the semicircular canals with consequent bending of the cupula and stimulation of the hair cells
   D. Perilymph over hair cells that have their processes embedded in the tectorial membrane

43. **The direction of nystagmus is vertical when a subject is rotated:**
   A. After warm water is put in one ear
   B. With the head tipped sideways
   C. After cold water is put in both ears
   D. With the head tipped backwards

44. **Nerve fibers from utricle and saccule end predominantly in:**
   A. Superior division of vestibular nucleus
   B. Medial division of vestibular nucleus
   C. Lateral division of vestibular nucleus
   D. Spinal cord bypassing the vestibular nucleus

45. Receptors concerned with labyrinthine righting reflexes are:

A. Muscle spindle
B. Proprioceptors in the neck
C. Hair cells in the cochlea
D. Otolithic organs

46. The hair cells in the saccule undergo depolarization when:

A. The stereocilia are pushed towards kinocilium
B. The stereocilia are pushed away from the kinocilium
C. The stereocilia are bent perpendicular to their axis with kinocilium
D. The stereocilia are stretched upwards

47. An individual's orientation in space depends in part on input from the following receptors except:

A. Vestibular receptors
B. Rods and cones in retina
C. Proprioreceptors in joints
D. Hair cells in organ of corti

48. Caloric stimulation produces all of the following except:

A. Sweating
B. Nystagmus
C. Vertigo
D. Nausea

49. Which of the following is not involved in the static equilibrium?

A. Utricle
B. Saccule
C. Lateral vestibular nucleus
D. Semicircular canals

50. All of the following cranial nerves are involved in vestibulo-occular reflex except:

A. 2nd cranial nerve
B. 3rd cranial nerve
C. 4th cranial nerve
D. 6th cranial nerve

ANSWERS

1 D	2 B	3 C	4 B	5 A	6 C	7 C	8 A
9 A	10 B	11 B	12 A	13 D	14 D	15 A	16 D
17 C	18 A	19 B	20 C	21 A	22 C	23 D	24 D
25 C	26 C	27 B	28 A	29 D	30 C	31 C	32 A
33 A	34 D	35 B	36 B	37 A	38 D	39 C	40 A
41 C	42 C	43 B	44 C	45 D	46 A	47 D	48 A
49 D	50 A						

Biochemistry-I

1. **A patient of (Herpes) Zoster oticus develop complication as meningitis. Apart from confirming the diagnosis by serological test, CSF examination of the patient will also show:**
   A. Pressure elevation
   B. Increased protein
   C. Increased cell count
   D. All the above

2. **Increased level of which Immunoglobulin (in nasal discharge) will help in the diagnosis of allergic rhinitis?**
   A. IgA
   B. IgD
   C. IgE
   D. IgM

3. **Glue like glassy white to yellow secretion which obstruct the nasal luman seen in cystic fibrosis which can be diagnosed by increased level of sodium chloride > 45 mEq/L in?**
   A. Nasal secretion
   B. Blood
   C. Sweat
   D. Urine

4. **For the diagnosis of subdural abscess, CSF examination was done. All finding are true in CSF examination except:**
   A. Moderate increase in cell count
   B. Increased pressure
   C. Increased protein
   D. Increased sugar level

5. **For acute tonsillitis, all the following tests are done except:**
   A. ESR estimation
   B. Renal function test
   C. Serum amylase
   D. CKMB estimation

6. **For the diagnosis of dermatomyositis all the following tests will help in the diagnosis except:**
   A. Urine for creatine
   B. Serum for GOT
   C. Blood urea
   D. Serum LDH

7. **What is true for the diagnosis of pharyngoesophagitis (Plummer-Vinson diseases)?**
   A. Extremely low serum iron level
   B. Normal serum iron level
   C. Low GOT level in serum
   D. High GOT level in serum

8. **For the diagnosis of chronic recurrent parotitis, which of the following statement is true?**
   A. Raised saliva amylase
   B. Raised serum amylase
   C. Raised pancreatic amylase
   D. Low pancreatic amylase

9. **Which statement is not true for Sjögren disease, increased level of?**
   A. Sodium chloride
   B. Albumin
   C. IgA, IgG and IgM
   D. IgA, IgG and IgE

10. **For the diagnosis of Sialadenosis (parotid gland inflammation), following biochemical parameter of saliva are true except:**
    A. Decreased lysozyme
    B. Increased protein
    C. Normal flow of parotid secretion
    D. Decreased IgA

11. **For the diagnosis of sialadenitis, following biochemical parameters of saliva are true *except*:**
    A. Increased lysozyme
    B. Increased protein (albumin)
    C. Decreased flow of parotid secretion
    D. Strongly decreased IgA

12. **A patient with complaint of tiredness, weight gain and cold intolerance provisionally diagnosed as a case of hypothyroidism. Following parameters will help in diagnosis *except*:**
    A. Decreased serum Triiodothyronine (T_3)
    B. Decreased serum Thyronine (T_4)
    C. Low serum cholesterol
    D. Increased TSH level

13. **The following tests are required to confirm the diagnosis of hyperthyroidism *except*:**
    A. Serum growth hormone
    B. Serum T_4
    C. Serum T_3
    D. Serum TSH

14. **Middle-aged female with H/O weight loss, irritability, sweating and sensitive to heat was diagnosed as a case of primary hyperthyroidism. Which of the following test is used as screening test?**
    A. Serum T_3
    B. Serum T_4
    C. Serum TSH
    D. Serum cholesterol

15. **One of the complication of middle ear infection is meningitis. Meningitis can be diagnosed by CSF examination with following parameters *except*:**
    A. Raised cell count
    B. Increased sugar level
    C. Increased protein level
    D. Reduced chloride level

16. **In case of facial paralysis which of the following most appropriate biochemical test will help to say cause is systemic?**
    A. Thyroid profile
    B. Blood sugar
    C. Blood urea
    D. Serum creatinine

17. **For the diagnosis of cerebrospinal rhinorrhea the following test will be positive with fluid from nasal cavity *except*:**
    A. Mucus detection test
    B. Test for albumin
    C. Fehling test
    D. Rothera's test

18. **8-year-old female child presented with history of chronic sinusitis and multiple nasal polypi. She had recurrent attack of chest infection and malabsorption syndrome. Which one of the following test would be useful for diagnosis?**
    A. Sweat chloride test
    B. IgE estimation
    C. Estimation of angiotensin converting enzyme
    D. ESR

19. **Amount of saliva secreted per day is:**
    A. 50 - 500 ml
    B. 500 - 1000 ml
    C. 1000 - 1500 ml
    D. 1500 - 2000 ml

20. **Sjögren's syndrome can be diagnose by all the following test *except* increased level of:**
    A. Sodium
    B. IgA and IgG
    C. Phosphate
    D. Lactoferrin and albumin

21. **To diagnose cerebrospinal fluid otorrhea, when origin is in question and fluid is scant. Which one from the following is the confirmatory test of choice, increased level of:**
    A. CSF for protein estimation ↑
    B. Detection of β_2 transferrin by immunoelectrophoresis ↑
    C. CSF for glucose estimation ↑
    D. Subarachnoid administration of fluorescein / isotopes ↑

22. **Which are the following blood test will help in the diagnosis of sarcoidosis an inflammatory lesion of nose?**
    A. Angiotensin converting enzyme
    B. Blood urea
    C. Serum creatinine
    D. Blood sugar

23. Which of the following will help in the diagnosis of Wegener's granulomatosis (an inflammatory lesion of nose)?
    A. Angiotensin converting enzyme
    B. Blood urea and creatinine
    C. Serum protein
    D. Blood sugar

24. To diagnose the cancer of mouth floor which of the following biochemical test should be done?
    A. Liver function test
    B. Gastric function test
    C. Endocrine function test
    D. Pancreatic function test

25. For the diagnosis of hematemesis, which of the following test will help?
    A. Gastric function test
    B. Liver function test
    C. Renal function test
    D. Pancreatic function test

26. For neonatal respiratory distress, which of the following biochemical test will help in diagnosis (most of the time)?
    A. Blood lecithin   B. Blood sphingomyelin
    C. Serum cholesterol D. Blood sugar

27. For confirmation of subclinical hyperthyroidism, which group of the tests will help?
    A. Undetectable TSH, high free T_4
    B. Undetectable TSH, normal free T_4 and high T_3
    C. Undetectable TSH, normal free T_4 and normal T_3
    D. Undetectable TSH, High T_4 and high T_3

28. 24-hour urine catecholamine estimation done and found high. Increased urine catecholamine will help to diagnose which tumor:
    A. Tumor of external ear
    B. Glomus tumor
    C. Tumor of cerebellopontine
    D. Tumor of nasal cavity

29. 10-year-old child presented with history of nasal obstruction. On examination nasal polyps are detected. To confirm the diagnosis which of the following test should be done?
    A. Culture of nasal smear
    B. Immunoglobulin study
    C. Sweat chloride test
    D. Blood sugar

30. For the diagnosis of hypothyroidism which following group of the tests will help:
    A. Normal TSH, normal T_4 and decreased T_3
    B. Normal TSH, decreased T_4 and decreased T_3
    C. Increased TSH, decreased T_4 and decreased T_3
    D. Increased TSH, normal T_4 and normal T_3

Multiple response type:
Write 'A' if 1,2,3 are correct, 'B' if 1 and 3 are correct, 'C' if 2 and 4 are correct and 'D' if all four are correct.

31. AIDS can be diagnosed by which of the following test:
    A. ELISA   B. Western blot test
    C. CD_4 T-cell count D. P-24 antigen

32. For evaluation the sense of taste, which are the solutions in various concentration used?
    A. Sodium chloride
    B. Citric acid
    C. Quinine sulphate
    D. Cane sugar

33. Mumps (parotitis) is a disease of parotid gland, which of the following statements are true for the diagnosis?
    A. Transient elevation of serum amylase
    B. Transient elevation of urine amylase
    C. Transient elevation of serum diastase
    D. Transient elevation of urine diastase

34. Apart from audiogram which of the following biochemical test will help in diagnosis of sensory neural hearing loss?
    A. Blood sugar
    B. Thyroid profile
    C. Blood urea
    D. Serum creatinine

35. Olfactory function may be assessed by which of the following biochemical tests (in absence of identifiable cause)?
    A. Thyroid stimulation hormone estimation
    B. Fasting blood glucose
    C. Renal function test
    D. Gastric function test

36. For fungal sinusitis diagnosis, which of the following biochemical tests will be helpful?
    A. Blood glucose
    B. Blood urea and creatinine estimation
    C. Immunoglobulin (IgE and IgG) estimation
    D. Thyroid function test

37. Which of the following tests are useful in the diagnosis of Wagener's granulomatosis (an inflammatory lesion of nose)?
A. Blood urea
B. Serum creatine
C. Urine analysis
D. Estimation of angiotensin converting enzyme

38. For Graves' disease which of the following tests will help in diagnosis?
A. Undetectable TSH
B. High free T_4
C. High 123 I uptake
D. Normal TSH

39. For the diagnosis of hyperparathyroidism, estimation of which of the following parameters will help?
A. TSH
B. PTH
C. Free T_4 and T_3 level
D. Serum calcium

Write (T) for True and (F) for False against each statements (Multiple true false responce type: more than one response may be correct)

40. For taste disturbance following taste test are done:
A. Caffeine or quinine for bitter
B. Citric acid for sour
C. Sucrose for sweet
D. Sodium chloride for salty

41. For Hashimoto's thyroiditis (early phase) comment for following test:
A. Test for thyroid antibodies positive
B. Serum calcitonin is increased
C. Serum TSH level is normal
D. Free T_4 level is normal

42. Important screening test for allergic rhinitis is examination of nasal discharge for increase level of:
A. IgA   B. IgD
C. IgE   D. IgM

43. For diagnosis of the hypothyroidism, following parameters was analyzed. Comment on them :
A. Decreased serum triiodothyronine (T_3)
B. Decreased serum thyronine (T_4)
C. Low serum cholesterol
D. Increased TSH level

Bibliography
1. Hans Heins Naumann: Differential Diagnosis in Otorhinolaryngology; First edition, 1995.
2. PL Dhingra: Disease of Ear, Nose and Throat; Third edition.
3. Mohd Maqbool: Textbook of Ear, Nose and Throat diseases; Ninth edition.
4. Alper, Myers and Eibling: Decision making in Ear, Nose and Throat disorders.
5. Ted L Tewfik: Congenital anomalies of the Ear, Nose and Throat.

ANSWERS

1 D	2 C	3 C	4 D	5 D	6 C	7 A	8 B
9 D	10 B	11 D	12 C	13 A	14 B	15 B	16 B
17 D	18 A	19 C	20 C	21 B	22 A	23 B	24 A
25 B	26 D	27 C	28 B	29 C	30 C	31 D	32 D
33 D	34 D	35 A	36 B	37 A	38 A	39 C	

40 A[T],B[T],C[T],D[T] 41 A[T],B[T],C[F],D[T] 42 A[F],B[F],C[T],D[F] 43 A[F],B[F],C[T],D[F]

Biochemistry -II

1. **The carbohydrate reserve in human body is:**
   A. Starch
   B. Cellulose
   C. Glycogen
   D. Insulin

2. **The repeating unit in hyaluronic acid is:**
   A. Glucuronic acid and galactose
   B. Glucuronic acid and galactosamine
   C. Glucuronic acid and glucosamine
   D. Glucuronic acid and N-acetyl glucosamine

3. **A fatty acid which is not synthesized in human body and has to be supplied in the diet:**
   A. Palmitic acid
   B. Oleic acid
   C. Linoleic acid
   D. Stearic acid

4. **The triacyl glycerol present in plasma lipoproteins are hydrolyzed by:**
   A. Lingual lipase
   B. Pancreatic lipase
   C. Co-lipase
   D. Lipoprotein lipase

5. **The calorific value of lipid is:**
   A. 4.0 K cal/gm
   B. 6.0 K cal/gm
   C. 9.0 K cal/gm
   D. 5.4 K cal/gm

6. **Rancidity of butter is prevented by the addition of:**
   A. Vitamin D
   B. Tocopherols
   C. Biotin
   D. Copper

7. **Which of the following is a sulfur containing essential amino acid?**
   A. Cysteine
   B. Cystine
   C. Methionine
   D. Homocysteine

8. **The serum antibody responsible for fighting gram +ve pyogenic bacteria is:**
   A. IgD
   B. IgE
   C. IgG
   D. IgA

9. **Which of the following immunoglobulin can cross the placenta?**
   A. IgM
   B. IgG
   C. IgA
   D. IgE

10. **Which of the immunoglobulin class has reaginic antibody?**
    A. IgG
    B. IgD
    C. IgE
    D. IgM

11. **Retinal is reduced to retinol by the enzyme retinene reductase in presence of which coenzyme:**
    A. FMN
    B. $NADPH^+H^+$
    C. $NADH^+H^+$
    D. FAD^+

12. **Increased carbohydrate consumption increases the dietary requirement for:**
    A. Thiamine
    B. Riboflavine
    C. Pyridoxine
    D. Folic acid

13. **Pyridoxal-phosphate is a cofactor for which of the following enzymatic reactions?**
    A. Decarboxylation reaction
    B. Phosphate group transfer
    C. Transmethylation reaction
    D. Dehydrogenase reaction

14. **The disease pellagra is due to a deficiency of:**
    A. Vitamin B_6
    B. Nicotinic acid
    C. Pantothenic acid
    D. Folic acid

15. **A biochemical indication of vitamin B_{12} deficiency can be obtained by measuring the urinary excretion of:**
    A. Pyruvic acid
    B. Lactic acid
    C. Malic acid
    D. Methyl malonic acid

16. To prevent rickets in a case of chronic renal disorders, which of the following substances should be administered?
    A. Cholecalciferol
    B. Ergocalciferol
    C. 25-hydroxy cholecalciferol
    D. 1, 25-di-hydroxy cholecalciferol

17. Which of the following vitamins is associated with synthesis of coagulation factor prothrombin?
    A. Retinal
    B. Tocopherol
    C. Menadione
    D. Ascorbic acid

18. The best test for acute pancreatitis in the presence of mumps is:
    A. Virus isolation
    B. Serum amylase
    C. Urinary amylase
    D. Serum lipase

19. Which of the following enzyme typically elevated in alcoholism?
    A. Serum ALP
    B. Serum GOT
    C. Serum gamma GT
    D. Serum LDH

20. Patients with hepatocellular jaundice tend to have:
    A. Lower serum ALP, LDH and AST activity
    B. Lower serum ALP, higher LDH and AST activity
    C. Higher serum ALP, LDH and AST activity
    D. Higher serum ALP, lower LDH and AST activity

21. If results of the serum bilirubin, serum ALP, LDH and AST determinations suggest obstructive jaundice, the best confirmatory test would be the estimation of:
    A. Serum ALT
    B. Serum 5-nucleotidase
    C. Serum protein electrophoresis
    D. Serum pseudocholinesterase

22. Which enzyme estimation will be helpful in differentiating the elevated serum ALP due to obstructive jaundice not due to bone disorders?
    A. Serum AST
    B. Serum ALT
    C. Serum LDH
    D. Serum 5-nucleotidase

23. Cardiac muscle contains which of the following CK-isoenzyme?
    A. MM and BB only
    B. MM, BB and MB
    C. MM only
    D. MB only

24. On the third day following onset of acute myocardial infarction, which enzyme estimation will have the best predictive value?
    A. Serum AST
    B. Serum CK
    C. Serum ALT
    D. Serum LDH

25. Serum AST activity is not characteristically elevated as the result of:
    A. Myocardial infarction
    B. Muscular dystrophies
    C. Peptic ulcer
    D. Infectious hepatitis

26. On which day following acute myocardial infarction the estimation of serum AST will be of greatest significance?
    A. First day
    B. Second day
    C. Third day
    D. Fourth day

27. Rise of which serum enzyme activity in four-eight hours after acute myocardial infarction is characteristically seen?
    A. AST
    B. ALT
    C. LDH
    D. CK

28. Cyanide is poisonous as it stops respiration because of its:
    A. Inhibition of TCA cycle
    B. Inhibition of myoglobin
    C. Formation of complex with Hb
    D. Inhibition of syndrome evidence

29. Bilirubin formed in reticuloendothelial cells is transported to liver in combination with:
    A. Albumin
    B. Globulin
    C. Haptoglobin
    D. Ceruloplasmin

30. In liver cells, bilirubin is conjugated with:
    A. Cholic acid
    B. Glycine
    C. Glucuronic acid
    D. Iduronic acid

31. In the normal resting state of humans, most of the blood glucose is consumed by:
    A. Liver
    B. Brain
    C. Adipose tissue
    D. Muscles

32. The following metabolic abnormalities occur in diabetes mellitus *except:*
    A. Increased plasma free fatty acids
    B. Increased pyruvate carboxylase activity
    C. Decreased lipogenesis
    D. Decreased gluconeogenesis

33. **Which of the following hormones is not involved in carbohydrate metabolism?**
    A. Cortisol   B. Glucagon
    C. Vasopressin   D. Growth hormone

34. **The lipoprotein with the fastest electrophoretic mobility and the lowest triglycerides content is:**
    A. VLDL   B. LDL
    C. HDL   D. Chylomicrons

35. **All of the following tissues are capable of using ketone bodies except:**
    A. Brain   B. Red blood cells
    C. Cardiac muscle   D. Skeletal muscle

36. **The major source of cholesterol in arterial smooth muscle cells is from:**
    A. LDL   B. HDL
    C. Chylomicrons   D. VLDL

37. **Ketone bodies are synthesized from fatty acid oxidation by which of the following organ:**
    A. Skeletal muscle   B. Kidney
    C. Erythrocytes   D. Liver

38. **Which of the following lipoproteins would contribute to a measurement of plasma cholesterol in a normal individual following a 12 hour fast?**
    A. Chylomicrons and VLDL and LDL
    B. VLDL and LDL and HDL
    C. VLDL and LDL
    D. LDL and HDL

39. **All statements regarding ketone bodies are true except:**
    A. They may result from starvation
    B. They are formed in kidneys
    C. They may be excreted in urine
    D. They are present in high concentration in uncontrolled diabetes mellitus

40. **All are true about phenylketonuria except:**
    A. Deficiency of phenylalanine hydroxylase
    B. Mental retardation
    C. Increased urinary excretion of p-hydroxy phenyl pyruvic acid
    D. Decrease of serotonin formation

41. **The rate of excretion of certain substances in 24-hr sample of urine can be used to estimate the rate of muscle protein loss. Which of the following substance falls into this category?**
    A. Urea
    B. Uric acid
    C. 3-methyl histidine
    D. Ergothioneine

42. **Alkaptonuria is an inherited disorder due to deficiency of the enzyme:**
    A. Transaminase
    B. Homogentisate oxidase
    C. Phenylalanine hydroxylase
    D. Cystathionine synthase

43. **Nonsense codon brings about:**
    A. Initiation of protein synthesis
    B. Termination of protein synthesis
    C. Elongation of polypeptide chains
    D. Post-translational modification of proteins

44. **In the process of transcription the flow of genetic information is from:**
    A. DNA to DNA   B. RNA to RNA
    C. RNA to DNA   D. DNA to RNA

45. **The anticodon region is an important part of the structure of:**
    A. r-RNA   B. t-RNA
    C. m-RNA   D. micro-RNA

46. **Another name for reverse transcriptase is:**
    A. DNA dependent DNA polymerase
    B. DNA dependent RNA polymerase
    C. RNA dependent DNA polymerase
    D. RNA dependent RNA polymerase

47. **Translation results in formation of:**
    A. m-RNA   B. t-RNA
    C. r-RNA   D. a protein molecule

48. **A drug which prevents uric acid synthesis by inhibiting the enzyme xanthine oxidase is:**
    A. Aspirin   B. Allopurinol
    C. Colchicines   D. Probenecid

49. **Hearing loss without mental retardation is present:**
    A. MPS I—Hurler's syndrome
    B. MPS II—Hunter's syndrome
    C. MPS III—Sanfilippo's syndrome
    D. MPS V—Scheie's syndrome

50. **Which of the following is synthesized by lipo-oxygense pathway:**
    A. Prostaglandins   B. Leukotrienes
    C. Prostacyclins   D. Thromboxanes

ANSWERS

1	C	**2**	D	**3**	C	**4**	D	**5**	C	**6**	B	**7**	C	**8**	C
9	B	**10**	C	**11**	B	**12**	A	**13**	A	**14**	B	**15**	D	**16**	D
17	C	**18**	D	**19**	C	**20**	C	**21**	B	**22**	D	**23**	D	**24**	D
25	C	**26**	B	**27**	D	**28**	D	**29**	A	**30**	C	**31**	B	**32**	D
33	C	**34**	C	**35**	B	**36**	A	**37**	D	**38**	B	**39**	B	**40**	D
41	C	**42**	B	**43**	B	**44**	D	**45**	B	**46**	C	**47**	D	**48**	B
49	D	**50**	B												

Pharmacology

1. In the treatment of head and neck cancers, the drug which can be given into the arterial blood of the tumor is:
   A. Cyclophosphamide
   B. Floxuridine
   C. Bleomycin
   D. Methotrexate

2. In head and neck cancer which of the following regimen is the current treatment of choice:
   A. Fluorouracial and cisplatin
   B. Methotrexate and cisplatin
   C. Vincristine and dactinomycin
   D. Radioiodine and cisplatin

3. Renal toxicity is the commonest toxic manifestation of:
   A. Taxol
   B. Leukovorin
   C. MESNA
   D. Cisplatin

4. Pulmonary fibrosis is a serious adverse reaction due to:
   A. Cisplatin
   B. Fluorouracil
   C. Vincristine
   D. Bleomycin

5. All of the following drugs are useful in treating head and neck cancer *except*:
   A. L-Asparaginase
   B. Hydroxy urea
   C. Vincristine
   D. Paclitaxel

6. In head and neck cancer chemotherapy cardiomyopathy is the adverse reaction due to the following agent:
   A. Bleomycin
   B. Doxorubicin
   C. Vincristine
   D. Cisplatin

7. The anticancer agent able to synchronize tumor cells into a radiation sensitive phase of the cell cycle is:
   A. Vinorelbine
   B. Doxorubicin
   C. Fluorouracil
   D. Hydroxy urea

8. Drug useful for surgical antimicrobial prophylaxis during oropharyngeal interventions:
   A. Cefazolin
   B. Ampicillin
   C. Gentamicin
   D. Doxycycline

9. Drug of choice in acute otitis media and sinusitis:
   A. Gentamicin
   B. Amoxicillin
   C. Benzathine penicillin
   D. Doxycycline

10. Ototoxic antibiotics are all the following *except:*
    A. Ofloxacin
    B. Moxalactam
    C. Sparfloxacin
    D. Trovafloxacin

11. All of the following are fluoroquinolones *except*:
    A. Moxifloxacin
    B. Moxalactam
    C. Sparfloxacin
    D. Trovafloxacin

12. Drug useful in oropharyngeal candidasis:
    A. Griseofulvin
    B. Amphotericin-B
    C. Zidovudine
    D. Nafliquine

13. Drugs useful in Group A, *Streptococcus pyogenes* infection of throat does not include:
    A. Penicillin-G
    B. Amoxicillin
    C. Cephalosporin
    D. Doxycycline

14. All of the following drugs are useful in sinusitis due to *Moraxella catarrhalis except*:
    A. Gentamicin
    B. Trimethoprim-Sulfamethoxazole
    C. Ciprofloxacin
    D. Tetracycline

15. All of the following drugs useful in Corynebacterium diphtheriae laryngotracheitis *except*:
    A. Benzyl penicillin and gentamicin
    B. Penicillin-G and Rifampicin
    C. Azithromycin
    D. Tetracycline

16. Antiviral agent useful in mucocutaneous herpes is:
    A. Acyclovir
    B. Famiciclovir
    C. Valacyclovir
    D. Penciclovir

17. Antiretroviral agents include all *except*:
    A. Stavudine
    B. Squinavir
    C. Zalcitabine
    D. Foscarnet

18. Antiseptic highly effective against gram-positive and gram-negative organisms does not include:
    A. Hexachlorophene
    B. Povidone iodine
    C. Sodium chlorite
    D. Chlorhexidine

19. Antiseptic useful as mouth wash and rinse is:
    A. Povidone iodine
    B. Chlorhexidine
    C. Glutaraldehyde
    D. Sodium hypochlorite

20. Antiemetic useful in chemotherapy induced nausea and vomiting includes all *except*:
    A. Ondansetron
    B. Dexamethasone
    C. Haloperidol
    D. Lansoprazole

21. Prokinetic agent useful in gastroesophageal reflex disease is:
    A. Droperidol
    B. Sucralfate
    C. Metoclopramide
    D. Omeprazole

22. Prokinetic agent which may cause extrapyramidal effects is:
    A. Domperidone
    B. Metoclopramide
    C. Bisacodyl
    D. Diphenhydramine

23. Receptor implicated in the mediation of emesis is:
    A. Serotonin-3
    B. Serotonin-1D
    C. Serotonin-1B
    D. Serotonin-2

24. Somatostatin analog useful in treating symptoms of GIT carcinoid tumor is:
    A. Domiperidone
    B. Octreotide
    C. Cisapride
    D. Metaclopramide

25. Drugs useful in migraine include all *except*:
    A. Ergotamine
    B. Aspirin
    C. Sumatriptan
    D. Diazepam

26. Sumatriptan useful in migraine acts as:
    A. Serotonin 1-A and 1-B antagonist
    B. Serotonin 1-C and 1-D antagonist
    C. Serotonin 1-B and 1-D agonist
    D. Serotonin 3 antagonist

27. Drugs useful in the prophylaxis of migraine include all *except*:
    A. Amitryptyline
    B. Phenelzine
    C. Prazosin
    D. Propranolol

28. New drugs under trail for migraine include all *except*:
    A. Nitric oxide inhibitor
    B. Bradykinin antagonist
    C. Platelet activating factor antagonists
    D. Substance-P-antagonists

29. The local anesthetic not useful as a topical anesthetic is:
    A. Lidocaine
    B. Mepivacaine
    C. Tetracaine
    D. Cocaine

30. Why 0.005% phenylephrine is combined with local anesthetic injection?
    A. To prolong the action
    B. To counteract the hypotension
    C. To prevent headache
    D. To produce blood less field of surgery

31. What is eutectic mixture?
    A. Procaine 2.5% + Lidocaine 2.5%
    B. Lidocaine 2.5% + Prilocaine 2.5%
    C. Mepivacaine 2.5% + Procaine 2.5%
    D. Cocaine 2.5% + Procaine 5%

32. Advantage of eutectic mixture of anesthetics is:
    A. Cream topically applied for skin graft harvesting
    B. As spinal anesthesia
    C. As anesthetic spray
    D. As buccal tablet

33. Local anesthetic useful only as topical dusting powder is:
   A. Lidocaine
   B. Mepivacaine
   C. Benzocaine
   D. Dibucaine

34. General anesthetic useful for endoscopy when co-operation of the patient is essential:
   A. Ether + Atropine
   B. Thiopentone + Halothane
   C. Ketamine + Diazepam
   D. Droperidol + Fentanyl

35. Antimotion sickness drug available as transdermal patch:
   A. Scopolamine
   B. Ondonsetron
   C. Atropine
   D. Buprenorphine

36. Drugs producing loss of hearing include all of the following *except*:
   A. Frusemide
   B. Etomidate
   C. Streptomycin
   D. Tobramycin

37. Antitubercular drug effective in the treatment of tuberculosis in HIV infected patients:
   A. Rifabutin
   B. Rifampicin
   C. Streptomycin
   D. Amidarone

38. In MDR tuberculosis drug useful:
   A. Isoniazid + Rifampicin + Ofloxacin
   B. Rifampicin + Isoniazid + Pyrazinamide
   C. Ethambutol + Streptomycin + Isoniazid
   D. Pyrazinamide + Ethambutol + Isoniazid

39. Antitubercular drug which is ototoxic and nephrotoxic:
   A. Isoniazid
   B. Ethambutol
   C. Rifampicin
   D. Amikacin

40. Antibiotic associated diarrohea can be treated with:
   A. Ampicillin + Chloramphenicol
   B. Streptomycin + Ampicillin
   C. Vancomycin + Metronidazole
   D. Tetracycline + Chloramphenicol

41. Which of the following is a long acting local anesthetic?
   A. Lidocaine
   B. Bupivacaine
   C. Procaine
   D. Tetracaine

42. Drug useful locally for epistaxis:
   A. Penicillin soaked guaze pack
   B. Adrenaline soaked guaze pack
   C. Lidocaine soaked cotton pack
   D. Vitamin K soaked guaze pack

43. Which of the following herb can be advised to an 80 yrs old man complaining of forgetfulness, frequent ringing in ears and vertigo?
   A. Garlic
   B. Peppermint
   C. Ginger
   D. Ginkgo

44. Which of the following vitamin can mask the symptoms of pernicious anemia?
   A. Vitamin B_{12}
   B. Niacin
   C. Folic acid
   D. Vitamin C

45. Which of the following describes the side effects of cyclosporine therapy for preventing graft rejection?
   A. Leucopenia
   B. Nephrotoxicity
   C. Hemorrhagic cystitis
   D. Hypoglycemia

46. Which of the following interleukins can be beneficial in AIDS treatment?
   A. IL-2
   B. IL-8
   C. IL-4
   D. IL-3

47. Which of the following is a phase specific antimalignant agent:
   A. Cyclophosphamide
   B. Busulphan
   C. Azathioprine
   D. MESNA

48. Which of the following is a cycle nonspecific antimalignant:
   A. Methotrexate
   B. Vincristine
   C. Paclitaxel
   D. Cyclophosphamide

49. Which of the following is a immunosuppressant hormone:
   A. Growth hormone
   B. Parathyroid
   C. Corticosteroid
   D. Estradiol

50. Drug of choice in tropical eosinophilia is:
   A. Ivermectin
   B. Diethyl carbamazine
   C. Suramin
   D. Piperazine

ANSWERS

1 B	2 A	3 D	4 D	5 A	6 A	7 D	8 A
9 B	10 C	11 B	12 B	13 D	14 A	15 D	16 A
17 D	18 C	19 B	20 D	21 C	22 B	23 A	24 B
25 D	26 D	27 C	28 C	29 C	30 A	31 B	32 A
33 A	34 C	35 D	36 C	37 A	38 A	39 D	40 C
41 B	42 B	43 D	44 C	45 B	46 A	47 C	48 D
49 C	50 B						

Pathology

1. All of the following statements about juvenile angiofibroma are true *except*:

   A. Common in adolescent males
   B. Presents with bilateral nasal block
   C. Histologically benign, but clinically malignant
   D. Metastasis occur

2. Most common organism isolated from cases of ozaena:

   A. *Staphylococcus pyogenes*
   B. *Klebsiella pneumoniae*
   C. *Corynebacterium diphtheriae*
   D. *Cocobacillus fetidus of Perez*

3. Most common pathogen isolated from chronic maxillary sinusitis is:

   A. *Actinomyces israeli*
   B. *Bacteroides*
   C. *Hemophilus influenzae*
   D. *Staphylococcus aureus*

4. Most common organism associated with orbital cellulites following chronic sinusitis is:

   A. *Actinomyces israeli*
   B. *Escherichia coli*
   C. *Mycobacterium tuberculosis*
   D. *Nocardia madurae*

5. Nasopharyngeal carcinoma is associated with:

   A. CMV   B. EBV
   C. HBV   D. HPV

6. Lethal midline granuloma is most commonly a neoplasm of:

   A. B cells   B. Dendritic cells
   C. NK cells   D. T cells

7. Which of the following is *not true* of olfactory neuroblastoma?

   A. Membrane bound secretory granules on E/M
   B. S-100 Positive
   C. Shows 11:22 translocation
   D. Tumor of neuroendocrine origin

8. Which of the following is *not* a feature of singers nodule?

   A. Bilateral lesions
   B. Causes progressive hoarseness
   C. More common in men
   D. Malignant change common

9. The following are features of acoustic neuroma *except*:

   A. Commonly arises from vestibular division of VIII nerve
   B. Metastases common
   C. Most common neoplasm of temporal bone
   D. Usually unilateral

10. Which of the following statements is *not true* of Inverted papilloma?

   A. Arises from lateral wall of nose
   B. Associated with nasal polyposis and allergy
   C. Commonly affects adult men
   D. Most common benign neoplasm of nose and paranasal sinuses

11. Which of the following features is of prognostic significance in olfactory neuroblastoma?

   A. Cytologic atypia
   B. Mitotic rate
   C. Presence or absence of tumor necrosis
   D. Vascularity

12. **Most common malignant mesenchymal tumor of nose is:**
    A. Fibrosarcoma
    B. Leiomyosarcoma
    C. Malignant fibrous histiocytoma
    D. Rhabdomyosarcoma

13. **Hereditary angioneurotic edema of larynx is characterized by the following *except:***
    A. Deficiency of serum complement factor C1inhibitors
    B. Low levels of C1, C4 and C2
    C. Colicky pain
    D. Urticaria

14. **Which of the following statements about Jugulotympanic paragangliomas is *not true*?**
    A. Distant metastasis common
    B. Female preponderance
    C. Slow growth
    D. Usually arises from paraganglion in wall of jugular bulb

15. **Most common site of occurrence of nasal glioma is:**
    A. Nasopharynx
    B. Nose
    C. Paranasal sinus
    D. Subcutaneous nodule near nasal bridge

16. **Most common site of occurrence of carcinoma of paranasal sinuses is:**
    A. Ethmoidal sinus
    B. Frontal sinus
    C. Maxillary sinus
    D. Sphenoid

17. **The most common type of adenocarcinoma of upper respiratory passages is:**
    A. Acinic cell tumor
    B. Adenoid cystic carcinoma
    C. Malignant mixed tumor
    D. Mucoepidermoid carcinoma

18. **Most common malignant neoplasm of nasopharynx is:**
    A. Adenocarcinoma
    B. Keratinizing squamous cell carcinoma
    C. Leiomyosarcoma
    D. Poorly differentiated squamous cell carcinoma

19. **Most common tumor metastasizing to upper respiratory tract is:**
    A. Breast carcinoma B. Colonic cancer
    C. Lung cancer   D. Renal cell carcinoma

20. **Mikulicz cells are seen in:**
    A. Mucormycosis   B. Rhinophyma
    C. Rhinoscleroma   D. Rhinosporidiosis

21. **Which of the following *does not* correlate with recurrence of papillomatosis of nasal cavity?**
    A. Epithelial mucous droplets
    B. Mitotic activity in original papillae
    C. Nuclear atypia
    D. Sinus involvement

22. **Most common nonepithelial neoplasm of upper respiratory tract is:**
    A. Angiofibroma
    B. Myxoma
    C. Ossifying fibroma
    D. Rhabdomyoma

23. **Destructive necrotizing otitis media in a diabetic results from:**
    A. *Hemophilus influenzae*
    B. *Pseudomonas aeruginosa*
    C. *Staphylococcus aureus*
    D. *Streptococcus pneumoniae*

24. **Most common malignant tumor of salivary gland is:**
    A. Acinic cell carcinoma
    B. Adenoid cystic carcinoma
    C. Mucoepidermoid carcinoma
    D. Squamous cell carcinoma

25. **Most common site of metastatic involvement of temporal bone is:**
    A. Internal auditory canal
    B. Mastoid
    C. Petrous apex
    D. Tegrem tympani

26. **The following statement about otosclerosis are true *except:***
    A. Affects adolescents and young adults
    B. Exclusively occurs in temporal bone
    C. Male preponderance
    D. Presents as slow progressive conductive hearing loss

27. **Most common tumor of middle ear is:**
    A. Acoustic neuroma
    B. Adenoma
    C. Adenocarcinoma
    D. Paraganglioma

28. **"Orphan Anne eye" or ground glass nuclei are seen in:**
    A. Anaplastic carcinoma of thyroid
    B. Follicular carcinoma of thyroid
    C. Medullary carcinoma of thyroid
    D. Papillary carcinoma of thyroid

29. **Which of the following thyroid cancers has better prognosis?**
    A. Follicular variant of papillary carcinoma
    B. Follicular carcinoma of thyroid
    C. Medullary carcinoma of thyroid
    D. Papillary carcinoma of thyroid

30. **Which of the following variants of papillary carcinoma of thyroid has excellent prognosis?**
    A. Diffuse sclerosing variant
    B. Encapsulated variant
    C. Follicular variant
    D. Tall cell variant

31. **The following statement regarding follicular carcinoma of thyroid are true *except*:**
    A. Cold nodules on scinti scan
    B. Regional lymph nodes usually involved
    C. Second most common cancer of thyroid
    D. Slowly progressive painless nodules

32. **Which of the following is *not* a feature of medullary carcinoma of thyroid?**
    A. Amyloid production
    B. Association with germ line RET protoncogene activation
    C. Association with ret/ptc translocation
    D. Origin from parafollicular C cells

33. **Increased risk of sinonasal carcinoma is associated with:**
    A. Asbestos workers
    B. Coal miners
    C. Nickel refiners
    D. Uranium miners

34. **Which of the following primary tumors most commonly metastasize to thyroid?**
    A. Breast carcinoma
    B. Carcinoma lung
    C. Melanoma
    D. Renal cell carcinoma

35. **Which of the following thyroid neoplasms is most likely to undergo clear cell change?**
    A. Follicular adenoma
    B. Follicular carcinoma
    C. Hurthle cell adenoma
    D. Papillary carcinoma

36. **Which of the following malignant neoplasms of thyroid have good prognosis?**
    A. Follicular carcinoma
    B. Hurthle cell carcinoma
    C. Medullary carcinoma
    D. Papillary carcinoma

37. **Which of the following features of papillary carcinoma of thyroid does not worsen the prognosis?**
    A. Age at onset
    B. Aneuploidy
    C. Cervical node metastasis
    D. Insular, epidermoid or anaplastic foci

38. **The most common histologic type of esophageal malignancy is:**
    A. Adenocarcinoma
    B. Lymphoma
    C. Malignant melanoma
    D. Squamous cell carcinoma

39. **Most common location of laryngeal carcinoma is:**
    A. Glottis
    B. Infraglottic
    C. Supraglottic
    D. Transglottic

40. **Most common histologic type of laryngeal cancer is:**
    A. Adenocarcinoma
    B. Small cell carcinoma
    C. Squamous cell carcinoma
    D. Verrucous carcinoma

41. **Most common malignant tumor of trachea is:**
    A. Adenocarcinoma
    B. Carcinoid tumor
    C. Small cell carcinoma
    D. Squamous cell carcinoma

42. **Average 5-year survival rate for supraglottic laryngeal cancers is:**
    A. 90% and above   B. 80%
    C. 65%   D. 40%

43. **Most common cause of secondary hyperparathyroidism is:**
    A. Non pituitary neoplasms
    B. Pituitary neoplasms
    C. Trauma
    D. Postpartum pituitary necrosis

44. **Most sensitive screening test for suspected hypothyroidism is estimation of:**
    A. T3   B. T4
    C. TRH   D. TSH

45. **The single most important risk factor for esophageal cancer is:**
    A. Barrett's esophagus
    B. Obesity
    C. *Helicobacter pylori* infection
    D. Tobacco exposure

46. **Overall 5-year survival rate in cases of adenocarcinoma of esophagus is:**
    A. Less than 20%   B. 30-50%
    C. 51- 65%   D. Less than 65%

47. **Squamous cell carcinoma of esophagus is rarely associated with:**
    A. Amplification of cmyc
    B. APC mutation
    C. P161 NK4 mutation
    D. P53 mutation

48. **A reversible process associated with crico-pharyngeal atresia is:**
    A. Amyotropic lateral sclerosis
    B. Gastroesophageal reflux disease
    C. Muscular dystrophy
    D. Pharyngoesophageal motility disorders

49. **Most common cause of hematemesis is:**
    A. NSAID use   B. Peptic ulcer disease
    C. Sepsis   D. Steroid therapy

50. **Severe more protracted course of recurrent respiratory papillomatosis is most commonly associated with:**
    A. HPV 6   B. HPV 11
    C. HPV 16   D. HPV 36

51. **The usual cause of pharyngocutaneous fistula is:**
    A. An error in surgical technique
    B. Delayed wound healing
    C. Infection
    D. Malnutrition

52. **Most common cause of congenital midline mass is:**
    A. Dermoid cyst
    B. Hemangioma
    C. Laryngocoele
    D. Thyroglossal duct cyst

53. **Principal clinical manifestation of painless thyroiditis is:**
    A. Infiltrative dermopathy
    B. Infiltrative ophthalmopathy
    C. Lidlag
    D. Palpitation and tachycardia

54. **Most common cause of a white patch over the lateral aspect of the tongue is:**
    A. Lichen planus
    B. Oral hairy leukoplakia
    C. Squamous cell carcinoma in situ
    D. Syphilis

55. **Malignant minor salivary gland tumors commonly occur at:**
    A. Base of tongue   B. Cheek
    C. Maxillary antrum D. Palate

56. **Most common bilateral malignant salivary gland tumor is:**
    A. Acinic cell tumor
    B. Adenoid cystic carcinoma
    C. Malignant Mixed tumor
    D. Mucoepidermoid carcinoma

57. **Apoptosis is characterized by all of the following *except*:**
    A. Cell shrinkage
    B. Chromatin condensation
    C. Formation of cytoplasmic blebs
    D. Inflammatory reaction in tissue

58. Schauman's body is seen in:
   A. Tuberculosis
   B. Silicosis
   C. Sarcoidosis
   D. Schistosomiasis

59. The most common Karyotype encountered in Klinefelter's syndrome is:
   A. 47 XXY / 48 XXY
   B. 46 XY / 47 XXY
   C. 47 XXY
   D. 49 XXXXY

60. Which of the following is an unequivocal marker of the malignant neoplasm?
   A. Metastasis
   B. Increased mitotic activity
   C. Anaplasia
   D. Rapidity of growth

61. Squamous cell carcinoma of cervix and anogenital region is associated with:
   A. HPV type 16 and 18
   B. HPV type 1
   C. HPV type 7
   D. HPV type 4

62. The following statements regarding Burkitt's lymphoma are true except:
   A. More than 90% African tumors carry EBV genome.
   B. It is neoplasm of B lymphocytes.
   C. It is the most common childhood tumor in Central Africa and New Guinea
   D. Antibody titers against viral caspid antigens are not elevated.

63. Which of the tumor is associated with Polycythemia?
   A. Cerebellar hemangioma
   B. Pancreatic carcinoma
   C. Bronchial adenoma
   D. Thymoma

64. CA-125 is a tumor maker associated with:
   A. Carcinoma breast
   B. Carcinoma colon
   C. Ovarian carcinoma
   D. Pancreatic carcinoma

65. Tertiary syphilis most commonly involves:
   A. CNS   B. Aorta
   C. Bone   D. Testes

66. Warthin-Finkeldey giant cells are characteristically seen in:
   A. Measles   B. Mumps
   C. Infectious   D. Rabies

67. Werneckie – Korsakoff syndrome is associated with deficiency of:
   A. Riboflavin   B. Thiamine
   C. Niacin   D. Cyanacobalamin.

68. The most common malignant neoplasm in children younger than one year of age is:
   A. Neuroblastoma
   B. Retinoblastoma
   C. Leukemia
   D. Ewing's sarcoma

69. In which type of Hodgkin's disease is 'Lacunar cell' primarily encountered?
   A. Lymphocyte predominant type
   B. Lymphocytic depletion type
   C. Nodular sclerosing type
   D. Mixed cellularity type

70. Infiltrates of gingiva are commonly seen in:
   A. Acute monocytic leukemia
   B. Acute promyelocytic leukemia
   C. Acute myelomonocytic leukemia
   D. Acute erythro leukemia

71. Raspberry tongue is usually seen in:
   A. Scarlet fever   B. Measles
   C. Mumps   D. HIV infection

72. Koplick's spots are characteristically seen in:
   A. Scarlet fever
   B. Infectious mononucleosis
   C. Measles
   D. Diphtheria

73. Most common malignant tumor of salivary glands is:
   A. Mucoepidermoid carcinoma
   B. Adenoid cystic carcinoma
   C. Acinic cell carcinoma
   D. Malignant mixed tumor

74. **Anticoagulant *not* used for collection of blood for transfusion purposes is:**
    A. ACD
    B. CPD
    C. CPD-Adenine
    D. EDTA

75. **The maximum amount of blood collected from a donor at a time is:**
    A. 425 ml
    B. 300 ml
    C. 600 ml
    D. 250 ml

76. **Red colored urine showing no RBC on microscopy but showing positive Benzidine test suggests:**
    A. Hemoglobinuria
    B. Hematuria.
    C. Porphyria.
    D. Dyes and drugs.

77. **Methanol in Leishman's stain acts as a:**
    A. Mordant
    B. Preservative
    C. Differentiating agent
    D. Fixative

78. **Transudative peritoneal fluid is obtained in the following conditions *except*:**
    A. Congestive cardiac failure
    B. Constrictive pericarditis.
    C. Tuberculosis
    D. Cirrhosis

79. **Osmotic fragility of RBC is decreased in:**
    A. Spherocytosis
    B. Thalassemia
    C. Congenital non phagocytic hemolytic anemia
    D. Acquired hemolytic syndrome.

80. **In the diagnosis of DIC the most important test is:**
    A. Detection of fibrin monomer
    B. Elevated levels of fibrin degradation products
    C. Decreased levels of fibrinogen
    D. Decreased FDP levels

81. **Desmin is a marker for:**
    A. Epithelial cells
    B. Muscle cells
    C. Glial cells
    D. Neural cells

82. **Transplantation of tissues between genetically nonidentical members of the same species is known as:**
    A. Autograft
    B. Isograft
    C. Allograft
    D. Xenograft

83. **ENL reaction is commonly seen in:**
    A. Lepromatous leprosy
    B. Tuberculoid leprosy
    C. Borderline tuberculoid leprosy
    D. Borderline lepromatous leprosy

84. **Which of the following is an obligate intracellular parasite?**
    A. *Mycobacterium leprae*
    B. *Mycobacterium tuberculosis*
    C. *Mycobacterium bovis*
    D. *Mycobacterium avium*

85. **The ideal storage temperature for blood samples is:**
    A. 4 to 6° C
    B. 8 to 10° C.
    C. – 4 to – 6° C
    D. 33 to 36° C.

86. **The stain used to demonstrate amyloid in gross specimens at autopsy is:**
    A. Congo red
    B. Thioflavine T
    C. PAS
    D. van Gieson's stain.

87. **Virchow's triad explains the pathogenesis of:**
    A. Thrombosis
    B. Carcinogenesis
    C. Fat embolism
    D. Infarction

88. **Change of one type of mature epithelium to another type of mature epithelium is known as:**
    A. Metaplasia
    B. Dysplasia
    C. Anaplasia
    D. Hypoplasia

89. **"Sago Spleen" is seen in:**
    A. Sarcoidosis.
    B. Amyloidosis.
    C. Chronic venous congestion
    D. Gaucher's disease

90. **"Heart failure cells" are seen in:**
    A. Lungs
    B. Heart
    C. Spleen
    D. Liver

91. **Teratoma arises from:**
    A. Totipotential cell
    B. Ectoderm
    C. Mesoderm
    D. Endoderm

92. **Schilling's test is used to diagnose:**
    A. Folate deficiency
    B. B_{12} deficiency
    C. Iron deficiency
    D. Riboflavine deficiency

93. Polycythemia is suspected when the hematocrit value is:
- A. More than 60%.
- B. Less than 45%.
- C. 35%
- D. 29%

94. "Soap Bubble" appearance on X-ray is characteristically seen in:
- A. Osteosarcoma
- B. Osteoclastoma
- C. Osteoblastoma
- D. Osteochondroma

95. "Codman's triangle on X-ray is seen in:
- A. Osteosarcoma
- B. Osteoclastoma
- C. Chondrosarcoma
- D. Ewing's sarcoma

96. The characteristic cell of a granuloma is:
- A. Macrophage
- B. Polymorph
- C. Lymphocyte
- D. Plasma cell

97. Stain used for reticulocyte count is:
- A. Wright's stain.
- B. Giemsa stain.
- C. Brilliant cresyl blue.
- D. Leishman's stain.

98. The anticoagulant of choice for determination of hematocrit is:
- A. Double oxalate
- B. Sodium citrate
- C. Potassium oxalate
- D. Sodium oxalate

99. The most common fungal infection of oral cavity in immunocompromised individuals is:
- A. Moniliasis
- B. Nocardiosis
- C. Histoplasmosis
- D. Actinomycosis

100. "Cor bovinum" is term used to describe heart in:
- A. Syphilis
- B. Myocarditis
- C. Hypertension
- D. Cardiomyopathy

101. The tumor marker for colonic cancer is:
- A. Carcinoembryonic antigen.
- B. Chorionic gonadotropin
- C. Alpha fetoprotein
- D. Progesterone

102. Wilson's disease is assosciated with abnormal metabolism of:
- A. Copper
- B. Magnesium
- C. Calcium
- D. Iron

103. Unidirectional movement of leukocytes across chemical gradient is known as:
- A. Chemotaxis.
- B. Chemokinesis.
- C. Diapedesis.
- D. Phagocytosis.

104. Hemorrhagic or red infarct is commonly seen in:
- A. Spleen
- B. Kidney
- C. Heart
- D. Lungs

105. Antibody present in the serum of an individual of blood Group B is:
- A. Anti A
- B. Anti B
- C. Both Anti A and Anti B.
- D. None.

106. Enzymatic fat Necrosis is associated with elevated serum levels of:
- A. SGPT
- B. SGOT
- C. Amylase
- D. Alkaline phosphatase

107. Lymphoid leukemoid reaction is *not* seen in:
- A. Tuberculosis
- B. Pertusis
- C. Pneumonia
- D. Viral infections

108. Leukopenia with relative lymphocytosis is seen in:
- A. Tuberculosis
- B. Typhoid
- C. Hepatitis
- D. Pertusis

Bibiliography
1. Ed. Steven G Silverberg: Principles and Practice of Surgical Pathology; II Edition, Churchill Livingstone, 1990.
2. Ed. Juan Rosai: Harcourt Brace and Co Asia PTE Ltd; Ackerman's Surgical Pathology VIII edition, 1996.
3. Ed. Kumar, Abbas & Fausto, Elsevier, Robbins and Cotran: Pathologic Basis of Disease; 7th edition, 2004
4. Ed. Christopher D. H. Fletcher: Diagnostic Histopathology of Tumors; Churchill Livingstone, 1995.

ANSWERS

1 D	2 B	3 C	4 B	5 B	6 C	7 C	8 D
9 B	10 B	11 C	12 D	13 D	14 A	15 D	16 A
17 B	18 D	19 D	20 C	21 B	22 A	23 B	24 C
25 C	26 C	27 D	28 D	29 D	30 B	31 B	32 C
33 C	34 C	35 C	36 D	37 C	38 D	39 A	40 C
41 C	42 C	43 B	44 D	45 A	46 A	47 B	48 B
49 B	50 B	51 A	52 D	53 D	54 B	55 D	56 A
57 D	58 C	59 C	60 A	61 A	62 D	63 A	64 C
65 D	66 A	67 B	68 A	69 C	70 C	71 A	72 C
73 C	74 D	75 C	76 A	77 A	78 C	79 A	80 D
81 D	82 A	83 B	84 A	85 A	86 A	87 A	88 A
89 B	90 A	91 A	92 B	93 A	94 B	95 A	96 A
97 C	98 A	99 A	100 A	101 A	102 C	103 A	104 D
105 A	106 C	107 C	108 B				

Microbiology

1. **Which one of these is not a prominent cause of acute sinusitis?**
   - A. *Streptococcus pneumoniae*
   - B. *Haemophilus influenzae*
   - C. *Moraxella catarrhalis*
   - D. *Mycoplasma pneumoniae*

2. **Which one of these is not a prominent cause of bacterial nosocomial sinusitis?**
   - A. *Staphylococcus aureus*
   - B. *Hemophilus influenzae*
   - C. *Pseudomonas aeruginosa*
   - D. *Klebsiella pneumoniae*

3. **Which one of these is an important cause of peritonsillar abscess?**
   - A. Fusobacterium
   - B. *Hemophilus influenzae*
   - C. *Pseudomonas aeruginosa*
   - D. *E.coli*

4. **Thrush is cause by:**
   - A. *Candida albicans*
   - B. Trichophyton rubrum
   - C. *Histoplasma capsulatum*
   - D. Pencillium SP

5. **Paul Bunnel test is used for the serodiagnosis of:**
   - A. Rickettsiosis
   - B. Infectious mononucleosis
   - C. Rheumatoid arthritis
   - D. Chicken pox

6. **Which type of haemolysis is produced by *Streptococcus pyogenes*?**
   - A. α - haemolysis
   - B. β - haemolysis
   - C. γ - haemoloysis
   - D. None of the above.

7. **β-haemolytic streptococci is divided based on lancefield grouping into:**
   - A. 17 groups
   - B. 19 groups
   - C. 21 groups
   - D. 23 groups

8. **CAMP test is used for the identification of:**
   - A. group A streptococci
   - B. group B streptococci
   - C. group C streptococci
   - D. group G streptococci

9. ***Streptococcus pyogenes* is differentiated from other streptococcus based on the sensitivity to:**
   - A. Penicillin
   - B. Tetracycline
   - C. Bacitracin
   - D. Ampicillin

10. **Lancefield grouping of β-Haemolytic streptococci is based on group specific:**
    - A. Carbohydrate
    - B. Protein
    - C. Lipoprotein
    - D. Lipopolysaccharide

11. **One of the following is not a surface protein antigen useful in serological typing of *Streptococcus pyogenes*:**
    - A. M Protein
    - B. T Protein
    - C. R Protein
    - D. K Protein

12. **One of the following is a major virulence factor of *Streptococcus pyogenes*:**
    - A. T Protein
    - B. R Protein
    - C. M Protein
    - D. Group specific carbohydrate

13. **In acute rheumatic fever of adults the ASO test is considered to be positive if the titre is:**
    - A. ≥ 50 Todd units/ml
    - B. ≥ 100 Todd units/ml
    - C. ≥ 150 Todd units/ml
    - D. ≥ 200 Todd units/ml

14. As per the lance field grouping, *Streptococcus agalactiae* belongs to:
    A. group A streptococci
    B. group B streptococci
    C. group C streptococci
    D. group D streptococci

15. One of the following organism is an important cause of infective endocarditis:
    A. *Streptococcus agalactiae*
    B. *Streptococcus dysgalactial*
    C. *Streptococcus viridans*
    D. *Streptococcus equisimilis*

16. *Streptococcus pyogenes* cell wall protein cross reacts with:
    A. Meninges   B. Synovial fluid
    C. Myocardium   D. Cardiae valves

17. Streptococcus pyogenes cell wall carbohydrate cross reacts with:
    A. Meninges   B. Synovial fluid
    C. Myocarduim   D. Cardiae valves

18. The susceptibility of a person to scarlet fever can be tested by:
    A. Schick test   B. Frei test
    C. Dick test   D. Casonis' test

19. The rash that occurs is scarlet fever is due to the sore throat and the production of one of the toxins by *Streptococcus pyogenes is*:
    A. Erythrogenic toxin
    B. Streptokinase
    C. Streptodornase
    D. Hyaluronidase

20. The number of biotypes of *corynebacterium diphtherium is*:
    A. 2   B. 4
    C. 3   D. 5

21. The intracytoplasmic granules of *corynebacterium diphtherium is*:
    A. Polyphosphate granules
    B. Poly - β- hydroxybutyrate granules
    C. Glycogen granules
    D. Sulphur granules

22. The medium used for the cultivation of *C. diphtheriae* is:
    A. Crystal violet blood agar
    B. Macconkey agar
    C. Deoxycholate citrate agar
    D. Loeffler's serum slope.

23. The toxin produced by *C.diphtheriae* is:
    A. Endotoxin   B. Enterotoxin
    C. Exotoxin   D. None of the above

24. "Chinese letter" morphology is seen in stained smears of:
    A. *Streptococcus pyogenes*
    B. *Hemophilus influenzae*
    C. *Corynebacterium diphtheriae*
    D. *Staphylococcus aureus*

25. The toxin produced by C.diphtheriae can be detected by:
    A. Ascolis thermoprecipitation test
    B. Eleks test
    C. Weil-felix test
    D. CAMP test

26. The causative agent of myringitis bullosa is a:
    A. Bacteria   B. Fungi
    C. Virus   D. Protozoa

27. The common cause of deafness in childhood is due to:
    A. Bleeding disorders B. Hypertension
    C. ASOM   D. CSOM

28. The etiological agent of rhinosporidiosis is a:
    A. Fungi   B. Bacteria
    C. Virus   D. Protozoa

29. One of the following infections can lead to bony septal perforation:
    A. Malaria   B. Syphilis
    C. Tuberculosis   D. Cysticercosis

30. Todd Hewitt broth medium is used for the culture of:
    A. *Streptococcus*   B. *Meningococcus]*
    C. *C.diphtheriae*   D. *H. influenzae*

31. Diphtheria is also known as:
    A. Weils disease
    B. Bilharziasis
    C. Bretonneaus disease
    D. Trench fever

32. **The mode of action of diphtheria toxin is:**
    A. Inhibition of protein synthesis
    B. Inhibition of DNA synthesis
    C. Inhibition levels of CAMP
    D. Altering the acetylcholine release

33. **The most common etiological agent of subacute bacterial endocarditis is:**
    A. group A β-hemolytic streptococcus
    B. group B β-hemolytic streptococcus
    C. group C β-hemolytic streptococcus
    D. streptococcus viridans

34. **In a schictest a test does of diphtheria toxin is injected in one arm and the diphtheria toxoid as a control in the other arm. Erythema and induration appears in both arms in 6-24 hours, reaches maximum in size by 48-72 hours and disappears by 96 hours. This indicates:**
    A. Negative reaction   B. Positive reaction
    C. Pseudo reaction   D. Combined reaction

35. **Diphtheria toxin has an affinity for which of the following tissues?**
    A. Heart muscle   B. Nerve endings
    C. Adrenal glands   D. All of the above

36. **A positive sehick test for diphtheria indicates that the person is:**
    A. Non hypersensitive and immune
    B. Suscepitble and non-hypersensitive
    C. Immune and hypersensitive.
    D. Nonimmune and hypersensitive

37. **A negative shick test indicates that the person is:**
    A. Nonhypersensitive and immune
    B. Susceptible and hypersensitive
    C. Immune and hypersensitive
    D. Susceptible and non-hypersensitive

38. **Snail track ulcers or mucous patches in the oropharynx is characteristics of:**
    A. Primary syphilis   B. Secondary syphilis
    C. Latent syphilis   D. Tertiary syphilis

39. **The causative agent of vincents angina is:**
    A. *Treponema pallidum* and *Leptotrichia buccalis*
    B. *Troponema vincentii* and *Leptospira icterohemorrhagiae*
    C. *Troponema vincentii* and *Leptotrichia buccalis*
    D. *Borrelia recurrentis* and *Leptospira icterohemorrhagiae.*

40. **Hemophilus influenzae is divided into different serotypes based on one of the cellular components:**
    A. Cell wall   B. Flagella
    C. Fimbriae   D. Capsule

41. **The number of serotypes hemophilus influenzae is divided into based on capsular antigen:**
    A. 2   B. 4
    C. 6   D. 8

42. **Most infections of hemophilus influenzae are caused by strains belonging to capsular:**
    A. serotype A   B. serotype B
    C. serotype C   D. serotype D

43. **Accessory growth factors required for the growth of hemophilus influenzae is:**
    A. Only X factor
    B. Only V factor
    C. Both X and V factor
    D. None of the above

44. **The phenomenon of satellitism is exhibited by hemophilus influenzae on:**
    A. Choclate agar   B. Nutrient agar
    C. Macconkey agar   D. Blood agar

45. **Hemophilus influenzae causes the following infections:**
    A. Epiglottitis   B. Pneumonia
    C. Meningitis   D. All the above

46. **Which stage is the most infective in whooping cough?**
    A. Carrier stage   B. Catarrhal stage
    C. Paroxysmal stage   D. Convalescent stage

47. **The most ideal specimen for the cultivation of B.pertussis is:**
    A. Sputum   B. Bronchoalveolar lavage
    C. Post nasal swab   D. Per nasal swab

48. **One of the following phases is used for the vaccine preperation of B.petrussis is:**
    A. Phase I   B. Phase II
    C. Phase III   D. Phase IV

49. **The most virulent form of B.pertussis is in:**
    A. Phase I   B. Phase II
    C. Phase III   D. Phase IV

50. **The least virulent form of B.pertussis is in:**
    A. Phase I   B. Phase II
    C. Phase III   D. Phase IV

51. **The pertussis component is present in DPT vaccine as:**
    A. Toxoid
    B. Live attenuated vaccine
    C. Killed vaccine
    D. DNA recombinant vaccine

52. **The number of serotypes of rhinoviruses are:**
    A. Twenty
    B. Forty
    C. Sixty
    D. More than one hundred

53. **All the following viruses can cause common cold** *except:*
    A. Rhinoviruses
    B. Coronaviruses
    C. Parainfluenza viruses
    D. Arboviruses

54. **The antigens of rhinoviruses can be demonstrated from the nasal washing by:**
    A. Complement fixation test
    B. ELISA test
    C. Agglutination test
    D. Precipitation test

55. **Polioviruses can be isolated from one of the specimens:**
    A. Blood   B. CSF
    C. Throat swab   D. Sputum

56. **The following serotypes of adenoviruses are commonly associated with respiratory infections:**
    A. Serotype 35 - 42   B. Serotype 25 - 34
    C. Serotype 10 - 42   D. Serotype 1 - 7

57. **One of the most important complications of mumps is:**
    A. Hepatosplenomegaly
    B. Paralysis
    C. Diarrhoea
    D. Orchitis.

58. **Kopliks spots are a characteristics feature in one of the following infections:**
    A. Influenza   B. Mumps
    C. Measles   D. Rhinovirus infection

59. **MMR vaccine is a:**
    A. DNA recombinant vaccine
    B. Killed vaccine
    C. Live attenuated vaccine
    D. Subunit vaccine

60. **Parainfluenza virus responsible for upper respiratory tract infection can be diagnosed from the exfoliated cells aspirated from respiratory tract by:**
    A. Immunofluorescent staining
    B. PCR
    C. Complement fixation test
    D. Neutralization test

ANSWERS

1 D	2 B	3 A	4 A	5 B	6 B	7 C	8 B
9 C	10 A	11 D	12 C	13 D	14 B	15 C	16 C
17 D	18 C	19 A	20 C	21 A	22 D	23 C	24 C
25 B	26 C	27 D	28 A	29 B	30 A	31 C	32 A
33 D	34 C	35 D	36 B	37 A	38 B	39 C	40 D
41 C	42 B	43 C	44 D	45 D	46 B	47 D	48 A
49 A	50 D	51 C	52 D	53 D	54 B	55 C	56 D
57 D	58 C	59 C	60 A				

Section 2
Otorhinolaryngology (ENT) and, Head and Neck Surgery

Otology

1. **Pinna develops from:**
   - A. Four mesodermal tubercles
   - B. Six ectodermal tubercles
   - C. Six mesodermal tubercles
   - D. Two ectodermal and four mesodermal tubercle

2. **The tympanic membrane develops from:**
   - A. Ectoderm
   - B. Mesoderm
   - C. Endoderm
   - D. All of the above

3. **Malleus and Incus develops from:**
   - A. Meckels cartilage
   - B. Reichters cartilage
   - C. Tympanic ring
   - D. Tubotympanic recess

4. **The obliquity of the TM with loss of meatus is:**
   - A. 15°-20°
   - B. 25°-30°
   - C. 35°-40°
   - D. 45°-55°

5. **The inner surface of TM is supplied by:**
   - A. Auriculotemporal nerve
   - B. Tympanic plexus
   - C. Greater auricular nerve
   - D. Arnolds nerve

6. **Which of the following is a part of tympanic plexus?**
   - A. Jacobsons nerve
   - B. Arnolds nerve
   - C. Auditory nerve
   - D. Auriculotemporal nerve

7. **Which part of the middle ear is formed by Tegmen tympani?**
   - A. Medial wall
   - B. Lateral wall
   - C. Roof
   - D. Floor

8. **The vibratory surface area of the tympanic membrane is:**
   - A. 45 sq.mm
   - B. 55 sq.mm
   - C. 65 sq.mm
   - D. 75 sq.m

9. **The lever ratio between handle of malleus and body of Incus is:**
   - A. 1.3
   - B. 1.8
   - C. 2.3
   - D. 2.8

10. **The round window is closed by:**
    - A. Basilar membrane
    - B. Ressieners membrane
    - C. Tectorial membrane
    - D. Secondary TM

11. **In adult the mastoid antrum lies at a depth of:**
    - A. 10 mm
    - B. 15 mm
    - C. 20 mm
    - D. 25 mm

12. **The hydraulic ratio in middle ear is:**
    - A. 9:1
    - B. 12:1
    - C. 15:1
    - D. 18:1

13. **The length of basilar membrane is:**
    - A. 25 mm
    - B. 35 mm
    - C. 45 mm
    - D. 55 mm

14. **The number of fibers in cochlear nerve is:**
    - A. 5 to 10 thousands
    - B. 15 to 25 thousands
    - C. 35 to 50 thousands
    - D. 60 to 80 thousands

15. The thickness of TM is:
    A. 0.075 to 0.1 mm   B. 0.1 to 0.5 mm
    C. 0.5 to 1 mm   D. 0.5 to 1 cm

16. Which of the following statement regarding promontory is not true?
    A. It overlies the basal turn of cochlea
    B. Horizontal part of facial nerve lies above it
    C. The tympanic recess lies above and in front of it
    D. Round window lies below and behind the promontory

17. The transverse diameter of the tympanic cavity at the narrowest point is:
    A. 1 mm   B. 2 mm
    C. 4 mm   D. 8 mm

18. Which nerve passes through the canal of Huguier?
    A. Chorda tympani
    B. Greater superficial petrosal
    C. Lesser superficial petrosal
    D. Deep petrosal

19. Prussak's space lies between the:
    A. Head of malleus and pars flaccida
    B. Neck of malleus and pars tensa
    C. Neck of malleus and shrapnells membrane
    D. Handle of malleus and shrapnells membrane

20. The length of internal auditory meatus is:
    A. 0.5 cm   B. 1 cm
    C. 2 cm   D. 4 cm

21. The resting electrical potential in scala media is:
    A. +5 millivolts   B. –5 millivolts
    C. +80 millivolts   D. –80 millivolts

22. The electrical potential difference between cornea and retina is around:
    A. +100 to –100 millivolts
    B. +100 to +300 millivolts
    C. +100 to +300 microvolts
    D. +300 to +1300 microvolts

23. Normal duration of nystagmus in caloric tests is:
    A. 30 to 60 seconds   B. 60 to 90 seconds
    C. 90 to 120 seconds   D. 2 to 3 minutes

24. The normal protrusion of auricle is about:
    A. 10° to 15°   B. 15° to 20°
    C. 20° to 30°   D. 30° to 35°

25. Otoliths are crystals of:
    A. Calcium carbonate
    B. Calcium bicarbonate
    C. Calcium sulphate
    D. Calcium phosphate

26. The length of bony cochlea is:
    A. 15 mm   B. 25 mm
    C. 35 mm   D. 45 mm

27. The narrowest part of facial canal is:
    A. 2 mm above stylomastoid foramen
    B. 4 mm above stylomastoid foramen
    C. 6 mm above stylomastoid foramen
    D. 8 mm above stylomastoid foramen

28. A 100 fold increase in intensity of sound is equivalent to a change of:
    A. 10 db   B. 20 db
    C. 50 db   D. 100 db

29. The average compliance range in normal impedence audiometry ias:
    A. 0.4 ml   B. 0.6 ml
    C. 0.8 ml   D. 1 ml

30. In cortical ERA a large negative(N2) peak is obtained at:
    A. 50 msec   B. 100 msec
    C. 175 msec   D. 200 msec

31. The ductus reuniens connect:
    A. Saccule with scala media
    B. Saccule with utricle
    C. Saccule with scala tympani
    D. Saccule with scala vestibuli

32. Which type of curve in Bekesy audiometry is diagnostic of nonorganic lesion?
    A. type II   B. type III
    C. type IV   D. type V

33. The incidence of acellular(sclerotic mastoid) is:
    A. 10%   B. 20%
    C. 25%   D. 30%

34. Fowler's test is positive in:
    A. Conductive deafness
    B. Cochlear deafness
    C. Retrocochlear deafness
    D. Central deafness

35. Recruitment is positive in:
   A. Conductive deafness
   B. Cochlear deafness
   C. Nerve deafness
   D. Central deafness

36. Place theory was proposed by:
   A. Rutherford   B. Helmhotz
   C. VonBekesy   D. Waver

37. Flat or dome shaped tympanogram is found in:
   A. Secretory otitis media
   B. Otosclerosis
   C. Eustachian tube obstruction
   D. Ossicular disruption

38. ABLB test is otherwise known as:
   A. Fowlers test   B. Reger test
   C. Carharts test   D. Differential limen test

39. Jerger's curve is related to:
   A. Speech audiometry   B. CERA
   C. BERA   D. Bekesy audiometry

40. Which noise is used for masking?
   A. Broadband sound
   B. Narrowband filtered sound
   C. Subsonic sound
   D. Supersonic sound

41. Which vestibular nucleus is known as Deiter's nucleus?
   A. Medial   B. Lateral
   C. Superior   D. Inferior

42. P.B and spondy words are used in:
   A. PTA
   B. Peep show audiometry
   C. Speech audiometry
   D. Impedence audiometry

43. Which of the following statement regarding Facial recess is true?
   A. Lies lateral to *Chorda tympani* and medial to vertical part of facial nerve
   B. Medial to *Chorda tympani* and lateral to horizontal part of facial nerve
   C. Medial to *Chorda tympani* and medial to horizontal part of facial nerve
   D. Medial to *Chorda tympani*, lateral to vertical part of facial nerve and below short process of incus

44. Which of the following statement regarding sinus tympani is true?
   A. Lies behind the oval and round window and medial to pyramid
   B. Behind oval window and lateral to pyramid
   C. Above round window and lateral to pyramid
   D. Below oval window and medial to pyramid

45. Which of the following statement regarding Trautman's triangle is true?
   A. Lies between superior petrosal and lateral sinus and behind the solid angle
   B. Between inferior petrosal and superior petrosal sinus
   C. Between superior petrosal and straight sinus
   D. Between inferior petrosal and lateral sinus

46. Carhart's notch is found at:
   A. 2000 Hz in bone conduction
   B. 2000 Hz in air conduction
   C. 4000 Hz in air conduction
   D. 4000 Hz in bone conduction

47. In noise pollution the maximum hearing loss is at the frequency of:
   A. 2-4 kHz   B. 4-6 kHz
   C. 6-8 kHz   D. 8-10 kHz

48. Which of the following waves on the BERA are the best measure of auditory acuity?
   A. 1st and 2nd   B. 2nd and 3rd
   C. 3rd and 4th   D. 4th and 5th

49. The child turns the head towards sound source at:
   A. Birth   B. 3 months
   C. 6 months   D. 1 year

50. The percentage of words normally repeated by the patient to determine SRT is:
   A. 20%   B. 25%
   C. 50%   D. 100%

51. Which of the following statement regarding electrocochleography is not true?
   A. Transtympanic thin needle electrode is place on the promontory and posterior to oval window.
   B. No masking is required
   C. Anesthesia does not affect the result
   D. Most information are from apical coil of cochlea

52. Which of the following statement regarding CERA is not true?

A. Pure tones are used at ½ to 2 seconds interval

B. A train of 30 to 60 pulse is necessary

C. A large negative peak (N1) is obtained at 200 - 250 msec.

D. A small positive (P1) peak is obtained at 50 - 60 msec.

53. Which of the following statement regarding overtone is not true?

A. The harmonics inherent in the sound (overtone determines the timbre

B. Overtones are simple multiples of the frequency of the lowest note

C. Also known as the simple multiples of the frequency of the fundamental note

D. They are simple multiples of the intensities of the lowest note

54. The stapedius muscle contract bilaterally at an intensity of sound stimulus above:

A. 40 dB   B. 50 dB

C. 70 dB   D. 90 dB

55. All the following are objective audiometry *except*:

A. Impedence audiometry

B. Bekesy audiometry

C. CERA

D. BERA

56. Which of following tuning fork test is used to detect NOHL?

A. Rinnes test   B. Weber's test

C. Chimani-Moose test   D. ABC test

57. Which of the following infection may cause unilateral sensorineural deafness?

A. Mumps   B. Measles

C. Rubella   D. Toxoplasmosis

58. Occulogyric reflex (OGR) is present at:

A. Birth   B. 4 wks

C. 8 wks   D. 16 wks

59. The critical pressure difference between middle ear and nasopharynx in barotrauma is:

A. 30 mm Hg   B. 60 mm Hg

C. 90 mm Hg   D. 120 mm Hg

60. Which of the following statement regarding the relationship between consonant and vowel in hearing and speech is not true?

A. Vowels sounds are roughly below 1500 Hz

B. Consonant sounds are usually above 1500 Hz

C. Vowels are relatively powerful sound and consonants are weak

D. Vowels are interspersed among consonants to give specific meaning to words.

61. Compare Table A with Table B:

Table A	Table B
A. Place Theory	1. Rutherfotd
B. Telephone Theory	2. Helmholtz
C. Volley Theory	3. Von Bekesy
D. Travelling wave Theory	4. Wever

62. Complications of CSOM versus CSF findings (Table A vs B):

Table A	Table B
A. Meningitis	1. Normal CSF pressure and contents
B. Lateral sinus thrombosis	2. Clear CSF with slight pleocytosis and ↑sed proteins
C. Brian abscess	3. ↑sed CSF proteins, polymorphs and pressure ↓ed CSF sugar and chloride with turbid CSF
D. Subdural abscess	4. ↑ed CSF pressure with normal sugar.

63. Types of deafness versus Bekesy audiogram (Table A vs B):

Table A	Table B
A. Conductive deafness	1. The continuous tracing drops abruptly away from the pulsed tracing before 500 Hz.
B. Sensory deafness (cochlear)	2. The continuous tone is heared better than pulsed fore
C. Nerve deafness	3. The continuous and pulsed tone tracing overlap throughout
D. Non organic deafness	4. The continuous and pulsed tone tracing overlap at low frequency but the continuous tracing drops below the pulsed tone between 500 and 1000 Hz and then runs parallel to it.

64. **Tympanometry – Compare Table (A) with (B):**

Table A	Table B
A. Otosclerosis	1. Increased compliance with normal pressure
B. Secretory otitis media	2. Normally shaped graph with decreased compliance
C. Eustachian tube obstruction.	3. Maximum compliance at negative pressure
D. Ossicular disruption	4. Flat or Dome shaped tympanogram

65. **Recruitment – Compare Table (A) with (B):**

Table A	Table B
A. Fowlers' test	1. Monoaural loudness balance test
B. Reger's test	2. ABLB test
C. SISI test	3. Measures the change in the intensity of a sound just sufficient to produce a perceptible alteration of loudness
D. Difference Limen test	4. A score of more than 60% is typical of cochlear deafness

66. **The most common type of dysplasia in congenital deafness is:**
   A. Michale type
   B. Mondini type
   C. Scheibe type
   D. Alexander type

67. **Which of the following statement regarding vestibular receptor organ is not true?**
   A. The special sensory epithelium in the semicircular canal is ampulary cristae
   B. The specialized epithelium in utricle and saccule is known as macula
   C. The macula of the utricle is in vertical plane and that of saccule is in horizontal plane
   D. Their epithelium is formed of cells surmounted by long hairlets

68. **Which of the following statement regarding vestibular haircells is not true?**
   A. The type I cells are rounded and flask-shaped
   B. They type II cells are cylindrical
   C. The type I cells resemble morphologically to the inner hair cells
   D. The type II cells have nerve chalice

69. **Which of the following statement regarding cochlear hair cells is not correct?**
   A. The outer hair cells contain 70-100 steriocilia
   B. The inner hair cells are present on the inner side of the inner rod
   C. The outer hair cells are columnar in shape
   D. The arrangement of steriocilia in inner and outer hair cells are like double 'V' and triple 'W' respectively.

70. **Which of the following statement regarding decibel is correct?**
   A. It is a simple ratio between two different intensities of sound
   B. It is equal to the logarithm of the simple ratio of intensities of two sounds.
   C. It is equal to logarithm of the simple ratio of sounds to the base 10
   D. It equals to 10 times the logarithm of the simple ratio of the sounds to the base 10

71. **The sound level used in clinical audiometry are related to a reference intensity pressure of:**
   A. 0.24 dyne cm^{-2} B. 0.0024 dyne cm^{-2}
   C. 0.00024 dyne cm^{-2} D. 0.0042 dyne cm^{-2}

72. **A 100 fold increase in the intensity of sound is equivalent to a change of:**
   A. 10 dB   B. 20 dB
   C. 50 dB   D. 100 dB

73. **In clinical work the threshold of normal hearing is defined as:**
   A. 0 dB   B. –5 dB
   C. 1 dB   D. –1 dB

74. **From a distance of 1 meter, a whisper has an intensity of:**
   A. 10 dB   B. 20 dB
   C. 30 dB   D. 40 dB

75. **Which of the following statements regarding overtone is not true?**
   A. It determine the quality if the sound
   B. It is the harmonics inherent in the sound which determine the timber
   C. Overtones are simple multiple of the frequency of the lowest note
   D. Overtones are simplest multiple of the intensity of the lowest fundamental note

76. **Jerger's curve is related to:**
    A. Bekesy audiometry
    B. Puretone audiometry
    C. Speech audiometry
    D. Impedance audiometry

77. **Which of the following wave in cortical evoked response audiometry is often prominent in young children?**
    A. P_1 B. N_1
    C. P_2 D. N_2

78. **Masking must always be applied to the better ear when the difference of the threshold is atleast:**
    A. 10 dB   B. 20 dB
    C. 30 dB   D. 40 dB

79. **Which of the following electrical activities measured by electrocochleography?**
    A. Cochlear microphonic
    B. Action potential
    C. Summation potential
    D. All of the above

80. **The percentage of word correctly repeated by the patient to determine normal speech reception threshold is:**
    A. 25%   B. 50%
    C. 75%   D. 100%

81. **Which of the following statement regarding various audiometric finding in different types of deafness is not true?**
    A. SISI score is high in cochlear deafness
    B. Tone decay is present in conductive deafness
    C. Speech discrimination is poor in nerve deafness
    D. Recruitment is present in sensory deafness

82. **Which of the following statement regarding electrocochleography is not true?**
    A. A transtympanic thin needle electrode is placed on the promontory
    B. This electrode lies just anterior to the oval window
    C. No masking is required and anesthesia does not affect the result
    D. Most of the information comes from the basal coil cochlea

83. **Which of the following statement regarding acoustic reflex threshold (ART) is not true?**
    A. Frequency between 500 Hz and 400 Hz are best used clinically.
    B. In normal ear the ART for pure tone is more than the ART for noise stimuli
    C. In conductive deafness the ART may be unobtainable.
    D. The ART for puretone alone can be used to predict the hearing acuity

84. **Which of the following audiometry maybe having the most promising use differentiating between cochlear and retrocochlear deafness?**
    A. Speech audiometry
    B. Evoked response audiometry
    C. Beckesy audiometry
    D. Impedance audiometry

85. **All the following audiometry are grouped under electric response audiometry (ERA) *expect:***
    A. Psychogalavinc skin response audiometry (PGSR)
    B. Cortical evoked response audiometry (CERA)
    C. Brainstem evoked response audiometry (BERA)
    D. Transtympanic electrocochleography.

86. **Which of the following statement regarding cortical electric response audiometry (CERA) is not true?**
    A. Electrodes are placed on the vertex and on the ear lobe or mastoid.
    B. Puretone are used at 1/2 to 2 seconds interval
    C. A small positive peak (P1) is obtained at 50 to 60 msec.
    D. A large negative peak (N1) is obtained at 200 to 250 msec.

87. **Which of the following statements regarding CERA is true?**
    A. There is no definite criteria for using CERA data for otoneurological diagnosis
    B. It does not give an accurate objective measure of the puretone audiogram in adult and older children.
    C. Passive co-operation of the patient is not essential movement does not blur the response.
    D. It takes only about 5 minutes to perform the test.

88. **Hearing tests used for screening young children and retardates in STYCAR are:**
   A. Reflex tests
   B. Behavioral tests
   C. Performance tests
   D. Objectives tests

89. **Conditioned audiometry is done to defect deafness:**
   A. Children
   B. Malingerers
   C. Pshyosomatic personality
   D. None of the above

90. **All the following are advantages of a body-worn model hearing aid except:**
   A. Great power is available
   B. Maximum application with minimum feedback
   C. Ability to produce stereophonic effect
   D. Ability to incorporate induction coil

91. **The frequency range for average recruitment in hearing aid is:**
   A. 20 to 20,000 Hz
   B. 500 to 4000 Hz
   C. 70 to 7,400 Hz
   D. 256 to 512 Hz

92. **Specific acoustic resistance of any medium depends on:**
   A. Density
   B. Elasticity
   C. Density of stiffness
   D. None of the above

93. **The minimum conductive hearing loss which can be detected by Rinne's test is:**
   A. 5 dB
   B. 10 dB
   C. 15 dB
   D. 25 dB

94. **The minimum conductive deafness that can be detected by Weber's test is:**
   A. 5 dB
   B. 10 dB
   C. 15 dB
   D. 25 dB

95. **Absolute bone conduction (ABC test is lengthened) in:**
   A. Otosclerosis
   B. Menier's disease
   C. Acoustic neuroma
   D. Presbyacusis

96. **All the following conditions can cause fluctuating deafness except:**
   A. Menier's disease
   B. Perilymph fistula
   C. Cogan's syndrome
   D. Otosclerosis

97. **Dysacousia present in Vogt-Koyanagi-Harada syndrome has all the features except:**
   A. Deafness develops before blindness
   B. It is usually bilateral
   C. Frequently associated with tinnitus and vertigo
   D. Otological symptoms begins to improve after few weeks as tinnitus and vertigo subsides

98. **Diagnostic finding of acoustic neuroma in pure tone audiometry is:**
   A. Sudden dip at 1,000 Hz in bone conduction
   B. Sudden dip at 2,000 Hz in bone conduction
   C. Sudden dip at 2,000 Hz in air and bone conduction (AC and BC)
   D. Sudden dip at 4,000 Hz in AC and BC

99. **Cochlear implants were first used in prelingually deaf children in 1980 by:**
   A. House
   B. Clark
   C. Shambaugh
   D. None of the above

100. **The neural element most likely to be stimulated by cochlear electrode is:**
   A. Spiral ganglion
   B. Inner hair cells
   C. Outer hair cells
   D. None of the above

101. **In intracochlear implant the electrode is placed in:**
   A. Scala media
   B. Scala tympani
   C. Scala vestibuli
   D. None of the above

102. **The average spiral ganglion cells in normal ear is around:**
   A. 10,000
   B. 20,000
   C. 30,000
   D. 50,000

103. **All the following systemic defects are found in LEOPARD syndrome except:**
   A. Electrocardiographic defect
   B. Occular hypotelorism
   C. Pulmonary stenosis
   D. Renal defect

104. Deafness association with mucopolysachha- ridosis includes all the following syndromes *except:*
    A. Hullgren's syndrome
    B. Hurler's syndrome
    C. Hunter's Syndrome
    D. Sanfilippo's syndrome

105. All the following syndrome causing deafness have chromosomal abnormality *except:*
    A. Turner's syndrome
    B. Noonan's syndrome
    C. Klinefelter's syndrome
    D. Cri-du-chat- syndrome

106. The correct noise limit specification in the school be:
    A. 10 to 20 dB   B. 20 to 30 dB
    C. 30 to 40 dB   D. 40 to 50 dB

107. The correct percentage of hearing loss at 45 dB, as per the Los Angeles Foundation of otology is:
    A. 20%   B. 30%
    C. 40%   D. 50%

108. Erythroblastosis fetalis typically causes loss that centers around:
    A. 1,000 to 2,000 Hz   B. 2,000 to 3,000 Hz
    C. 3,000 to 5,000 Hz   D. 4,000 to 5,000 Hz

109. Which type CROS hearing aid is used when the ear that better hearing is normal?
    A. High CROS   B. Mini CROS
    C. Power CROS   D. Focal CROS

110. The nucleus multichannel device cochlear implant was developed at:
    A. Melbourne   B. London
    C. Los Angeles   D. Paris

ANSWERS

1 B	2 D	3 A	4 D	5 B	6 A	7 C	8 D
9 A	10 D	11 B	12 D	13 B	14 C	15 A	16 C
17 B	18 A	19 C	20 B	21 C	22 D	23 C	24 C
25 A	26 C	27 D	28 B	29 B	30 B	31 A	32 D
33 B	34 B	35 B	36 B	37 A	38 A	39 D	40 B
41 B	42 C	43 D	44 A	45 A	46 A	47 D	48 D
49 C	50 C	51 D	52 C	53 D	54 C	55 B	56 C
57 A	58 D	59 C	60 D	61 A-2, B-1, C-4, D-3		62 A-3, B-1, C-2, D-4	
63 A-3, B-4, C-1, D-2		64 A-2, B-4, C-3, D-1		65 A-2, B-1, C-4, D-3		66 C	67 C
68 D	69 A	70 D	71 C	72 B	73 B	74 C	75 D
76 A	77 D	78 D	79 D	80 B	81 B	82 B	83 D
84 B	85 A	86 D	87 A	88 B	89 A	90 C	91 B
92 C	93 C	94 A	95 A	96 D	97 A	98 D	99 A
100 A	101 B	102 D	103 D	104 A	105 B	106 C	107 B
108 C	109 B	110 A					

Rhinology

1. The bridge of the nose is formed by:
A. Nasal bone
B. Nasal spine of frontal bone
C. Frontal process of maxilla
D. None of the above

2. Septal cartilage is otherwise known as:
A. Greater alar cartilage
B. Lesser alar cartilage
C. Quadrilateral cartilage
D. Lower lateral cartilage

3. Middle turbinate is formed by:
A. Vomer
B. Ethmoid
C. Maxilla
D. None of the above

4. Superior meatus is confined to:
A. Anterior 1/3 of the lateral wall of nasal cavity
B. Posterior 1/3 of the lateral wall of nasal cavity
C. Anterior 2/3 of the lateral wall of nasal cavity
D. Posterior 2/3 of the lateral wall of nasal cavity

5. Nasolacrimal duct opens to:
A. Anterior end of inferior meatus
B. Posterior end of inferior meatus
C. Anterior end of middle meatus
D. Posterior end of middle meatus

6. Frontonasal duct opens into the:
A. Inferior meatus
B. Middle meatus
C. Superior meatus
D. Sphenoethmoidal recess

7. All the following bones form the bony part of the nasal septum *except:*
A. Vomer
B. Perpendicular plate of ethmoid
C. Crest of maxilla
D. Cribiform plate of ethmoid

8. The main sensory supply of nose is derived from:
A. Facial nerve
B. Vidian nerve
C. Maxillary nerve
D. None of the above

9. The parasympathetic supply of nose is through:
A. Greater superficial petrosal nerve
B. Lesser superficial petrosal nerve
C. Deep petrosal nerve
D. Olfactory nerve

10. The olfactory nerve contains around:
A. 5 fillaments
B. 10 fillaments
C. 20 fillaments
D. 50 to 100 fillaments

11. The eddies are formed by the:
A. Inspired air around middle meatus
B. Inspired air around middle turbinade
C. Expired air around middle turbinade
D. Expired air around middle meatus

12. The cavernous sinus is related to:
A. Frontal sinus
B. Anterior ethmoidal sinus
C. Posterior ethmoidal sinus
D. Sphenoid sinus

13. The drug of choice in trigeminal neuralgia is:
A. Aspirine
B. Phenobarbitone
C. Ergotamine
D. Carbamzepine

14. Hypersomia is a feature of:
A. Hypertrophic rhinitis
B. Vasomotor rhinitis
C. Rhinitis medicomentosa
D. Hysterical neurosis

15. **Sphenoid sinus is best seen in:**
    A. Submentovertical view
    B. Occipitofrontal view
    C. Occipitomental view
    D. Oblique view

16. **All the following statements regarding rhinophyma are true *except*.**
    A. It occurs almost exclusively in males
    B. It is due to hypertrophy of sebaceous gland
    C. The tip of the nose is usually affected
    D. It is more common during adolescence

17. **All the following statement regarding congenital choanal atresia are true *except*:**
    A. It is due to persistence of bucconasal membrane
    B. Membranous type are more common than bony
    C. Unilateral atresia are more common than bilateral
    D. Comple atresia is more common than implete

18. **The most important consideration in maxillo-facial injury is:**
    A. Arrest of bleeding
    B. Management of shock
    C. Maintenance of airway
    D. Management of associated head injury

19. **CSF rhinorrhea is common in trauma to the fracture of:**
    A. Frontal bone
    B. Ethmoid
    C. Sphenoid
    D. None of the above

20. **The commonest fracture in injury to nose and PNS is:**
    A. Maxilla
    B. Ethmoid
    C. Sphenoid
    D. Nasal bone

21. **All the following statement regarding Guerines fracture are true *except*:**
    A. It is otherwise known as Le Fort's type II
    B. It involves the central middle third of the face.
    C. The fracture line runs between upper alveolus and maxilla
    D. It is found in head on crushes due to heavy blow

22. **All the following structures are the contents of pterygopalatine fossa *except*:**
    A. Third part of maxillary artery
    B. Maxillary nerve
    C. Sphenopalatine garglion
    D. Pterygoid plexus

23. **The color of the olfactory epithelium is:**
    A. Pink
    B. Red
    C. Yellow
    D. Pinkish red

24. **The incidence of conchal pneumatization in sphenoid sinus is:**
    A. 1%
    B. 10%
    C. 20%
    D. 40 to 60%

25. **Rhinolith may contain the following salt *except*:**
    A. Calcium sulphate
    B. Calcium phosphate
    C. Calcium carbonate
    D. Magnesium phosphate

26. **The most common virus in coryza is:**
    A. Influenza virus
    B. Parainfluenza virus
    C. Rhino virus
    D. Respiratory syncitial virus

27. **Repeated digital trauma to nose causes epistaxis due to bleeding from:**
    A. Retrocollumular vein
    B. Anterior facial vein
    C. Sphenopalatine artery
    D. Sphenopalatine vein

28. **The length of nasal cavity in adult is:**
    A. 5 cm
    B. 7.5 cm
    C. 10 cm
    D. 15 cm

29. **In septal hematoma, blood mainly accumulates in:**
    A. Submucous layer
    B. Subperichondrial layer
    C. Subperiosteal layer
    D. None of the above

30. **Chondrocyts in avascular cartilage die in:**
    A. 1 day
    B. 3 days
    C. 5 days
    D. 7 days

31. **The concept of SMR operation was popularized by:**
    A. Killian
    B. Cottle
    C. Mezenbaum
    D. Galloway

32. **The concept of septoplasty was popularized by:**
    A. Freer
    B. Cottle
    C. Killian
    D. None of the above

33. **All the following components are part of young's syndrome** *except:*

    A. Obstructive azoospermia
    B. Primary ciliary diskinesia
    C. Bronchiectasis
    D. Sinusitis

34. **All the following components are part of pick wickian syndrome** *except:*

    A. Excessive day time somnolence
    B. Morbid obesity
    C. Left heart failure
    D. Elevated PCO_2

35. **Death in Wegener granulomatosis is usually due to:**

    A. Renal failure
    B. Respiratory failure
    C. Heart failure
    D. Cardiorespiratory failure

36. **All the following statement regarding Stewart's granulma are false** *except:*

    A. Presence of focal glomerulonephritis
    B. Presence of systemic vascullitis
    C. Steriod and crystotoxic drugs is given
    D. Radiotherapy is the treatment of choice

37. **The diagnostic titre of the IgG antibody to VCA in nasopharyngeal cancer (NPC) is:**

    A. 1/5   B. 1/10
    C. 1/80   D. 1/640

38. **The diagnostic titre of IgG antibody to EA in NPC is:**

    A. 1/5   B. 1/10
    C. 1/80   D. 1/640

39. **The antibody titre of practical value in the serological screening for NPC in endemic region is:**

    A. IgA/EA   B. IgG/EA
    C. IgA/VCA   D. IgG/VCA

40. **All the following statement regarding the HLA genetic markers in NPA are true** *except:*

    A. The major histocompatability gene complex is on the short arm of chromosome 5
    B. I comprises of 6 recognized loci
    C. There are at least 18 recognized alleles at HLA-A Locus and 32 at HAL – B locus
    D. Each alleles determines an antigen

41. **All the following statement regarding HLA haplotype AW 19-B17 in NPC are true** *except:*

    A. Short term survival
    B. Mostly older onset (> 30 yr)
    C. High VCA/EA titres and low ADCC titres
    D. Most patients die within two years

42. **All the following statement regarding the differential HLA frequency distribution in NCP are true** *except:*

    A. BW-46 is confined to older patients (> 30 year)
    B. BW 17 / BW 48 is associated with both old and young patients
    C. B11 and B13 are associated with decreased risk
    D. B13 is associated with younger patients

43. **The relative risk with haplotype A2–BW46 in NPC is:**

    A. 1.5 time   B. 1.9 time
    C. 2.2 times   D. 3.4. times

44. **Transantral ethmoidectomy is otherwise known as:**

    A. Lynch – Howarth operation
    B. Janson – Horgan operation
    C. Patterson's operation
    D. Denker's operation

45. **External frontoethmoidectomy is otherwise known as:**

    A. Jansen–Horgan operation
    B. Canfield's operation
    C. Lynch – Howarth operation
    D. Mac-Neils operation

46. **All the following conditions are indications for external from to ethmoidectory** *except:*

    A. Definitive oncological treatment of sinus malignacy
    B. Recurrent ethmoidal polyps
    C. Orbital cellulits in acute ethmoiditis
    D. Mucocele of frontal sinus

47. **All the following statement regarding IgE are true** *except:*

    A. It is comprised of two heavy and two light chains
    B. The molecular weights of the above chains are 72,500 and 23,000 respectively
    C. The sedimentation coefficient is 11s.
    D. The carbohydrate of the molecule is 21%.

48. An odorant molecule has the following properties *except:*
    A. The molecular weight lies between 20 and 300
    B. The molecule is relatively apolar
    C. It is more soluble in water and less in lipid
    D. The relative number of the molecule decides the particular quality of smell

49. Identify the correct chemical and pure odorant below, with matching smell:
    A. Trimethyle amine – Fishy
    B. Phynyle ethanole – Sweaty
    C. 1-Valeric acid – Rose water
    D. Methane – Roasted popcorn

50. Identify the chemical and pure odorant below with mis matched smell:
    A. Methone – Minty
    B. Acetic acid – Vinegar
    C. 2-isobutyl-3-methoxypyrazine—Musky
    D. Dodecylmercaptan – Petrol like

51. All the following bones from the bony nasal pyramid *except:*
    A. Nasal bone
    B. Perpendicular plate of ethmoid
    C. Frontal process of maxilla
    D. Nasal spine of frontal bone.

52. Kiesselbach's plexus is formed by all the following arteries *except:*
    A. Sphenopalatine artery
    B. Greater palatine artery
    C. Anterior ethmoidal artery
    D. Posterior ethmoidal artery

53. All the following are complications of sinusitis *except:*
    A. Mucocele   B. Pyocele
    C. Meningocele   D. Meningitis

54. All the following statements regarding psudohypertention are tissue *except:*
    A. Caused by injury to medial canthal ligament
    B. Inter canthal distance is increased
    C. Interpupillary distance is normal
    D. Presence of visual disturbance

55. Encephalocele is:
    A. Herniation brain tissue
    B. Herniation of dura
    C. Herniation of brain tissue with dura
    D. None of the above

56. The venous plexus near the posterior end of inferior turbinate is known as:
    A. Woodruff's area
    B. Little's area
    C. Pterygoid plexus
    D. Keisselbach's plexus

57. Pharyngeal recess is otherwise known as:
    A. Sphenoethmoidal recess
    B. Frontal recess
    C. Fossa of Rossen muller
    D. Pyriform fossa

58. Nasal cholesteatoma is otherwise known as:
    A. Rhinitis sicca
    B. Rhinitis caseosa
    C. Rhinitis medicamentosa
    D. None of the above

59. Sodium chromoglycate acts by:
    A. Increasing mast cell permeability
    B. Decreasing mast cell permeability
    C. Stabilizing the mast cell permeability
    D. Decreasing the number of mast cells

60. Olfactory placodes develops in gestation at about:
    A. 3 weeks   B. 6 weeks
    C. 9 weeks   D. 12 weeks

61. The immunoglobulin present in nasal mucoma is primarily:
    A. IgA   B. IgG
    C. IgE   D. IgM

62. The origin of the cytokine (IL–1) in allergic inflammation is from:
    A. Mast cells   B. Macrophages
    C. T-cells   D. Eosinophils

63. Mast cells produces all the following cytokines *except:*
    A. IL-1   B. IL-4
    C. IL-5   D. IL-8

64. The predominant antibody in early immune response is:
    A. IgA   B. IgG
    C. IgM   D. IgE

65. The antibody found in large quantities on circulatory B cells is:
    A. IgA   B. IgG
    C. IgE   D. IgD

66. The only Ig that crosses the placenta is:
   A. IgG
   B. IgM
   C. IgE
   D. IgA

67. The major antibody of secondary (anamnestic) response is:
   A. IgA
   B. IgD
   C. IgE
   D. IgG

68. The type of allergic reaction in delayed hypersensitivity is:
   A. Type I
   B. Type II
   C. Type III
   D. Type IV

69. Thommen's postulate regarding effectiveness of allergen is on:
   A. Plant pollens
   B. Animal danders
   C. Moulds
   D. House dust

70. Based on embryologic precursors the first lamella of the ethmoid labyrinth in adult is:
   A. Ethmoid bulla
   B. Uncinate process
   C. Haitus semilunaris
   D. Middle turbinate

71. The length of uncinate process is around:
   A. 0.5 to 1 cm
   B. 1 to 1.5 cm
   C. 1.5. to 2 cm
   D. 2 to 2.5 cm

72. Onodi cell is a highly pneumatized:
   A. Anterior ethmoid cell
   B. Middle ethmoid cell
   C. Posterior ethmoid cell
   D. None of the above

73. Sphenoethmoid cell otherwise known as:
   A. Haller cell
   B. Agger nasi cell
   C. Onodi cell
   D. None of the above

74. The ethmoid cells extending along the medial orbital floor are known as:
   A. Hallar cells
   B. Onodi cells
   C. Aggernasi cells
   D. Concha Bullosa

75. All the following statement regarding nasal gliomas are true *except:*
   A. Consists of heterotrophic glial tissue
   B. No patent intracranial connection
   C. Do not transilluminate
   D. Positive Furstenburg's sign

76. The most common fungal infection of nose and PNS in USA is:
   A. Histoplasmosis
   B. Blastomycosis
   C. Cryptococcosis
   D. Rhinosporidiosis

77. Charcot – Leyden crystals are found in the Mucin of patients suffering from:
   A. Rhinosinusitis
   B. Allengic Rhinosinusitis
   C. NARES
   D. AFRS

78. The most common intracranial complication of sinusitis is:
   A. Meningitis
   B. Epidural abcess
   C. Subdural abcess
   D. Brain abcess

79. Wegener's triad consists of all the following features *except:*
   A. Necrotising granuloma of respiratory tract
   B. Glomerulonephritis
   C. Raised ESR
   D. Vasculitis

80. Antinuclear cytoplasmic antibody (c-ANCA) is found in:
   A. Wegener's granuloma
   B. Stewart's granuloma
   C. Fungal granuloma
   D. Rhinoscleroma

81. Churg-Strauss syndrome is characterized by all the following features *except:*
   A. Necrotising vasculitis
   B. Polyneuritis multiplex
   C. Asthma
   D. Hypereosinophilia

82. Smelling of non-existent odour is known as:
   A. Parosmia
   B. Phantosmia
   C. Dysosmia
   D. Chacosmia

83. All the following medications can produce rhinitis *except:*
   A. ACE inhibitors
   B. Betablockers
   C. Oral contraceptives
   D. Corticosteroids

84. Pregnancy tumor or granuloma gravidarum is otherwise known as:
   A. Sinonasal hemangioma
   B. Cavernous hemangioma
   C. Lobular capillary hemangioma
   D. Hemangiopericytoma

85. **The most common cause of death in relapsing polychondritis is:**
    A. Cardiac failure
    B. Pneumonia
    C. Renal failure
    D. Cardiorespiratory failure

86. **The mainstay therapy of relapsing polychondritis is:**
    A. Corticosteroids
    B. Cyclophosphamide
    C. Azathoprine
    D. Methotrexate

87. **All the following statemnets regarding angiocentric nasal T cell lymphoma are true** *except:*
    A. It is associated with E-B virus
    B. Common in Asia and China
    C. Presents as midline destructive lesion
    D. Chemotherapy is the treatment of choice

88. **All the following fungi can cause rhinocerebral mucomycosis** *except:*
    A. Rhizopus
    B. Nocardia
    C. Mucor
    D. Absidia

89. **Schneiderian papilloma is otherwise known as:**
    A. Ringertz tumor
    B. Inverted papilloma
    C. Transitional cell papilloma
    D. All the above

90. **The fungus responsible for acute invasive fungal sinusitis in 90% of cases is:**
    A. *Rhizopus oryzae*
    B. *Aspergillous flavus*
    C. *Aspergillous fumigatus*
    D. *Aspergillous niger*

91. **All the following features are present in fungal ball (mycetoma)** *except:*
    A. Noninvasive in nature
    B. Usually due to aspergillous fumigatus
    C. Patients are usually immunocompromised
    D. Recurrence is not common after surgery

92. **As per the Lederman's classification of tumors of nose and PNS all the following sites belong to suprastructure** *except:*
    A. Ethmoidal labyrinth
    B. Frontal sinus
    C. Sphenoid sinus
    D. Maxillary antrum

93. **The anatomical relation of Fossa of Rossen Muller with eustachian tube is that the later lies:**
    A. Anteriorly
    B. Posteriorly
    C. Posterolaterally
    D. Medially

94. **The actual surface area of nasopharynx is approximately:**
    A. $20\ cm^2$
    B. $30\ cm^2$
    C. $50\ cm^2$
    D. $70\ cm^2$

95. **Sinus of morgagni lies between the:**
    A. Base of skull and superior constrictor
    B. Superior and middle constrictor
    C. Middle and inferior constrictor
    D. None of the above

96. **Adenoid may be very small or absent in:**
    A. Familial hypogama globulinemia
    B. Wiskoff-Addrick syndrome
    C. All of the above
    D. None of the above

97. **The amount of water evaporated from the surface of nasal mucosa in 24 hours is:**
    A. 200 ml
    B. 500 ml
    C. 800 ml
    D. 1000 ml

98. **The mucous blanket in nasal mucosa moves at a speed of:**
    A. 5 to 10 mm per second
    B. 5 to 10 mm per minute
    C. 10 to 15 mm per second
    D. 10 to 15 mm per minute

99. **The amount of nasal secretion produced in 24 hours is:**
    A. 200 to 300 ml
    B. 300 to 500 ml
    C. 600 to 700 ml
    D. 800 to 1000 ml

100. **The nasal cilia at room temperature beat at:**
    A. 5 to 10 times per second
    B. 10 to 20 times per second
    C. 5 to 10 times per minute
    D. 10 to 20 times per minute

101. **The pH of nasal secretion is nearly constant at:**
    A. 6.5
    B. 7
    C. 7.4
    D. 7.5

102. **The amount of air the nose breathe every 24 hours is:**
    A. 200 cubic feet
    B. 500 cubic feet
    C. 800 cubic feet
    D. 1000 cubic feet

103. The radiator mechanism of the nose warm up the inspired cold air to near body temperature in:
    A. ¼ second
    B. ½ second
    C. 1 second
    D. 2 second

104. The most common malignant tumor involving the skin of the nose is:
    A. Melanoma
    B. Squamous cell carcinoma
    C. Basal cell carcinoma
    D. None of the above

105. Columellar septum is formed by the:
    A. Medial crura of the alar cartilages
    B. Lateral crura of the alar cartilages
    C. Quadrilateral cartilage
    D. None of the above

106. The fracture of the nasal septum resulting from blows from the front is known as:
    A. Guerine fracture
    B. Jarjaway fracture
    C. Chevallet fracture
    D. None of the above

107. The most common cause of nasal septal perforation is:
    A. Lupus
    B. Leprosy
    C. Tuberculosis
    D. Trauma

108. Whistling sound in nasal septal perforation is caused by:
    A. Large anterior perforation
    B. Large posterior perforation
    C. Small anterior perforation
    D. Small posterior perforation

109. Kemicetive antiozaena solution contains all the following *except:*
    A. Chloromycetin
    B. Potassium iodide
    C. Oestradiol
    D. Vitamin D_2

110. Destruction of anterior nasal spine is found in:
    A. Leprosy
    B. Syphilis
    C. Tuberculosis
    D. Sarcoidosis

111. Mucocele of the frontal sinus usually presents in 90% of cases on the:
    A. Superiomedial quadrant of orbit
    B. Inferiomedial quadrant of orbit
    C. Superiolateral quadrant of orbit
    D. Inferior lateral quadrant of orbit

112. Sphenoethmoidal mucocele may have similar clinical features as in:
    A. Superior orbital fissure syndrome
    B. Orbital apex syndrome
    C. All of the above
    D. None of the above

113. Samter's triad consists of all the following *except:*
    A. Nasal polyp
    B. Bronchial asthma
    C. Aspirin sensitivity
    D. Chronic sinusitis

114. Exposure to wood-dust is causative factor mainly for the adenocarcinoma of:
    A. Maxillary sinus
    B. Frontal sinus
    C. Sphenoid
    D. Ethmoid

115. The most common organism responsible for acute bacterial sinusitis is:
    A. Hemophyllus influenza
    B. Streptococcus pneumoniae
    C. Streptococcus viridanoe
    D. Staphylococcus aureus

116. Physaliferous cells on histology are characteristic of:
    A. Burkitt's lymphoma
    B. Hodgkin's lymphoma
    C. Non-Hodgkin lymphoma
    D. Chordoma

117. Which of the following industrial workers are prone to malignancy of nose and PNS?
    A. Chromium
    B. Vanadium
    C. Aluminium
    D. Platinum

118. The first radiological evidence of frontal sinus is present at age of:
    A. One year
    B. Two year
    C. Four years
    D. Six years

119. The first radiologic evidence of ethmoid sinus is present at the age of:
    A. One year
    B. Two years
    C. Three years
    D. Four years

120. The maximum number of cranial nerves affected in the orbital complication of sinusitis is:
    A. Orbital cellulitis
    B. Orbital abcess
    C. Superior orbital fissure syndrome
    D. Orbital apex syndrome

ANSWERS

1	A	2	C	3	B	4	B	5	A	6	C	7	D	8	C
9	A	10	C	11	C	12	D	13	D	14	D	15	A	16	D
17	B	18	C	19	B	20	D	21	A	22	D	23	C	24	A
25	A	26	C	27	A	28	B	29	B	30	B	31	A	32	B
33	B	34	C	35	A	36	D	37	D	38	C	39	C	40	A
41	B	42	D	43	D	44	B	45	C	46	A	47	D	48	C
49	A	50	C	51	B	52	D	53	C	54	D	55	C	56	A
57	C	58	B	59	C	60	A	61	A	62	B	63	A	64	C
65	D	66	A	67	D	68	D	69	A	70	B	71	C	72	C
73	C	74	A	75	D	76	A	77	D	78	A	79	D	80	A
81	B	82	B	83	D	84	C	85	A	86	A	87	D	88	B
89	D	90	A	91	C	92	D	93	D	94	C	95	A	96	C
97	D	98	B	99	C	100	B	101	B	102	B	103	A	104	C
105	A	106	B	107	C	108	C	109	B	110	A	111	A	112	C
113	D	114	D	115	B	116	D	117	A	118	D	119	A	120	D

Laryngology

1. **All the following statements regarding thyroid cartilage are true *except*:**
   - A. It develops from the fourth visceral arch
   - B. Begins to ossify at 25 yr of age
   - C. The angle of fusion is 120 degrees in male
   - D. Inferior cornu articulates with cricoid cartilage

2. **All the following statements regarding cricoid cartilage are false *except*:**
   - A. Develops from 6th arch
   - B. Its broad in front and narrow behind
   - C. It's thinner and weaker than thyroid cartilage
   - D. Anterior surface has a horizontal line

3. **The name of the cartilage formed in the aryepiglottic fold is:**
   - A. Cuneiform
   - B. Corniculate
   - C. Aretinoid
   - D. None of the above

4. **The cartilage of tritecea is formed by:**
   - A. Hypoepiglottic ligament
   - B. Thyroepiglottic ligament
   - C. Lateral thyrohyoid ligaments
   - D. Medial thyrohyoid ligaments

5. **Corniculate cartilage is otherwise known as:**
   - A. Cartilage of wrisburg
   - B. Cartilage of santorini
   - C. Arytenoid cartilage
   - D. Cricoid cartilage

6. **All the following regarding conus elasticus are true *except*:**
   - A. Its otherwise known as cricovocal membrane
   - B. It's the lower part of elastic membrane of larynx
   - C. It's mainly composed of yellow elastic tissue
   - D. It's attached above to the inferior border of cricoid cartilage

7. **All the following are extrinsic ligaments of larynx *except*:**
   - A. Median cricothyroid ligament
   - B. Median thyrohyoid ligament
   - C. Lateral thyrohyoid ligament
   - D. Hypoepiglottic ligament

8. **Thyrohyoid membrane is pierced by all the following structures *except*:**
   - A. External branch of superior laryngeal nerve
   - B. Internal branch of superior laryngeal nerve
   - C. Superior laryngeal artery
   - D. Superior laryngeal vein

9. **All the following are adductor muscles of larynx *except*:**
   - A. Lateral cricoarytenoid
   - B. Transverse portion of inter arytenoids
   - C. External portion of thyroarytenoids
   - D. Cricothyroid

10. **Vocalis muscle is a specialized part of:**
    - A. Cricothyroid
    - B. Thyroarytenoid
    - C. Lateral cricoarytenoid
    - D. posterior cricoarytenoid

11. **All the following muscles of larynx are intrinsic *except*:**
    - A. Thyrohyoid
    - B. Thyroarytenoid
    - C. Thyroepiglottic
    - D. Posterior cricoarytenoids

12. **The subglottic space lies between the:**
    A. True vocal cord and upper boundary of cricoid cartilage
    B. True vocal cord and lower boundary of cricoid cartilage
    C. False vocal cord and upper boundary of cricoid cartilage
    D. False vocal cord and lower boundary of cricoid cartilage

13. **All the following statements regarding recurrent laryngeal nerve are true *except*:**
    A. It's otherwise known as inferior laryngeal nerve
    B. It's anterior lateral branch is sensory
    C. It hooks around the subclavian artery on the right side
    D. It travels in the tracheoesophageal groove

14. **The loop of Galen is formed by:**
    A. Anterolateral and posteromedian branch of recurrent laryngeal nerve
    B. Anterolateral branch of recurrent laryngeal nerve and external laryngeal branch of superior laryngeal nerve
    C. Anterolateral branch of recurrent laryngeal nerve and internal laryngeal branch of superior laryngeal nerve
    D. Posteromedial branch of recurrent laryngeal nerve and external laryngeal branch of superior laryngeal nerve

15. **The delphian lymph node is found on the:**
    A. Thyrohyoid membrane
    B. Cricothyroid membrane
    C. Cricovocal membrane
    D. Cricotracheal membrane

16. **Which of the following statements regarding the saccule of larynx is false?**
    A. Its otherwise known as the Oilcan of larynx
    B. It's a conical shaped pouch with numerous mucous gland
    C. It ascends from posterior part of the ventricle
    D. It lies between inner surface of thyroid cartilage and the false vocal cord

17. **The length of the rima glottides in male is:**
    A. 1.5 cm   B. 2.5 cm
    C. 3.5 cm   D. 4.5 cm

18. **The length of glottis in female is:**
    A. 1.6 cm   B. 2.6 cm
    C. 3.6 cm   D. 4.6 cm

19. **The vocal cord vibration is best analyzed by:**
    A. Indirect laryngoscopy
    B. Direct laryngoscopy
    C. Microlaryngoscopy
    D. Stroboscopy

20. **Which of the following folds is sphincter of larynx?**
    A. Aryepiglottic fold
    B. Pharyngoepiglottic folds
    C. Median glossoepiglottic fold
    D. Lateral glossoepiglottic fold

21. **Which of the following statements regarding phonation is false?**
    A. Pitch is inversely proportional to the length of the cord
    B. Pitch is directly proportional to the tension of the cord
    C. Pitch is directly proportional to the loudness
    D. Pitch is inversely proportional to the air pressure

22. **The length of the adult vocal cord is:**
    A. 7-14 cm   B. 15-21 cm
    C. 22-25 cm   D. 25-30 cm

23. **Which of the following cartilage is like a Signet ring?**
    A. Thyroid   B. Cricoid
    C. Cuneiform   D. Corniculate

24. **Which of the following cartilage is pyramidal in shape?**
    A. Epiglottis   B. Arytenoid
    C. Cuneiform   D. Corniculate

25. **The lymphatic drainage of the vocal cord is to the:**
    A. Upper deep cervical node
    B. Lower deep cervical node
    C. Prelaryngeal lymph node
    D. None of the above

26. **Reinke's space is found in the:**
    A. True vocal cord
    B. False vocal cord
    C. Ventricles of larynx
    D. Saccule of larynx

27. **Mogiphonia is commonly found in:**
    A. Singer
    B. Teacher
    C. Preacher
    D. All of the above

28. **The safety muscles of larynx is:**
    A. Posterior cricoarytenoid
    B. Lateral cricoarytenoid
    C. Interarytenoid
    D. Cricothyroid

29. **The internal tensor muscle of the vocal cord is:**
    A. Cricothyroid
    B. Thyroepiglottic
    C. Aryepiglottic
    D. Vocalis

30. **The external tensor muscle of vocal cord is:**
    A. External portion of thyroarytenoid
    B. Internal portion of thyroarytenoid
    C. Cricothyroid
    D. Transverse portion of interarytenoids

31. **The only abductor muscle of the vocal cord is:**
    A. Lateral cricoarytenoid
    B. Posterior cricoarytenoid
    C. Cricothyroid
    D. Inter arytenoid

32. **Puberphonia is commonly founding:**
    A. Adolescent females
    B. Adolescent male
    C. Adult male
    D. Adult female

33. **The focal length of the lens used for microlaryngoscopy is:**
    A. 100 mm
    B. 200 mm
    C. 300 mm
    D. 400 mm

34. **All the following statements regarding laryngeal ventricles are true *except:***
    A. This is the site of primitive air sac
    B. It's the space between true and false vocal cords
    C. Commonest site of malignancy in larynx
    D. This is the site for potential origin of laryngocele

35. **The commonest site for vocal nodule is:**
    A. Anterior 1/3rd and posterior 2/3rd of vocal cord
    B. Anterior 2/3rd and posterior 1/3rd of vocal cord
    C. Anterior commissure
    D. Posterior commissure

36. **The commonest organism found in acute epiglottitis is:**
    A. *Streptococcus pyogenes*
    B. *Streptococcus viridians*
    C. *Klebsiella*
    D. Haemophilus influenza

37. **All the following regarding laryngismus stridulous are true *except*:**
    A. Commonly found in 2 yrs old child with rickets
    B. May be associated with celiac disease
    C. Hypoventilation and alkalosis may be present
    D. Presence of carpopedal spasm

38. **Acute supraglottic laryngitis is otherwise known as:**
    A. Laryngismus stridulous
    B. Laryngitis stridulosa
    C. Acute epiglottitis
    D. None of the above

39. **The commonest fungal disease of larynx is:**
    A. Blastomycosis
    B. Histoplasmosis
    C. Mucormycosis
    D. Candidiasis

40. **The commonest cause of laryngeal perichondritis is:**
    A. Tuberculosis
    B. Leprosy
    C. Malignancy
    D. Radiation

41. **The most common cause of laryngeal stridor in children is:**
    A. Acute laryngitis
    B. Acute laryngotracheobronchitis
    C. Laryngeal papilomatosis
    D. Laryngomalacia

42. **Cylindrical epiglottis is found in:**
    A. Tuberculous laryngitis
    B. Acute epiglottitis
    C. Laryngomalacia
    D. None of the above

43. **Turban shaped epiglottis is found in:**
    A. Tuberculous laryngitis
    B. Acute epiglottitis
    C. Lupus of larynx
    D. Syphilitic laryngitis

44. Red pepper granulation of larynx is found in:
   A. Tuberculous laryngitis
   B. Leprotic laryngitis
   C. Lupus of larynx
   D. Mycosis of larynx

45. Mouse nibbled appearance of vocal cord is seen in:
   A. Cancer of larynx
   B. Tuberculous laryngitis
   C. Syphilitic laryngitis
   D. All of the above

46. Commonest site of infection in tuberculous laryngitis is:
   A. Anterior commissure
   B. Epiglottis
   C. Inter arytenoid region
   D. None of the above

47. Mouth eaten ulcer is found in:
   A. Patchy dermia of larynx
   B. Contact ulcer of vocal cord
   C. Keratosis of larynx
   D. Tuberculous laryngitis

48. Arthritis of cricoarytenoid joint is found in:
   A. Rheumatic arthritis
   B. Rheumatoid arthritis
   C. Perichondritis of larynx
   D. All of the above

49. Contact ulcer or Kiss ulcer of larynx is due to:
   A. Sexually transmitted diseases
   B. Kissing disease
   C. Vocal abuse
   D. None of the above

50. Emergency laryngotomy is done through the:
   A. Thyrohyoid membrane
   B. Cricothyroid membrane
   C. Cricovocal membrane
   D. Cricotracheal membrane

51. The commonest laryngeal mass is:
   A. Papilloma
   B. Vocal nodule
   C. Vocal polyp
   D. Malignancy

52. Vocal polyp is commonly found in the:
   A. Anterior commissure
   B. Posterior commissure
   C. Junction of anterior 1/3rd and posterior 2/3rd of vocal cord
   D. Junction of anterior 2/3rd and posterior 1/3rd of vocal cord

53. Chondroma of larynx is mostly found in:
   A. Thyroid cartilage
   B. Cricoid cartilage
   C. Arytenoid cartilage
   D. Cuneiform cartilage

54. All the following conditions of larynx are not premalignant *except:*
   A. Malignant papilomatosis
   B. Solitary papilloma
   C. Contact ulcer
   D. Intubation granuloma

55. The commonest benign growth of larynx is:
   A. Chondroma
   B. Myoma
   C. Solitary Papilloma
   D. Multiple Papilomatosis

56. The treatment of choice for multiple papilomatosis of larynx is:
   A. Interferon   B. Autogenous vaccine
   C. Cryosurgery   D. Laser surgery

57. Supra vital staining is done by:
   A. Methylene blue   B. Toludine blue
   C. Sudan black   D. Methylene Green

58. The male to female sex ratio of laryngeal malignancy is:
   A. 2:1   B. 4:1
   C. 8:1   D. 16:1

59. The incidence of lymph node metastasis of cervical node in supraglottic growth is:
   A. 10 %   B. 20 %
   C. 40 %   D. 60 %

60. The most commonest type of laryngeal cancer is:
   A. Supraglottic   B. Glottic
   C. Subglottic   D. Transglottic

61. The treatment of choice for stage 1 glottic cancer is:
A. Radiotherapy
B. Chemotherapy
C. Partial laryngectomy
D. Total laryngectomy

62. T 1N1 M1 laryngeal cancer corresponds to:
A. Stage 1
B. Stage 2
C. Stage 3
D. Stage 4

63. T4N0 M0 laryngeal cancer corresponds to:
A. Stage 1
B. Stage 2
C. Stage 3
D. Stage 4

64. Blom singers prosthesis is fitted between:
A. Larynx and trachea
B. Larynx and pharynx
C. Trachea and esophagus
D. Trachea and pharynx

65. Ortner's syndrome is found in:
A. Mitral stenosis
B. Mitral regurgitation
C. Aortic stenosis
D. Aortic regurgitation

66. Position of vocal cord in combined paralysis of superior and recurrent laryngeal nerve is:
A. Median
B. Paramedian
C. Cadaveric
D. None of the above

67. Functional aphonia is diagnozed in case of:
A. Bilateral adductor palsy
B. Bilateral abductor palsy
C. Unilateral abductor palsy
D. None of the above

68. A slaky wavy cord is due to:
A. Unilateral recurrent laryngeal nerve palsy
B. Bilateral recurrent laryngeal nerve palsy
C. Superior laryngeal nerve palsy
D. None of the above

69. The voice is rough and tires quickly in:
A. Superior laryngeal nerve palsy
B. Unilateral recurrent laryngeal nerve palsy
C. Bilateral recurrent laryngeal nerve palsy
D. None of the above

70. Smokers of above 40 yrs of age are more prone to develop cancer larynx by:
A. 4 times
B. 8 times
C. 16 times
D. 32 times

71. The incidence of lymphatic metastasis in glottic cancer is about:
A. 4%
B. 8%
C. 16%
D. 20%

72. The incidence of glottic cancer is around:
A. 15%
B. 30%
C. 45%
D. 65%

73. All the following are etiological factors for acute hemorrahagic laryngitis except:
A. Violent coughing
B. Shouting
C. Weight lifting
D. Beta hemolytic streptococcal infection

74. All the statements regarding contact ulcer are true except:
A. It's otherwise a contagious disease
B. It's otherwise known as "kiss ulcer"
C. Referred otalgia may be found
D. Vocal fatigue appears early

75. All the statements regarding quincke's edema of larynx are true except:
A. It's a type of angioneurotic edema
B. It may be due to drug allergy
C. Idiosyncracy to food is also a factor
D. Mental excitement is not a factor

76. The area of the glottis in the newborn is around:
A. 8 sq.mm
B. 16 sq.mm
C. 24 sq.mm
D. 32 sq.mm

77. The length of the vocal cord at birth is:
A. 3 mm
B. 5 mm
C. 7 mm
D. 9 mm

78. The length of the adult vocal cord in male is:
A. 14-15 mm
B. 15-16 mm
C. 17-21 mm
D. 22-25 mm

79. Subglottic stenosis is diagnosed when the diameter of the cricoid ring is around:
A. 1.5 mm
B. 2.5 mm
C. 3.5 mm
D. 4.5 mm

80. **All are contraindications for horizontal partial Laryngectomy** *except*:
    A. Fixation of vocal cord
    B. Involvement of interarytenoid space
    C. Tumour crossing the ventricle and involving the true vocal cord
    D. Involvement of epiglottis

81. **The length of the vocal cord in adult female is:**
    A. 11 to 12 mm   B. 13 to 14 mm
    C. 15 to 16 mm   D. 17 to 18 mm

82. **All the statements given below regarding aphasia are correct** *except*:
    A. Conduction aphasia is associated with left perisylvian lesions
    B. Wernicke's aphasia is generally associated with lesions of the posterior region of left superior temporal gyrus
    C. Transcortical sensory aphasia is associated with left hemispheric lesion involving posterior portion of middle temporal gyrus
    D. Broca's aphasia is associated with area 40

83. **Broca's aphasia is due to involvement of area:**
    A. 22   B. 39
    C. 40   D. 44

84. **Wernicke's aphasia is due to involvement of area:**
    A. 22   B. 39
    C. 40   D. 45

85. **The commonest cause of unilateral abductor (incomplete) palsy on left side is:**
    A. Thyroid surgery
    B. Laryngeal carcinoma
    C. Esophageal carcinoma
    D. Bronchogenic carcinoma

86. **The commonest symptom of gastro esophageal reflux laryngitis {GERD} is:**
    A. Dysphonia   B. Dysphagia
    C. Vocal fatigue   D. Heart burn

87. **Congenital laryngeal cyst occurs most commonly in:**
    A. Supraglottic area   B. Glottic area
    C. Subglottic   D. None of the above

88. **Treatment of OSAS is required if the RDI per hour of sleep is more than:**
    A. 5   B. 10
    C. 15   D. 20

89. **The main stay of therapy in OSAS is:**
    A. Protryptyline   B. Tracheotomy
    C. U3P   D. CPAP

90. **The larynx of the newborn lies at the vertebral level of:**
    A. C1 – C2   B. C2 – C3
    C. C3 – C4   D. C4 – C5

91. **All the following statements regarding trachea are correct** *except*:
    A. It begins at C6 and divides at T5 vertebrae level
    B. Transverse diameter is 15 mm and anteroposterior diameter is 20 mm
    C. Length of trachea is about 10–12 cm
    D. It's lined by pseudostratified ciliated columnar epithelium

92. **The lingular division of bronchus is a segmental branch of:**
    A. Right upper lobe bronchus
    B. Right lower lobe bronchus
    C. Left upper lobe bronchus
    D. Left lower lobe bronchus

93. **The dead space in tracheostomy is reduced by:**
    A. 10% to 20%   B. 20% to 30%
    C. 30% to 50%   D. 50% to 70%

94. **The angle formed by right main bronchus is:**
    A. 15 degrees   B. 25 degrees
    C. 35 degrees   D. 45 degrees

95. **The angle formed by left main bronchus is:**
    A. 25 degrees   B. 45 degrees
    C. 65 degrees   D. 75 degrees

96. **All the following statements regarding tracheal rings are correct** *except*:
    A. The total number of rings is between 16 and 20
    B. The number of rings in cervical position is between 6 to 7
    C. Cartilaginous part of the ring occupies anterior 1/3rd of the circumference
    D. They may get calcified at old age

97. **The commonly used size of bronchoscope in adults is:**
    A. 7 mm × 40 cm   B. 7 mm × 30 cm
    C. 4 mm × 30 cm   D. 4 mm × 40 cm

98. The commonest cause of "Scabberd" Trachea is:

A. Enlarged mediastinal lymph node
B. Enlarged thymus
C. Metastatic neck mass
D. Goitre

99. All the following statements regarding malignant tumors are true *except*:

A. Adenocarcinoma of bronchus is more frequent in males than females
B. Secondary invasions are more common than primary tumours in trachea

C. Superior lobe bronchus is more affected
D. Oat cell varient is a type of anaplastic carcinoma of bronchus

100. All the following statements regarding malignant tumours of bronchial tree are true *except*:

A. Atypical pneumonia may be the first indication of the presence of carcinoma of bronchus
B. Horner's syndrome is seen in pancoast tumor
C. Hilar lymph node metastasis involves only the left recurrent laryngeal nerve
D. The usual and earliest lymphatic spread is often to the mediastinal lymph nodes

ANSWERS

1 C	2 A	3 A	4 C	5 B	6 D	7 A	8 A
9 D	10 B	11 A	12 B	13 B	14 D	15 A	16 C
17 B	18 A	19 D	20 A	21 D	22 B	23 B	24 B
25 D	26 A	27 D	28 A	29 D	30 C	31 B	32 B
33 D	34 C	35 A	36 D	37 C	38 C	39 A	40 D
41 D	42 C	43 A	44 A	45 B	46 C	47 C	48 D
49 C	50 B	51 C	52 A	53 B	54 B	55 D	56 D
57 B	58 C	59 C	60 B	61 A	62 D	63 D	64 C
65 A	66 C	67 A	68 C	69 A	70 D	71 A	72 D
73 D	74 A	75 D	76 C	77 C	78 C	79 C	80 D
81 C	82 D	83 D	84 A	85 D	86 A	87 A	88 D
89 D	90 A	91 C	92 D	93 C	94 B	95 D	96 C
97 A	98 D	99 A	100 D				

Pediatric Otolaryngology -I

1. **Emperipolesis is pathognomonic of:**
   A. Castleman's Disease
   B. Rosai-Dorfman Disease
   C. Melkerson-Rosanthal Syndrome
   D. Cherubism.

2. **Which of the branchial arch is actually absent in human beings?**
   A. Third arch   B. Fourth arch
   C. Fifth arch   D. Sixth arch

3. **Hyoid bone is formed from which of the following branchial arches:**
   A. First and second arch
   B. Second and third arch
   C. Third and fourth arch
   D. Fourth and fifth arch

4. **Which of the following is correct regarding thyroglossal fistula?**
   A. It can manifest with a sinus opening lateral to midline
   B. Excision of hyoid bone is unnecessary for suprahyoid fistulae
   C. The inner opening of the fistula is located in the floor of mouth
   D. It is embryonically related to tuber cinerium

5. **An 8-year-old boy presents with bilateral cervical lymphadenopathy and splenic deposits due to Hodgkin's lymphoma. What is the stage of disease according to Ann-Arbor classification?**
   A. II E
   B. II S
   C. III E
   D. III S

6. **Jaw involvement is common in:**
   A. African lymphoma
   B. American lymphoma
   C. Mediterranean lymphoma
   D. None of the above.

7. **In a child with Non-Hodgkin's lymphoma which of the following investigation is mandatory:**
   A. CSF analysis
   B. Echocardiography
   C. Spirometry
   D. Urine analysis

8. **Which of the following is not a complication of treatment for stage II Hodgkin's lymphoma of neck in a child?**
   A. Thyroid cancer
   B. Breast cancer
   C. Leukemia
   D. Hepatocellular cancer

9. **Which of the following drug is a chemo-therapeutic adjuvant in head and neck lymphoma?**
   A. Desferoxamine
   B. Somatostatin
   C. Allopurinol
   D. Clofibrate

10. **Prenatal demonstration of cystic hygroma in a fetus in ultrasonography should raise the suspicion of:**
    A. Down's syndrome
    B. Klinefelter's syndrome
    C. Turner's syndrome
    D. Apert's syndrome

11. **Which of the following is useful in the treatment of cystic hygroma of neck?**

    A. OK 234
    B. OK 432
    C. KO 234
    D. KO 432

12. **Cervical sinus of His is related to:**

    A. First branchial fistula
    B. Second branchial fistula
    C. Third branchial fistula
    D. Fourth branchial fistula

13. **All the following are differential diagnosis for sternomastoid tumor in a child; *except*:**

    A. Teratoma
    B. Lymphoma
    C. Lateral aberrant thyroid
    D. Neuroblastoma

14. **Treatment of mycobacterium avium intracellulare scrofulaceum (MAIS) lymphadenitis of neck in a 7-Year-old child is:**

    A. Surgical excision with antitubercular drugs (ATT)
    B. Surgical excision without ATT
    C. ATT with out surgical excision
    D. Any of the above.

15. **Cat-scratch disease of neck is caused by:**

    A. Endolimax nana
    B. Rochalimea henselae
    C. Negleria fowleri
    D. Branhamella catarrhallis

16. **Which of the following is true of epignathus?**

    A. It is a tumor
    B. It is a malformation of jaw
    C. It is a parasite
    D. None of the above

17. **Ideal endotracheal tube for neonates with laryngotracheoesophageal cleft is:**

    A. Southoral tube
    B. Jackson-Rees Tube
    C. Donahoe-Hendren Tube
    D. Minnesota tube

18. **Levaditi's myotomy is a treatment for:**

    A. Achalasia cardia
    B. Esophageal atresia
    C. Cricopharyngeal spasm
    D. Nut cracker esophagus

19. **Primary anastomosis is discouraged in which type of tracheoesophageal anomaly:**

    A. Esophageal atresia (EA without tracheo Esophageal Fistula (TEF)
    B. EA + distal TEF
    C. EA + proximal TEF
    D. EA + TEF of both ends.

20. **Treatment of tracheomalacia is:**

    A. Tracheoplasty
    B. Aortopexy
    C. Tracheal splinting
    D. Tissue engineered trachea

21. **Chest X-ray of a child with bronchial foreign body may show any of the following *except*:**

    A. Ipsilateral hyperinflation
    B. Contralateral hyperinflation
    C. Ipsilateral collapse
    D. Contralateral collapse

22. **Tissue engineered trachea is useful in the treatment of:**

    A. Tracheomalacia
    B. Tracheal atresia
    C. Tracheoesophageal cleft
    D. All of the above.

23. **Youngest patient of rhinosporidiosis described in literature was:**

    A. 3 Days
    B. 3 weeks
    C. 3 months
    D. 3 Years

24. **Torticollis is seen in which of the following syndrome:**

    A. Klippel-Trenaunay syndrome
    B. Sandifer's syndrome
    C. Turner's syndrome
    D. Robin's syndrome

25. **Pathognomonic symptom of neonate with unilateral choanal atresia is:**

    A. Feeding difficulty in ipsilateral breast of mother
    B. Feeding difficulty in contralateral breast of mother
    C. Cyclical breathing pattern
    D. Cheyne – stokes breathing pattern.

26. **Nasal polyp in a child should raise the suspicion of:**

    A. Familial polyposis coli
    B. Peutz – Jegher Syndrome
    C. Cystic fibrosis
    D. Addison's disease

27. **Which of the following will be absent in an infant with Kartagener's syndrome:**
    - A. Chronic maxillary sinusitis
    - B. Recurrent respiratory infection or cough
    - C. Situs in versus
    - D. Recurrent otitis media

28. **Which of the following is not a Stone's criterion to diagnose inhalation burns of trachea:**
    - A. Singed vibrissae
    - B. Soot in pharynx
    - C. Microulcers in trachea
    - D. Restlessness.

29. **Hearing aids are recommended in children with congenital deafness if the auditory threshold is above:**
    - A. 30 dB
    - B. 60 dB
    - C. 90 dB
    - D. None of the above

30. **Consonants affected by cleft palate include all except:**
    - A. D
    - B. K
    - C. B
    - D. J

31. **What is the correct size of endotracheal tube for a newborn baby of 2 kg weight?**
    - A. 3 mm
    - B. 3.5 mm
    - C. 4 mm
    - D. 4.5 mm

32. **In which of the following anomalies fetal surgery is indicated:**
    - A. Esophageal atreasia with TEF
    - B. Choanal atresia
    - C. Tracheal atresia
    - D. None of the above

33. **EXIT (Exuterointrapartum Tracheostomy) is used in the treatment of:**
    - A. Tracheoesophageal fistula
    - B. Diaphragmatic hernia
    - C. Bronchopulmonary sequestration
    - D. Phrenic nerve palsy

34. **Which of the following is a contraindication for tonsillectomy?**
    - A. Epidemic of poliomyelitis
    - B. Epidemic of Cholera
    - C. Epidemic of bird-flu
    - D. All of the above

35. **All are derivatives of first pharyngeal pouch except:**
    - A. Eustachian tube
    - B. Middle ear cavity
    - C. Mastoid air cells
    - D. Cochlea

36. **Which is true of pediatric tracheal papillomatosis?**
    - A. Caused by herpes virus
    - B. Malignant transformation is uncommon
    - C. Interferon therapy is curative
    - D. Papillomas may penetrate into mediastinum and erode great vessels

37. **Commonest cause of congenital vocal cord paralysis is:**
    - A. Arnold-Chiari Malformation
    - B. Obstetric iatrogenic injuries
    - C. Maternal medications
    - D. None of the above

38. **Complication of tracheoesophageal repair using Lanman-Height technique is:**
    - A. Tracheal stenosis at the site of fistula ligation
    - B. Peptic ulceration of the fistula site in trachea
    - C. Tracheomalacia
    - D. All of the above

39. **Which of the following is false regarding a coin impacted in cricopharynx?**
    - A. It can be removed by Foley catheter extraction
    - B. Possibility of underlying motility disorder of esophagus should be investigated
    - C. Orientation of coin in plain X-ray can differentiate it from laryngeal impaction of coin.
    - D. Metal detector is a better screening technique than plain X-ray.

40. **All the following are useful in diagnosing a safety pin impacted is esophagus except:**
    - A. Esophagoscopy
    - B. Metal detector
    - C. Plain radiographs
    - D. Esophagogram

41. **Which of the following is not a differential diagnosis of congenital nasal polyp?**
    - A. Meningoencephalocoele
    - B. Benign nasal polyp
    - C. Glioma
    - D. Hemangioma

42. **Which of the following is a not cause of true macroglossia?**
    A. Pierre-Robin Syndrome
    B. Down's Syndrome
    C. Beckwith-Wiedemann Syndrome
    D. Melkerson-Rosanthal Syndrome

43. **Which of the following is not a criteria in the Musgrov's rule of 10 in cleft lip surgery?**
    A. 10 weeks of age
    B. 10 Kg weight
    C. 10 g/dl hemoglobin
    D. 10,000/cmm WBC count

44. **Sialographic appearance of recurrent idiopathic parotitis in children is described as:**
    A. Chain of lakes appearance
    B. Sand storm appearance
    C. Dancing peacock appearance
    D. Hour – glass appearance

45. **Which of the following is not a recommended treatment of recurrent parotitis of children?**
    A. Parotid duct dilatation
    B. Radiotherapy
    C. Parotidectomy
    D. Sclerotherapy

46. **A 3-year-old male child presented with multiple cervical lymphadenopathy of 2 months duration. His father was a known patient of pulmonary tuberculosis 8 years before and completed chemotherapy for the same. The child had been given BCG vaccination at birth. Clinically lymphoma was suspected based on the consistency of node. His ESR was 6 mm/hr and Mantoux was 15 mm. Histopathology of lymph node biopsy was reported as nonspecific lymphadenitis. Which of the following is the best course of further management:**
    A. To sample additional lymph nodes by repeat biopsy
    B. To start empirical antitubercular drug therapy and to assess the response
    C. To give him 3 doses of radiotherapy each of 500 rads
    D. To do nothing but wait and watch him closely

47. **Which is incorrect regarding a child with Pierre – Robin Syndrome?**
    A. This child is more prone for otitis media
    B. Cleft palate to be repaired at 10 months before the child starts speaking
    C. Retrognathia may improve spontaneously with the growth of facial skeleton
    D. Macroglossia noted in these children is an illusion

48. **Embryonically soft palate develops from:**
    A. Primary palate
    B. Secondary palate
    C. Both of them
    D. None of them.

49. **Which of the following is not a treatment of parotid hemangioma?**
    A. Interferon therapy
    B. Sclerotherapy
    C. Radiotherapy
    D. Surgical excision

50. **Pinna of ear develops from which of the following embryonic structure?**
    A. Otic placode
    B. Auricular tubercle
    C. First and second branchial pouches
    D. All of the above

ANSWERS

1 B	2 C	3 B	4 A	5 D	6 A	7 A	8 D
9 C	10 C	11 B	12 D	13 C	14 B	15 B	16 A
17 C	18 B	19 A	20 B	21 D	22 B	23 C	24 B
25 A	26 C	27 A	28 C	29 A	30 D	31 B	32 C
33 B	34 A	35 D	36 B	37 D	38 C	39 B	40 D
41 B	42 A	43 B	44 B	45 C	46 A	47 B	48 B
49 D	50 B						

Pediatric Otolaryngology-II

1. **The commonest type of tracheo - oesophageal anomaly is:**
   A. Oesophageal atresia with distal TOF
   B. Oesophageal atresia with proximal TOF
   C. Oesophageal atresia with proximal and distal TOF
   D. Tracheo-oesophageal fistula (TOF) without oesophageal atresia

2. **The commonest system affected in tracheo - oesophageal anomaly is:**
   A. Cardiovascular system
   B. Gastrointestinal system
   C. Genitourinary system
   D. Respiratory system

3. **Single most common cardiac malformation in tracheo-oesophageal anomaly is:**
   A. Atrial septal defect
   B. Patent ductus arteriosus
   C. Ventricular septal defect
   D. Mitral valve stenosis

4. **The incidence of polyhydraminos in mothers of infant with oesophageal atresia is:**
   A. 10%   B. 20%
   C. 30%   D. 40%

5. **The diagnosis of achalasia is best confirmed by:**
   A. Oesophageal manometry
   B. Rigid oesophagoscopy
   C. Barium swallow X-ray of oesophagus
   D. Fibroptic flexible oesophagoscopy

6. **The commonest gastrointestinal anomaly in oesophageal atresia is:**
   A. Meckel's diverticulum
   B. Malrotation of midgut
   C. Duodenal atresia
   D. Congenital pyloric stenosis

7. **All the following drugs may be helpful in achalsia except:**
   A. Isosorbide dinitrate
   B. Amyl nitrate
   C. Prostaglandin E_2
   D. Atropine

8. **The name of surgical procedure for achalasia cardia is:**
   A. Ramstedt's operation
   B. Nissen fundoplication
   C. Dohlman's operation
   D. Heller's operation

9. **All the following syndromes with congenital deafness are autosomal dominant traits except:**
   A. Waardenburg's syndrome
   B. Alport's syndrome
   C. Treacher Collins syndrome
   D. Pendred's syndrome

10. **All the following syndromes with congenital deafness are autosomal recessive traits except:**
    A. Usher's syndrome
    B. Pierre-Robin syndrome
    C. Pendred's syndrome
    D. Jervell and Lange - Nielsen syndrome

11. **Congenital deafness with retinitis pigmentosa is found in:**
    A. Ballantyne syndrome
    B. Usher's syndrome
    C. Cogan's syndrome
    D. Cockayne's syndrome

12. **All the following statements regarding Cogan's syndrome are true except:**
    A. It is an autoimmune disease
    B. Non - syphilitic interstitial keratitis is found
    C. Usually manifests first in adolescence
    D. Causes conductive deafness

13. All the following statements are true regarding Refsum's disease *except:*
    A. It is an autosomal dominant disorder
    B. It is associated with retinitis pigmentosa
    C. Peripheral neuropathy is a feature
    D. Cerebellar ataxia is a feature

14. All the following statements are true regarding waardenburg's syndrome *except:*
    A. It is an autosomal dominant trait
    B. 20% of affected patients have white forelock
    C. 45% of affected patients have heterochromia iridia
    D. 90% cases have medial displacement of lateral canthus

15. Congenital deafness with bizarre ECG abnormality is found in:
    A. Crouzon's syndrome
    B. Fanconi's syndrome
    C. Norrrie's syndrome
    D. Jervell and Lange - Nielsen syndrome

16. The primary genetic defect in cystic fibrosis is in the:
    A. Short arm of chromosome No. 7
    B. Long arm of chromosome No. 7
    C. Long arm of chromosome No. 8
    D. Short arm of chromosome No. 8

17. The definitive diagnosis of cystic fibrosis is done by testing:
    A. Blood   B. Urine
    C. Sweat   D. CSF

18. Which of the following is found in excess in the sweat of the patient with cystic fibrosis:
    A. Potassium   B. Calcium
    C. Chloride   D. Sodium

19. The common neonatal presentation of cystic fibrosis:
    A. Peritonitis
    B. Obstructive jaundice
    C. Hepatosplenomegaly
    D. Meconeum ileus

20. The stridor in laryngomalacia disappears in most cases after:
    A. 2 to 3 months   B. 3 to 6 months
    C. 6 to 12 months D. 18 to 24 months

21. The commonest site of laryngeal web is:
    A. Anterior half of glottis
    B. Posterior half of glottis
    C. Supraglottis
    D. Subglottis

22. All the following statements regarding congenital vocal cord paralysis are true *except:*
    A. Unilateral palsy is found four times more than bilateral
    B. Diagnosis can be confirmed by laryngoscopy
    C. Accounts for 6% to 13% of all cases of congenital stridor
    D. Second most common cause of congenital stridor

23. The maximum number of inhaled foreign bodies are found in the age group of:
    A. 1 to 3 years   B. 2 to 6 years
    C. 6 to 8 years   D. 8 to 10 years

24. The most frightening and dangerous paediatric emergency due to respiratory infection is:
    A. Acute epiglottitis
    B. Acute laryngitis
    C. Acute laryngotracheobronchitis
    D. Laryngitis stridulosa

25. The commonest deep neck space infection in infancy is:
    A. Ludwig's angina
    B. Acute retropharyngeal abscess
    C. Chronic retropharyngeal abscess
    D. Parapharyngeal abscess

26. Classical "Thumb sign" in X-ray - lateral view of neck is found in:
    A. Acute epiglottitis
    B. Acute laryngitis
    C. Retropharyngeal abscess
    D. Parapharyngeal abscess

27. All the following statements regarding Choanal atresia are false *except:*
    A. 10% bony and 90% cartilaginous
    B. 90% bony and 10% cartilaginous
    C. 40% bony and 60% cartilaginous
    D. 60% bony and 40% cartilaginous

28. The commonest craniofacial defect found in children is:
    A. Apert's syndrome
    B. Carpenter syndrome
    C. Cruzon's syndrome
    D. Goldenhar syndrome

29. Which of following anomalies is not associated with choanal atresia:
    A. Coloboma
    B. Cardiac anomaly
    C. Genital hypoplasia
    D. Retinitis pigmentosa

30. All the statements regarding Treacher collins syndrome are true except:
    A. Otherwise known as Berry syndrome
    B. Associated with fish like mouth and birds like nose
    C. Antimongoloid slant of palpebral fissure
    D. Coloboma in the inner third of upper eyelid

31. Sturge - Weber syndrome is characterized by all the following factors except:
    A. Unilateral venous angiomatosis of leptomeninges
    B. Contralateral facial angiomatosis (Port - Wine stain)
    C. Ipsilateral gyriform calcification of cerebral cortex
    D. Ocular defect

32. Which of the following statement is not true regarding branchial fistula:
    A. It is anterior to sternomastoid
    B. Commonly found in upper one-third of neck
    C. Most fistula end well before pharynx
    D. Recurrent discharge is an indication for surgery

33. All the following statements regarding dysphagia lusoria are true except:
    A. It is due to congenital vascular anomaly
    B. Commonly found in infant
    C. Presence of chronic stridor and brassy cough
    D. Commonest anomaly in the arch of aorta

34. All the following are common causes of dysphagia lusoria except:
    A. Right aortic arch
    B. Double arch of aorta
    C. Right subclavian artery anomaly
    D. Common carotid artery anomaly

35. Which of the following statement is true regarding diagnostic bronchoscopy in dysphagia lusoria:
    A. Pulsatile swelling seen in right antero lateral tracheal wall
    B. Pulsatile swelling seen in right posterior wall of trachea
    C. Pulsatile swelling seen in left tracheal wall
    D. Non-pulsatile swelling seen in right tracheal wall

36. Tick (✓) the correct and cross (×) the incorrect statement given below regarding rhabdomyosarcoma:
    A. It is the most common variety of soft tissue sarcoma in childhood
    B. More than one-third arise in the head and neck region
    C. There seems to be a familial association between childhood rhabdomyosarcoma and maternal carcinoma of breast
    D. Three quarter of all paediatric cases are above ten years of age

37. Tick (✓) the correct and cross (×) the incorrect statement given below regarding rhabdomyosarcoma:
    A. A botryoid appearance is almost diagnostic
    B. The best chemotherapy is the triple drug regimen of vincristine, actinomycin - D and cyclophosphamide
    C. It is more common in male than female children in proportion 2:1
    D. Local control can be achieved by radio therapy in high proportion of cases

38. Tick (✓) the correct and cross (×) for incorrect statement given below regarding head and neck tumors in children:
    A. Non - Hodgkin's lymphoma is the commonest tumor excluding brain tumor
    B. Lymphoma constitute 10% of all malignancy in 0 to 14 years of age
    C. Hodgkin's disease is more common than non-hodgkin's lymphoma
    D. Most T-cell lymphoma arises in the mediastinum

39. **Tick (✓) the correct and cross (✗) for incorrect statement given below regarding head and neck Tumors in children:**
    A. Most non-Hodgkin's lymphoma have a follicular rather than diffuse pattern histopathologically
    B. Burkitt's lymphoma is a "B" cell lymphoma common in west african countries
    C. The so called "starry sky" appearance of histopathological study is not specific for Burkitt's lymphoma
    D. 50% non-Hodgkin's lymphoma present with nasopharyngeal symptoms

40. **All the following statements regarding Cri-Du-Chat syndrome are correct *except*:**
    A. The most striking feature is the characteristic high pitched "Mewing" stridor
    B. Diamond shaped rima glottidis on laryngoscopy
    C. There is a partial deletion of short arm of the sixth chromosome in group "B"
    D. Respiratory distress is uncomon and tracheostomy rarely required

41. **All the following statements regarding cherumbism are true *except*:**
    A. It was first described by Jones in 1933
    B. Females are affected twice as frequently as males
    C. The familial incidence is one of the characteristic feature
    D. It may be inherited as a dominant trait with variable expressivity

42. **The calvarial deformity causing scaphocephaly is otherwise known as:**
    A. Boat skull
    B. Tower skull
    C. Oblique skull
    D. Clover-Leaf skull

43. **Tower skull is otherwise known as:**
    A. Oxycephaly
    B. Brachycephaly
    C. Plagiocephaly
    D. Turricephaly

44. **All the statements regarding Hemifacial atrophy are correct *except*:**
    A. It is otherwise known as Parry - Romberg syndrome
    B. It classically starts in the first decade

C. It starts with atrophy of subcutaneous fat in the paramedian area of the face
    D. It may be associated with ipsilateral Jacksonian epilepsy

45. **All the following statements regarding cleft palate are true *except*:**
    A. Presence of rhinolalia aperta
    B. Velopharyngeal insufficiency is found in complete cleft palate
    C. The optimum time of repair is at 10 years of age
    D. Bifid uvula is feature of submucous cleft palate

46. **The commonest paranasal sinus affected in children is:**
    A. Maxillary sinus
    B. Frontal sinus
    C. Ethmoid sinus
    D. Sphenoid sinus

47. **Which of the following paranasal sinus is rudimentary or absent at birth:**
    A. Maxillary sinus
    B. Frontal sinus
    C. Ethmoid sinus
    D. Sphenoid sinus

48. **Which of the following statements regarding Letterer-Siwe disease is not true *except*:**
    A. It is a rare acute illness in infancy and early children
    B. This is a disease of reticuloendothelial system affecting spleen, liver and lymph nodes
    C. Pyrexia is usually accompanied by a purpuric rash and secondary hypochromic anaemia
    D. There is no skeletal lesion and the condition is not fatal

49. **All the following statements regarding Hand-Schuller-Christian disease are true *except*:**
    A. It belongs to a group of disease called Langerhans' Cell Histiocytosis or histiocytosis X
    B. It is less severe and more chronic form in children and young adult
    C. Proptosis and diabetes inspidus may be present
    D. Treatment is always surgical

50. **All the following statements regarding eosinophilic granuloma are true *except*:**
    A. It is a type of malignant granuloma
    B. It affects children and young adults
    C. Most often temporal or frontal bones are affected
    D. Otological manifestation may mimic tuberculous mastoiditis

ANSWERS

1 A	2 A	3 C	4 C	5 A	6 B	7 D	8 D
9 D	10 B	11 B	12 D	13 A	14 D	15 D	16 B
17 C	18 D	19 D	20 D	21 A	22 D	23 A	24 A
25 B	26 A	27 B	28 C	29 D	30 D	31 B	32 B
33 D	34 D	35 A					

36 A – ✓, B – ✓, C – ✓, D – ✗   37 A – ✓, B – ✓, C – ✗, D – ✗   38 A – ✓, B – ✓, C – ✗, D –

39 A – ✗, B – ✗, C – ✓, D – ✗   40 C   41 B   42 A   43 D   44 D

45 C   46 C   47 B   48 D   49 D   50 A

Head and Neck Surgery

1. **The most common skin lump in neck is:**
   - A. Lipoma
   - B. Melanoma
   - C. Dermoid cyst
   - D. Sebaceous cyst

2. **The commonest group of neck swellings seen in hospital are from:**
   - A. Thyroid
   - B. Lymph node
   - C. Salivary gland
   - D. Metastasis

3. **The most common swelling in neck encountered in general practice is:**
   - A. Goiter
   - B. Thyroid adenoma
   - C. Thyroglossal cyst
   - D. Infected lymph node

4. **The commonest cystic swelling in neck is:**
   - A. Cystic hygroma
   - B. Sebaceous cyst
   - C. Dermoid cyst
   - D. Branchial cyst

5. **All the following conditions are causes of enlarged lymph node in posterior triangle of neck** *except:*
   - A. Toxoplasmosis
   - B. Tonsillitis
   - C. Brucellosis
   - D. Infectious mononucleosis

6. **Bilateral neck node involvement is commonly seen in the malignancy of:**
   - A. Base of tongue
   - B. Fossa of Rosenmuller
   - C. Pyriform fossa
   - D. Supraglottic larnyx

7. **Salivary gland swelling associated with sarcoidosis and uveitis is known as:**
   - A. Mickulicz syndrome
   - B. Heerfordt's syndrome
   - C. Sjögren's syndrome
   - D. Sicca syndrome

8. **The commonest benign tumor of salivary gland is:**
   - A. Pleomorphic adenoma
   - B. Monomorphic adenoma
   - C. Oncocytoma
   - D. None of the above

9. **The commonest malignant tumor of salivary gland is:**
   - A. Adenocarcinoma
   - B. Squamous cell carcinoma
   - C. Acinar cell carcinoma
   - D. Adenoid cystic carcinoma

10. **The male to female sex ratio in Warthin's tumor is:**
    - A. 1:2
    - B. 2:1
    - C. 3:1
    - D. 7:1

11. **All the following statements regarding Warthin's tumor are true** *except:*
    - A. It is a type of monomorphic adenoma
    - B. It is otherwise known as papillary cystadenoma lymphomatosum
    - C. 10% of the tumors are bilateral
    - D. The peak age incidence is in the fourth decade

12. **The commonest midline congenital neck mass below hyoid is:**
    - A. Thyroglossal cyst
    - B. Dermoid cyst
    - C. Branchial cyst
    - D. Cystic hygroma

13. **All the following statements regarding muco-epidermoid tumors of salivary gland are true** *except:*
    - A. These are of variable malignacy
    - B. They can arise in any of the salivary glands
    - C. One out of ten involve the parotid gland
    - D. They are more predominant in males

14. **The incidence of pyriform fossa tumor in hypopharyngeal growth is:**
    A. 20%   B. 40%
    C. 60%   D. 80%

15. **80% of tumors of tongue arise in the:**
    A. Tip of tongue
    B. Lateral margin
    C. Base of tongue
    D. Dorsum of tongue

16. **All the following structures are preserved during functional neck dissection except:**
    A. Internal jugular vein
    B. Sternomastoid muscle
    C. Spinal accessory nerve
    D. Submandibular gland

17. **The sex incidence of postcricoid growth for female is:**
    A. 20%   B. 40%
    C. 50%   D. 90%

18. **All the following statements regarding postcricoid malignancy are false except:**
    A. Five year survival rule is around 50%
    B. Posterior wall of postcricoid region is more involved than anterior wall
    C. Lymph node metastasis is often bilateral in postcricoid growth
    D. It is more common in male than female.

19. **All the following statements regarding cancer of laryngopharynx are true except:**
    A. Incidence of lymphatic metastasis is highest in pyriform fossa growth
    B. The tumors of posterior pharyngeal wall are usually exophytic and in midline
    C. Tumor of the pyriform fossa often presents early
    D. Postcricoid growth may be associated with Patterson-Brown-Kelly syndrome.

20. **All the following arteries are branches of external carotid artery except:**
    A. Superior thyroid   B. Inferior thyroid
    C. Lingual   D. Facial

21. **The longest cranial nerve in the body is:**
    A. 5th CN   B. 7th CN
    C. 10th CN   D. 12th CN

22. **The largest cranial nerve in the body is:**
    A. 5th CN   B. 7th CN
    C. 8th CN   D. 10th CN

23. **The smallest cranial nerve in the body is:**
    A. 1st CN   B. 2nd CN
    C. 3rd CN   D. 4th CN

24. **The cranial nerve which travels the longest distance in the bony canal is?**
    A. 3rd CN   B. 5th CN
    C. 7th CN   D. 9th CN

25. **The cranial nerve having the largest number of autonomic ganglion is:**
    A. 3rd CN   B. 5th CN
    C. 7th CN   D. 12th CN

26. **The total number of skull bones is:**
    A. 18   B. 20
    C. 22   D. 25

27. **Match the parasympathetic ganglions in Table A with its trigeminal association in Table B:**

Table A	Table B
A. Ciliary ganglion	1. Maxillary division
B. Pterygopalatine ganglion	2. Ophthalmic division
C. Submandibular ganglion	3. Mandibular division
D. Otic ganglion	4. Trigeminal nerve trunk
E. Gasserian ganglion	5. Lingual nerve

28. **Semilunar ganglion is found in the:**
    A. Maxillary division of trigeminal nerve
    B. Mandibular division of trigeminal nerve
    C. Opthalmic division of trigeminal nerve
    D. Trigeminal nerve trunk

29. **Match the salivary glands in Table A with their ducts in Table B:**

Table A	Table B
A. Parotid gland	1. Duct of Rivinus
B. Submandibular gland	2. Whartons duct
C. Sublingual gland	3. Stenson's duct

30. **The duct of sublingual salivary gland is also known as:**
    A. Duct of Rivinus   B. Duct of Bartholin
    C. Both A and B   D. None of the above

31. **All the muscles of palate are supplied by the pharyngeal plexus *except*:**
    A. Levator Veli Palatini
    B. Tensor Veli Palatini
    C. Palatoglossus
    D. Palotopharyngeus

32. **All the following statements regarding cervical sympathetic ganglion are false *except*:**
    A. Inferior ganglion is the smallest
    B. Stellate ganglion is formed by fusion of middle and inferior ganglion
    C. Superior ganglion lies at the level of C6 vertebra
    D. Ansa subclavian is formed by middle and inferior ganglion.

33. **All the following statements regarding cervical sympathetic chain are correct *except*:**
    A. It does not receive any white rami communicants
    B. It sends out gray rami communicans
    C. Preganglionic fibres does not synapse with cervical ganglion
    D. Postganglionic fibers originate from the cervical ganglion

34. **The carotid plexus is formed by branches form:**
    A. Superior cervical ganglion
    B. Middle cervical ganglion
    C. Inferior cervical ganglion
    D. All of the above

35. **All the following statements regarding diagastric muscle are true *except*:**
    A. Anterior belly develops from the 1st branchial arch
    B. Posterior belly develops from the hyoid arch
    C. Anterior belly is supplied by the 5th cranial nerve
    D. Posterior belly is supplied by the 9th cranial nerve

36. **All the muscles of pharynx are supplied by pharyngeal plexus *except*:**
    A. Stylopharyngeous
    B. Salpingopharyngeus
    C. Palatopharyngeus
    D. Superior constrictor

37. **The least unconventional clinical staging system for head and neck cancer is:**
    A. TNM
    B. AJC
    C. STNMP
    D. S-A-C (Feinstein's)

38. **The wave length of CO_2 laser is:**
    A. 2.5 mewm
    B. 5.6 mewm
    C. 10.6 mewm
    D. 15.5 mewm

39. **The CO_2 laser is hemostatic for blood vessels of size with diametre of:**
    A. 0.05 mm
    B. 0.5 mm
    C. 0.1 mm
    D. 0.005 mm

40. **Mega voltage external radiation is usually delivered at does of:**
    A. 300 to 500 rads/mt
    B. 900 to 1000 rads/mt
    C. 2000 to 3,000 rads/mt
    D. 4000 to 5000 rads/mt

41. **Progressive pulmonary fibrosis is a side effect of:**
    A. Methotrexate
    B. Cyclophosphamide
    C. Vincristine
    D. Bleomycin

42. **Rhytidoplasty refers to:**
    A. Septoplasty
    B. Rhinoplasty
    C. Septorhinoplasty
    D. Face lift

43. **The earliest noticeable feature of aging face appears in:**
    A. Frontal region
    B. Circum oral region
    C. Periorbital region
    D. Nasolabial region

44. **All the following conditions are indication for trans-sphenoidal hypophysectomy *except*:**
    A. Breast cancer
    B. Severe diabetic retinopathy failing laser therapy
    C. Radiological evidence of enlarged sella turcica with suprasellar extension of the pituitary tumor
    D. Nelson's syndrome

45. **The classic 'Silent' site or clinical blind spot in head and neck, notorious for metastatic neck node is:**
    A. Pyriform fossa
    B. Nasopharynx
    C. Base of tongue
    D. Vallecula

46. **The incidence of primary tumors in head and neck producing metastatic neck mass is:**
    A. 25%
    B. 45%
    C. 65%
    D. 85%

47. **All the salivary tumours mentioned below are cold on technitium scan *except*:**
    A. Warthin's tumor
    B. Mixed cell tumor
    C. Mucoepidermoid tumor
    D. Oncocytoma

48. **The smallest and most fragile of all the cranial bone is:**
    A. Nasal bone   B. Lacrimal bone
    C. Ethmoid bone   D. Zygomatic bone

49. **The cranial bone resembling a bat with outstreched wings is:**
    A. Sphenoid   B. Ethmoid
    C. Maxilla   D. Temporal

50. **Match the items in Table A with Table B regarding the communications of pterygopalatine fossa:**

    Table A   Table B
    1. Pterygomaxillary   a. Infratemporal fossa
       fissure
    2. Infraorbital fissure   b. Middle cranial fossa
    3. Pterygoid canal   c. Orbital cavity
    4. Palatinovaginal   d. Foramen lacerum
       canal
    5. Greater palatine   e. Roof of nasal cavity
       canal
    6. Foramen rotundum   f. Roof of oral cavity
    7. Sphenopalatine   g. Nasal cavity
       foramen

51. **Partial pharyngectomy with partial laryngectomy is done for limited malignant growth involving:**
    A. Vallecula
    B. Epiglottis
    C. Apex of pyriform fossa
    D. All the above

52. **Total pharyngolaryngectomy is indicated for tumours spreading widely across the midline of posterior pharyngeal wall or shaving circumferential involvement of more than:**
    A. 20%   B. 30%
    C. 40%   D. 50%

53. **The best flap to repair the pharyngeal defect after total pharyngolaryngectomy is:**
    A. PMMC   B. Latismus dorsi
    C. Deltopectoral   D. None of the above

54. **The type of laryngectomy suitable for small carcinoma in the anterior part of the vocal cord is:**
    A. Lateral partial laryngectomy
    B. Frontolateral partial laryngectomy
    C. Supraglottic partial laryngectomy
    D. Total laryngectomy

55. **The surgery of choice for anteriorly placed growth involving both vocal cords is:**
    A. Total laryngectomy
    B. Frontolateral partial laryngectomy
    C. Lateral partial laryngectomy
    D. Supraglottic partial laryngectomy

56. **Lymph node metastasis are often bilateral in:**
    A. Nasopharyngeal malignancy
    B. Laryngeal malignancy
    C. Post cricoid maliganancy
    D. None of the Above

57. **For the repair of type II pharyngocutaneous fistula in most of the cases, the best distant flap is the medially based:**
    A. Deltopectoral flap   B. PMMC flap
    C. Latismus dorsi flap   D. Buccal flap

58. **The type of flap prefered for closure of type III pharyngocutaneous fistula is:**
    A. Revascularized foream flap based on radial artery
    B. Revascularized fore arm flap based on ulnar artery
    C. PMMC flap
    D. None of the above

59. **Which of the following statements regarding repair of pharyngocutaneous fistula is not true?**
    A. This is a complication after total laryngectomy
    B. Repair should not be undertaken ideally before 60 days
    C. Type I fistula is the one where both the epithelial surface can be provided locally
    D. Type II fistula is the one where both surfaces must be provided from a distance

60. **In an impeding pharyngocutaneous fistula, the leak of saliva from the postoperative wound is usually evident by:**
    A. 34 to 35th day   B. 7th to 10th day
    C. 15th to 21st day D. 25th to 30th day

61. **All the following incidences of lymph node meta stasis at presentation of supraglottic tumor are false except:**
    A. T_1 – 50 to 65%   B. T_2 – 30 to 40%
    C. T_3 – 40 to 55%   D. T_4 – 13 to 40%

62. **All the following statements regarding cervical metastasis in occult primary tumors are true** *except:*
    A. 50% of cases present with adenopathy
    B. Squamous cell is predominant histologic type
    C. 90% of the primaries are in head and neck regions
    D. Five year survival rate is 30%

63. **All the following statements regarding rhabdomyosarcoma are true** *except:*
    A. Most common soft tissue malignancy of head and neck in children
    B. Often present before the age of 10
    C. Rapid growth
    D. Five year survival rate is upto 50%

64. **The site of occurrence in order of frequency in paraganglioma is:**
    A. i. Carotid body ii. Intravagal iii. Jugulotympani iv. Laryngeal
    B. i. Jugulotympani ii. Carotid body iii. intravagal iv. Laryngeal
    C. i. Carotid body ii. Jugulotympani iii. intravagal iv. laryngeal
    D. i. Intravagal ii. Carotid body iii. Jugulotympani iv. Laryngeal

65. **All the following statements regarding paraganglioma are correct** *except:*
    A. 10% are multicentric
    B. 8% are associated with another malignancy
    C. 2 to 6% metastasize
    D. 20% hormonally active

66. **All the following statements regarding teratoma are true** *except:*
    A. Tumors of pluripotent embryonal cells
    B. 10% occur in head and neck
    C. Polyhydramnios is present in 18%
    D. Males more often affected

67. **All the following statements regarding teratoma are correct** *except:*
    A. Composed of all three germinal layers
    B. Usually not solid
    C. Often fatal
    D. Cellular differentiation allows recognition of organ structure

68. **All the following statements regarding epignathi are true** *except:*
    A. Composed of all three germinal layers
    B. Most differentiated of all forms
    C. Often fatal
    D. Rarely arises from midline and basi sphenoid

69. **All the following statements regarding the histogenesis of parotid tumors are true** *except:*
    A. Acinar cells – Squamous cells carcinoma
    B. Epithelial cells – Myoepithelial carcinoma
    C. Intercalated duct cell – Mixed tumor
    D. Excretory duct cell – mucoepidermoid carcinoma

70. **Of all the salivary gland tumors adenoidcystic carcinoma constitutes:**
    A. 6%   B. 12%
    C. 15%   D. 20%

71. **A scan with technitium 99 m reveals 'hot' nodule in:**
    A. Adenoidcystic carcinoma
    B. Warthin's tumor
    C. Acinous tumor
    D. Mucoepidermoid carcinoma

72. **Multiple endocrine neoplasia2 (MEN2) is associated with:**
    A. Follicular thyroid carcinoma
    B. Papillary thyroid carcinoma
    C. Medullary thyroid carcinoma
    D. Hurthle cell tumor

73. **Individuals with MEN2 will develop thyroid carcinoma in:**
    A. 20% of cases   B. 30% of cases
    C. 60% of case   D. 90% of cases

74. **The lifetime penetrance of medullary thyroid carcinoma in MEN2A is:**
    A. 15%   B. 30%
    C. 60%   D. 90%

75. **The lifetime penetration of medullary thyroid carcinoma in MEN2B is nearly:**
    A. 30%
    B. 60%
    C. 80%
    D. 100%

76. **Thyroidectomy is recommended in MEN2A at the age of:**
    A. 6 years   B. 16 years
    C. 30 years   D. 36 years

77. **Thyroidectomy is recommended in MEN 2B at:**
    A. Birth   B. 6 years
    C. 10 years   D. 16 years

78. **The incidence of carcinoma of esophagus is increased in patients with:**
    A. Achalasia
    B. Plummer – Vinson Syndrome
    C. Oculopharyngeal syndrome
    D. All of the above

79. **A biopsy which shows Zimmerman cells is suggestive of:**
    A. Hodgkins lymphoma
    B. Nonhodgkins lymphoma
    C. Rhabdomyosarcoma
    D. Hemangiopericytoma

80. **Gardner's syndrome or familial colonic polyposis is associated with:**
    A. Undifferentiated thyroid carcinoma
    B. Well-differentiated thyroid carcinoma
    C. Parafollicular cell tumor
    D. None of the above

81. **All the following statements regarding chordoma are correct except:**
    A. Rare skull base or nasopharyngeal malignancy
    B. Originates from the notochord remnant
    C. Histology demonstrates physaliferous cells with "Soap bubble" appearance
    D. Four year survival rate is 40%.

82. **Cancer of the head and neck, world wide, are the:**
    A. Third most common cancer
    B. Fourth most common cancer
    C. Fifth most common cancer
    D. Sixth most common cancer

83. **The most common sites of head and neck squamous cell carcinoma by far in the western world are:**
    A. Nose and paranasal sinuses
    B. Nose and nasopharynx
    C. Larynx and hypopharynx
    D. Oral cavity and oropharynx

84. **Cessation of smoking for 10 years leads to a gradual reduction of the risk of head and neck squamous cell carcinoma (HNSCC) by:**
    A. 30%   B. 50%
    C. 70%   D. 90%

85. **Protooncogenes have a more dominant role than tumor supressor genes in the development of:**
    A. Reticuloendothelial malignances
    B. Solid tumors
    C. All the above
    D. None of the above

86. **The most common chromosomal aberration detected on head and neck cancer is the loss of chromosome region:**
    A. 3p14   B. 3p21
    C. 3p22   D. 9p21

87. **In the TNM classification the suffix N$_{2a}$ indicates metastasis in:**
    A. Single ipsilateral lymph node
    B. Multiple ipsilateral lymph node
    C. Single contralateral lymph node
    D. Multiple contralateral lymph node

88. **In the current stage grouping for head and neck carcinomas as per the UICC (1997) stage IV a includes:**
    A. T4 N0M0   B. T4 N1M0
    C. Any TN2M0   D. All of the above

89. **The new inclusion for current stage grouping for head and neck cancer as per UICC (1997) is:**
    A. IV A   B. IV B
    C. IV C   D. All of the above

90. **Mid line nodes are considered:**
    A. Ipsilateral   B. Bilateral
    C. Contralateral   D. None of the above

91. **The limitations of T staging in TNM system includes:**
    A. Tumor size not related to prognosis
    B. Hard to assess clinical extent
    C. Debatable anatomical boundaries
    D. All of the above

92. **The cumulative incidence of synchronous primary in head and neck is about:**
    A. 5%   B. 10%
    C. 15%   D. 20%

93. The mainstay initial investigation in cervical lymphadenopathy is:
A. Biopsy   B. FNAC
C. X-ray   D. Blood test

94. The incidence of clinical occult metastatic lymph node detection by CT or MRI is:
A. 5 to 10%   B. 10 to 20%
C. 20 to 30%   D. 30 to 40%

95. The incidence of malignant adenopathy in the malignancy of PNS is:
A. 8%   B. 18%
C. 28%   D. 35%

96. Out of all malignant salivary gland tumors, mucoepidermoid carcinoma accounts approximately:
A. One-half   B. One-third
C. One-fourth   D. One-fifth

97. Hurthle cell carcinoma is a variant of:
A. Pupillary carcinoma
B. Medullary carcinoma
C. Follicular carcinoma
D. Anaplastic carcinoma

98. A previous history of Hashimotos thyroidits is almost always present in:
A. Papillary thyroid carcinoma
B. Follicular thyroid carcinoma
C. Medullary thyroid carcinoma
D. Thyroid lymphoma

99. The greatest likelihood of nodal spread in thyroid tumor is in:
A. Follicular carcinoma
B. Papillary carcinoma
C. Medullary carcinoma
D. Anaplastic carcinoma

100. In thyroid tumors, hematogenous spread is more common in:
A. Papillary carcinoma
B. Medullary carcinoma
C. Follicular carcinoma
D. Thyroid lymphoma

101. In thyroid tumors, calcification is found in 50% cases of:
A. Papillary carcinoma
B. Anaplastic carcinoma
C. Medullary carcinoma
D. Follicular carcinoma

102. The MRI magnetic field in most clinical scanners ranges from:
A. 0.5 to 1.5 Tesla   B. 1.5 to 2.5 Tesla
C. 2.5 to 3.5 Tesla   D. 3.5 to 4.5 Tesla

103. The limitation of N staging in TNM classification is:
A. There is no mention of levels
B. No immunological status
C. No mention of extra capsular spread
D. All of the above

104. The tumor quote "Seven times seven makeup your mind err you cut across langer's line" was told by:
A. McFee   B. Sir Harrold Gillies
C. Schobinger   D. Hayes Martin

105. All the following suture materials are non-absorbable except:
A. Prolene   B. Vicryl
C. Nurolon   D. Polybutesten

106. Which of the following suture material have the highest tensile strength and lasts longest?
A. Plain catgut   B. Chromic catgut
C. Poly dioxanone   D. Vicryl

107. The drainage from radical neck dissection within the first 24 to 48 hrs approximately measures:
A. 50 to 100 ml/ day
B. 200 ml/day
C. 300 ml/day
D. 400 ml/day

108. To prevent deep vein thrombosis in high risk head and neck cancer patients, periopertive and postoperative subcutaneous low molecular weight heparine should be given in the dose of:
A. 1000 units daily   B. 1500 units daily
C. 2500 units daily   D. 3500 units daily

109. All the following statements regarding adjuvant radio therapy in head and neck cancer are true except:
A. It is the elective postoperative irradiation
B. It includes prophylactic irradiation of clinically negative neck
C. It follows the complete surgical excision of the tumors
D. It also includes the irradiation of known residual disease following incomplete surgery

110. Teletherapy is otherwise known as:
    A. Interstitial radiotherapy
    B. External beam radiotherapy
    C. Intracavitary brachetherapy
    D. None of the abvoe

111. The energy of the photon beam of around 300 KV is known as:
    A. Orthovoltage   B. Super voltage
    C. Mega voltage   D. None of the above

112. Which of the following is not an advantage of megavoltage radiotherapy?
    A. Increased dose at depth
    B. Increased bone absorption
    C. Skin sparing
    D. Better precision

113. The bulk of radiotherapy is carried out using:
    A. Photons   B. Electrons
    C. Neutrons   D. Protons

114. The implant materials used on brachytherapy is/are:
    A. Radon   B. Calsium
    C. Iridium   D. All of the above

115. One rad is equivalant to:
    A. 0.001Gy   B. 0.01 Gy
    C. 0.1 Gy   D. 1.0 Gy

116. All the cytotoxic drugs given below used in head and neck cancer are alkylating agents except:
    A. Cyclophosphamide
    B. Itosfamide
    C. Nitrosureas
    D. Methotrexate

117. The cytotoxic drug carmustine or lomustine is a:
    A. Alkylating agent   B. Antimetabolite
    C. Plant derivative   D. Antibiotic

118. The most common cystic lesion of the jaw is:
    A. Dentigerous cyst   B. Radicular cyst
    C. Residual cyst   D. Eruption cyst

119. The most common odontogenic tumor is:
    A. Ameloblastoma
    B. Cementoma
    C. Complex odontoma
    D. Compound odontoma

120. All the following chemotherapeutic agents used in head and neck cancer belong to antimetabolite group except:
    A. Methotrexate   B. 6-Mercaptopurine
    C. 5-Fluorouracil   D. Vincristine

121. Which of the following chemotherapeutic agent used in head and neck cancer is an anticancer antibiotic?
    A. 6-thioguanine   B. Cisplatin
    C. Doxorubicin   D. Procarbozine

122. All the following chemotherapeutic agents used in head and neck cancer are antitumour antibiotics except:
    A. Actinomycin D   B. Bleomycin
    C. Doxorubicin   D. Melphalan

123. The usual route of administration of the following cytotoxic drugs used in head and neck cancer is by IV bolus except for:
    A. Doxorubicine   B. Bleomycine
    C. Methotrexate   D. Cyclophosphamide

124. Lung fibrosis is a major toxicity of:
    A. Bleomycin   B. Actiomycin – D
    C. Carboplatin   D. Vinblastin

125. Ototoxicity is a complication of:
    A. Methotrexate   B. Cisplatin
    C. Bleomycin   D. Cyclophosphamide

126. Folinic acid is used along with:
    A. Cisplatin   B. Bleomycin
    C. Methotrexate   D. Vincristine

127. Cytarabine is a:
    A. Alkylating agent
    B. Purine antagonist
    C. Pyrimidine antagonist
    D. Antitumor antibiotic

128. Neoadjuvant chemotherapy is given:
    A. Before radiotherapy
    B. During radiotherapy
    C. After radiotherapy
    D. Both after and before radiotherapy

129. The most common single chemotherapeutic drug is:
    A. Cyclophosphamide
    B. Methotrexate
    C. Vincristine
    D. 5-Flurouracil

130. **The most widely used drug combination in head and neck malignancy is:**
    A. Vincristine, bleomycin, methotrexate and 5-flurouracil
    B. Cisplatin, vincristine, Doxorubcin and 5-Flurouracil
    C. Cyclophosphamide, Vinblastine, Carboplatin and Chlorambucil
    D. Procarbazine, Cytarabine, Vincristine and Methotrexate

131. **The appropriate sequence of analgesic ladder used for pain control in cancer of head and neck cancer is:**
    A. Paracetamol, diclofenac, morphine and corpoxamol
    B. Diclofenac, morphine, paracetamol and corpoxamol
    C. Morphine, paracetomol, diclofenac and corpoxamol
    D. Paracetamol, diclofenac, corpoxamol and Morphine

132. **The incidence of major complications in head and neck surgery is around:**
    A. 5%   B. 10%
    C. 20%   D. 40%

133. **All the following major vessels are potential source of bleeding in head and neck surgery except:**
    A. External carotid artery
    B. Internal jugular vein
    C. External jugular vein
    D. Thyrocervical trunk

134. **When both the internal jugular veins are ligated, the intracranial pressure within 24 hrs rises?**
    A. Two fold   B. Three fold
    C. Four fold   D. Five fold

135. **Increased intracranial pressure shows all the following clinical features except:**
    A. Restlessness from headache
    B. Rise of pulse
    C. Rise of blood pressure
    D. Swelling and cyanosis of face

136. **Midline or contralateral lymphatic metastasis after treatment of head and neck cancer in epithelial site with bilateral lymphatic drainage is:**
    A. Epiglottis
    B. Hypopharynx
    C. Base to tongue
    D. All of the above

137. **All the following statements regarding Lhermitte's syndrome are true except:**
    A. It is due to demyelination of cervical spinal cord
    B. It may occur 12 weeks after neck irradiation
    C. Recovery occurs spontaneously
    D. Characterized by shooting pain down the arms and legs on neck extension

138. **Which of the following distant axial flaps represents work horses for 90% of cases in head and neck reconstruction?**
    A. Pectoralis major and lattismus dorsi
    B. Pectoralis major and sternomastoid
    C. Lattismus dorsi and trapezeius
    D. Lattismus dorsi and sternomastoid

139. **The reconstruction of choice for repairing large pharyngeal defect is by:**
    A. Lattismus dorsi flap
    B. Pectoralis major flap
    C. Rectus abdominis flap
    D. Free Jejunal flap

140. **The vascular pedicle in pectoralis major flap belongs to:**
    A. Type II   B. Type III
    C. Type IV   D. Type V

141. **The first attempt to quantity the performance status of patients with advanced cancer is by:**
    A. McNeil   B. Karnofsky
    C. DeSanto   D. DePippo

142. **The most popular method of percutaneous tracheostomy currently is:**
    A. Seldinger type
    B. Ciaglia type
    C. Minitracheostomy
    D. None of the above

143. **All the following are contraindication to percutaneous tracheostomy except in:**
    A. Children   B. Enlarged thyroid
    C. ICU   D. Bleeding diathesis

144. **The incidence of ICU patients requiring tracheostomy at any one time is approximately:**
    A. 3%
    B. 13%
    C. 23%
    D. 30%

145. All the following facts regarding presentation of thyroglossal cysts are true *except*:
A. 90% midline
B. 95% left side (in the remaining 10%)
C. 75% prehyoid
D. 25% have fistula

146. All the following clinical features are found in branchial cysts *except*:
A. 2/3 left and 1/3 right side
B. 2/3 lie anterior to upper 1/3 of sternomastoid
C. Persistent swelling 20% and intermittent swelling 80%
D. 70% clinically cystic and 30% solid

147. All the following clinical features are found in laryngocoele *except*:
A. Male : Female 1 : 5
B. 4/5 unilateral
C. 30% external and 20% internal
D. 1% contain a carcinoma

148. The causative organism of *Brucellosis* in cattle is by:
A. *Brucella melitensis*
B. *Brucella abortus*
C. *Brucella ovis*
D. *Brucella suis*

149. The most common primary lesions among parapharyngeal tumors are:
A. Neurogenic tumors
B. Paragangliomas
C. Salivary gland tumors
D. Vascular tumors

150. All the following facts regarding cartoid body tumor are true *except*:
A. High incidence in peru, colorado and Mexico city
B. 10% positive family history
C. 30% bilateral
D. Male : Female 1 : 5

151. The lymph nodes of the level V-group are found in:
A. Anterior triangle
B. Posterior triangle
C. Carotid triangle
D. Occipital triangle

152. The lymph nodes of the VI group are otherwise known as:
A. Visceral group
B. Middle jugular group
C. Lower jugular group
D. None of the above

153. The lymph nodes of the level VII are found in:
A. Upper anterior mediastinum
B. Lower anterior mediastinum
C. Middle mediastinum
D. Posterior mediastinum

As per the classic study of lindberg the probability of cervical metastasis (N) related to primary (T) staging in patients with head and neck squamous cell carcinoma (HNSCC) for the following primary sites. Tick (√) for correct answer and (×) for wrong answer:

154. Floor of mouth (   ) T_1 – No (89%) N_1 (9%) N_2-N_3 (2%)

155. Oral tongue (   ) T_2 – No (70%) N_1 (19%) N_2-N_3 (1%)

156. Nasopharynx (   ) T_4 – No (8%) N_1 (11%) N_2-N_3 (82%)

157. Softpalate (   ) T_3 – No (35%) N_1 (26%) N_2-N_3 (39%)

158. Base of tongue (   ) T_1 – No (30%) N_1 (15%) N_2-N_3 (55%)

159. Tonsillar Fossa (   ) T_1 – No (10%) N_1 (13%) N_2-N_3 (76%)

160. Supraglottic larynx (   ) T_2 – No (61%) N_1 (10%) N_2-N_3 (29%)

161. Hypopharynx (   ) T_2 – No (30%) N_1 (20%) N_2-N_3 (49%)

162. Hypopharynx (   ) T_4 – No (37%) N_1 (21%) N_2-N_3 (42%)

163. Retromolar trigone and anterior faucial pillar (   ) T_1 – No (88%) N_1 (2%) N_2-N_3 (9%)

164. Retromolar trigone and anterior faucial pillar (   ) T_1 – No (46%) N_1 (21%) N_2-N_3 (33%)

165. **Joint classification for regional cervical lymphadenopathy by UICC and AJC applied to all head and neck tumors *except:***
    A. Oral cavity and oropharynx
    B. Oral cavity and nasopharynx
    C. Nasopharynx and thyroid
    D. Thyroid and hypopharynx

166. **The radionuclides used for scanning is/are:**
    A. Gallium citrate
    B. Technetium – 99m
    C. Pentavalant DMSA
    D. All of the above

167. **The metabolic activity of cervical lymph node can be assessed by:**
    A. MRI
    B. SPECT
    C. PET
    D. USG

168. **All the following are treatment options for the N0 neck *except:***
    A. Elective surgery
    B. Elective radiotherapy
    C. Elective chemotherapy
    D. Policy of "Wait and See"

169. **All the following are indications for elective neck treatment *except:***
    A. Greater than 20 to 25% chance of subclinical neck disease
    B. Vigilant followup is not possible
    C. Clinical evaluation of the neck is difficult
    D. Imaging suggesting no occult nodal spread

170. **The primary site for a metastatic lymph node in posterior triangle, particularly in young person is:**
    A. Nose
    B. PNS
    C. Nasopharynx
    D. Laryngopharynx

171. **A cancer presenting with a neck node is more common in men than women in the ratio of:**
    A. M:F-1:2
    B. M:F-1:3
    C. M:F-1:4
    D. M:F-1:5

172. **The chance of living for 5 years in patients with an occult head and neck primary if treated properly is:**
    A. 15%
    B. 25%
    C. 50%
    D. 75%

173. **One of the criteria for the diagnosis of branchogenic carcinoma is no other primary should become evident in the follow-up for:**
    A. One year
    B. Two years
    C. Three years
    D. Five years

174. **Crile described the first classic radical neck dissection in the year:**
    A. 1906
    B. 1910
    C. 1916
    D. 1920

175. **The lymph node found in the Chaissaignac's triangle is:**
    A. Rouvier's node
    B. Henle's node
    C. Scalene's node
    D. Node of woods

176. **The most crippling long-term complication of radical neck dissection is:**
    A. Chylous fistula
    B. Pharyngocutaneous fistula
    C. Skull-base syndrome
    D. Shoulder's syndrome

177. **Type 3 modified radical neck dissection is also known as:**
    A. Comprehensive neck dissection
    B. Functional neck dissection
    C. Selective neck dissection
    D. All of the above

178. **Preservation of spinal accessory nerve is necessary in modified radical neck dissection:**
    A. Type I
    B. Type II
    C. Type III
    D. None of the above

179. **The non lymphatic structure (S) preserved in type 3 modified radical neck dissection is/are:**
    A. Spinal accessory nerve
    B. Internal jugular vein
    C. Sternocleidomastoid muscle
    D. All of the above

180. **The lymph node group removed on modified radical neck dissection are from level:**
    A. I–III
    B. I–IV
    C. I–V
    D. I–VI

181. **The most common primary head and neck malignancy is carcinoma of:**
    A. Oral cavity and oropharynx
    B. Oral cavity and hypopharynx
    C. Larynx and oral cavity
    D. Laryngopharynx and oropharynx

182. The inferior boundary of paraglottic space is:

A. Conus elasticus
B. Vocal cord
C. Vestibular fold
D. Aryepiglottic fold

183. The most common benign tumor of larynx is:

A. Chondroma
B. Papilloma
C. Neurofibroma
D. Hemangioma

184. The human papilloma virus (HPV) responsible for Juvenile papillomatosis of larynx belongs to type:

A. 6 and 7   B. 7 and 9
C. 6 and 9   D. 6 and 11

185. Microcarcinoma of vocal cord describes a superficial carcinoma of maximum size:

A. 5 x 5 x 5 mm
B. 10 x 5 x 5 mm
C. 15 x 15 x 13 mm
D. 10 x 10 x 3 mm

186. The incidence of lymph node metastasis in supraglottic carcinoma as per the UICC classification for N1 is as:

A. 49%   B. 33%
C. 28%   D. 18%

187. The most common site for distant metastasis in laryngeal cancer is:

A. Lung   B. Liver
C. Brain   D. None of the above

188. The parameter (s) to be checked during video stroboscopy is/are:

A. Fundamental frequency
B. Bilateral symmetry
C. Amplitude of vibration
D. All of the above

189. All the following facts regarding the surgical pathology of lip cancer are true except:

A. The lip is the most common site of cancer in mouth
B. Approximately 93% of the tumor present in lower lip
C. The most common tumor on lower lip is adenocarcinoma
D. The male to female ratio is 80 : 1

190. The most common tumor in the upperlip is:

A. Squamous cell carcinoma
B. Basal cell carcinoma
C. Adenocarcinoma
D. Verrucous carcinoma

191. Basal cell carcinoma in the upperlip is more common in female than male in the ratio of:

A. 2 : 1   B. 5 : 1
C. 10 : 1   D. 20 : 1

192. All the following flaps are used in lip reconstruction except:

A. Abbe Estlander flap
B. Karapandzic flap
C. Gillies fan flap
D. Platysma flap

193. The most suitable flap for reconstruction in tumor of the commisure is:

A. Abbeflap
B. Abbe Estlander flap
C. Karapandzic flap
D. Gillies flap

194. All the following site incidence of oral squamous carcinoma are true except:

A. Tongue – 35%
B. Floor of mouth – 30%
C. Alveolus – 20%
D. Buccal Mucousa – 15%

195. The most common site of tongue cancer is:

A. Dorsal surface
B. Ventral surface
C. Lateral border
D. Tip of the tongue

196. The approximate five year survival rate after curative treatment for oral cancer in stage I is:

A. 75 to 95%
B. 65 to 85%
C. 45 to 65%
D. 10 to 35%

197. The most common site for interstitial implantation of radionuclides in head and neck is:

A. Nasal cavity
B. Sinus cavity
C. Oral cavity
D. Buccal cavity

198. **The second most common site for oropharyngeal tumors is:**
   A. Lateral wall
   B. Base of tongue
   C. Soft palate
   D. Posterior wall

199. **The incidence of No neck at presentation of pyriform fossa carcinoma is:**
   A. 35%
   B. 70%
   C. 60%
   D. 55%

200. **All the following are inclusion criteria for primary radical radiotherapy in hypopharyngeal carcinoma except:**
   A. Vertical length of turnover should not exceed 5 cm
   B. Horizontal length should not exceed 6 cm
   C. Vocal cord must be mobile
   D. No neck nodes

201. **Approximately, the incidence of patients with hypopharyngeal carcinoma are not treatable at presentation is:**
   A. 15%
   B. 25%
   C. 40%
   D. 50%

202. **Tracheo-oesophageal Puncture (TEP), currently the surgical method of choice for voice restoration after laryngectomy was introduced by:**
   A. Singer and Issiki
   B. Singer and Blom
   C. Blom and Issiki
   D. Issiki and Woodman

203. **In 10% of pleomorphic adenomas of salivary gland, polysomy is found in the chromosome:**
   A. 17
   B. 18
   C. 19
   D. 20

204. **A high level of expression of Ki–67 nuclear antigen is a very strong adverse prognostic indicator in:**
   A. Pleomorphic adenoma
   B. Adenocarcinoma
   C. Adenoid cystic carcinoma
   D. Mucoepidermoid carcinoma

205. **The most common salivary gland tumor in children is:**
   A. Pleomorphic adenoma
   B. Mucoepidermoid tumor
   C. Acinic cell tumor
   D. Warthin's tumor

206. **The salivary gland tumor having a marked tendency to invade nerves with high frequency of pain is:**
   A. Adenocarcinoma
   B. Squamous cell carcinoma
   C. Lymphoepithelial carcinoma
   D. Adenoid cystic carcinoma

207. **Lymphoepithelial carcinoma is mostly associated with:**
   A. Asians
   B. Africans
   C. Europeans
   D. Scandinavians

208. **The gold standard for investigation of parotid tumors is:**
   A. FNAC
   B. Sialography
   C. CT Scan
   D. Incisonal biopsy

209. **All the following salivary gland tumors are of high grade malignancy except:**
   A. Oncocytic carcinoma
   B. Squamous cell carcinoma
   C. Undifferentiated carcinoma
   D. Acinic cell carcinoma

210. **All the following salivary gland tumors are of low grade malignancy except:**
   A. Salivary duct carcinoma
   B. Basal cell adenocarcinoma
   C. Mucinous adenocarcinoma
   D. Papillary cystadenocarcinoma

211. **The corner stone of investigation to detect cancer in solitary thyroid nodule is:**
   A. Open biopsy
   B. FNAC
   C. CT Scan
   D. USG

212. **The nerve found in the Joll's triangle is:**
   A. External branch of superior laryngeal
   B. Internal branch of superior laryngeal
   C. Anteromedial branch of inferior laryngeal
   D. Posteriomedial branch of inferior laryngeal

213. **Beahr's triangle is formed by:**
   A. Inferior thyroid artery, superior laryngeal nerve and common carotid artery.
   B. Superior thyroid artery, superior laryngeal nerve and internal carotid artery
   C. Inferior thyroid artery, common carotid artery and recurrent laryngeal nerve
   D. Superior thyroid artery, external carotid artery and superior laryngeal nerve

214. The incidence of papillary carcinoma in thyroid malignancy is:

A. 20%   B. 40%

C. 60%   D. 80%

215. The approximate frequency of cervical lymph-node involvement in Hodgkin's disease is:

A. 20%   B. 30%

C. 50%   D. 70%

216. The most common site of mucosal melanomas in head and neck is:

A. Oral cavity   B. Nasal and sinus cavity

C. Pharynx   D. Larynx

217. All the following cysts are nonodontogenic or fissural cysts except:

A. Nasolabial cyst

B. Radicular cyst

C. Median cyst

D. Nasopalatine cyst

218. Odontogenic keratocyst is otherwise known as:

A. Eruption cyst

B. Gingival cyst

C. Residual cyst

D. Primordial cyst

ANSWERS

1 D	2 A	3 D	4 C	5 B	6 A	7 B	8 A
9 D	10 D	11 D	12 A	13 D	14 C	15 B	16 D
17 D	18 C	19 C	20 B	21 C	22 A	23 D	24 C
25 B	26 C	27 A-2, B-1, C-5, D-3, E-4	28 D	29 A-3, B-2, C-1		30 C
31 B	32 D	33 C	34 A	35 D	36 A	37 D	38 C
39 B	40 B	41 D	42 D	43 C	44 C	45 B	46 D
47 A	48 B	49 A	50 1-a, 2-c, 3-d, 4-e, 5-f, 6-b, 7-g		51 D	52 D
53 A	54 A	55 B	56 C	57 A	58 A	59 D	60 B
61 C	62 A	63 D	64 C	65 D	66 D	67 B	68 D
69 A	70 A	71 B	72 C	73 D	74 D	75 D	76 A
77 A	78 D	79 D	80 B	81 D	82 D	83 C	84 C
85 A	86 D	87 A	88 D	89 D	90 A	91 D	92 C
93 B	94 B	95 B	96 C	97 C	98 D	99 B	100 C
101 B	102 A	103 D	104 B	105 B	106 C	107 B	108 D
109 D	110 B	111 A	112 B	113 A	114 D	115 B	116 D
117 A	118 B	119 A	120 D	121 C	122 D	123 B	124 A
125 B	126 C	127 C	128 A	129 B	130 A	131 D	132 C
133 C	134 D	135 B	136 D	137 D	138 A	139 D	140 D
141 B	142 A	143 D	144 B	145 D	146 C	147 A	148 B
149 C	150 D	151 B	152 A	153 A	154 √	155 √	156 ×
157 √	158 √	159 ×	160 √	161 √	162 ×	163 √	164 ×
165 C	166 D	167 C	168 C	169 D	170 C	171 C	172 C
173 D	174 A	175 C	176 D	177 D	178 A	179 D	180 C
181 C	182 A	183 B	184 D	185 D	186 D	187 A	188 D
189 C	190 B	191 B	192 D	193 B	194 D	195 C	196 A
197 C	198 B	199 A	200 B	201 B	202 B	203 A	204 C
205 B	206 D	207 A	208 C	209 D	210 A	211 B	212 A
213 C	214 D	215 D	216 A	217 B	218 D		

Syndromes and Synonyms

1. **All the following fungal infections are commonly found in Acquired Immuno Deficiency syndrome(AIDS)** *except:*
   A. Cryptococosis
   B. Histoplasmosis
   C. Blastomycosis
   D. Candidiasis

2. **As per the WHO clinical definition AIDS in adult is diagnosed by the presence of** *atleast:*
   A. One major with two minor signs
   B. One major with one minor signs
   C. Two major with one minor signs
   D. Two major with two minor signs

3. **All the following signs for clinical diagnosis of AIDS in adult as per WHO criteria are included in the major category** *except:*
   A. Weight loss   > 1 month
   B. Chronic diarrohea   > 1month
   C. Fever   > 1 month
   D. Persistent cough   > 1 month

4. **All the following features for clinical diagnosis of AIDS are included in the minor criteria** *except:*
   A. Generalized lymphadenopathy
   B. Recurrent herpes zoster infection
   C. Persistent cough for more than one month
   D. Persistent fever for more than one month

5. **All the following cutaneous lesions may be found in AIDS** *except:*
   A. Molluscum
   B. Psoriasis
   C. Kaposi's sarcoma
   D. Seborric dermatitis

6. **All the statements regarding Aarskog-Scott syndrome are correct** *except:*
   A. It is otherwise knows as Faciodigitogenital syndrome
   B. It is a X-linked disease
   C. It is characterized by Ante-verted nostril and ocular hypertension
   D. Narrow upper lips is also a feature

7. **Adair-Dighton's syndrome or osteogenesis Imperfecta tarda / congenita is characterized by all the following features** *except:*
   A. Brittle bones   B. Deafness
   C. Blue sclera   D. Retinitis pigmentosa

8. **Albers-Schönberg syndrome is characterized by all the following features** *except:*
   A. Facial palsy
   B. Brittle bone
   C. Anemia
   D. Retinopathy

9. **Apert's syndrome or acrocephally syndactyly is a characterized by all the following features** *except:*
   A. Autosomal recessive trait
   B. Maxillary hypoplasia
   C. Mid-digital syndactyly
   D. Flat fore head

10. **Alstorm's syndrome is characterized by all the following features** *except:*
    A. Retinitis pigmentosa
    B. Loss of peripheral vision
    C. Deafness
    D. Nystagmus

11. All the following features may be found in Arnold-Chiari syndrome *except:*
    A. Unilateral vocal cord palsy
    B. Hydrocephalus
    C. Meningomyelocecle
    D. Stridor

12. Albright's syndrome is characterized by all the following *except:*
    A. Secretory otitis media
    B. Anemia
    C. Chronic eczema
    D. Thrombocytic purpura

13. All the following feature may be found in Alport's syndrome *except:*
    A. Hemorrahagic nephritis
    B. Conductive hearing loss
    C. Keratoconus
    D. Hypertension

14. The cranial nerves affected in Avellis' syndrome are:
    A. 9th and 10th   B. 10th and 11th
    C. 11th and 12th   D. 9th, 10th and 11th

15. All the following statement regarding Avelli's syndrome are correct *except:*
    A. Involvement of nucleus ambigous
    B. Involvement of spinothalamic tract
    C. Laryngeal paralysis develops after palatal palsy
    D. Involvement of vagus and cranial accessory nerves

16. All the following features may be present in Barany's syndrome *except:*
    A. Deafness   B. Tinnitus
    C. Giddiness   D. Frontal headache

17. Ballantyne syndrome is characterized by all the following features *except:*
    A. Blue eyes
    B. Blonde hair
    C. Sensorineural hearing loss
    D. Retinitis pigmentosa

18. Behcet's syndrome is characterized by all the following features *except:*
    A. Orogenital ulcer
    B. Sero positive arthritis
    C. Erythema nodosum
    D. Uveitis and vasculitis

19. All the following statements regarding Bannworth's syndrome or Lymes disease are correct *except:*
    A. The causative organism is a virus
    B. Presence of meningo polyneuritis
    C. Erythema chronicum migrans is a feature
    D. There may be sore throat and stuffy nose

20. All the following statements regarding Bogorad's syndrome are correct *except:*
    A. It is otherwise known as crocodile tear
    B. It is characterized by increased lacrimation during eating
    C. The cause is faulty regeneration of facial nerve
    D. The treatment is vidian neurectomy

21. Bonner's syndrome is due to the lesion in the:
    A. Deiter's nucleus
    B. Nucleus ambigous
    C. Bechterew's nucleus
    D. Schwalbe's nucleus

22. All the following features may be present in Cogan's syndrome *except:*
    A. Deafness
    B. Vertigo
    C. Tinnitus
    D. Seropositive interstitial keratitis

23. CHARGE syndrome is associated with:
    A. Tracheo esophageal fistula
    B. Congenital choanal atresia
    C. Arnold-chiari malformation
    D. Cogan's disease

24. All the following features of Chrug-Straus syndrome *except:*
    A. Neutrophilia
    B. Vasculitis
    C. Necrotising granulomatosis
    D. Bronchial asthma

25. Itellis syndrome is seen in:
    A. CSOM   B. Mastoiditis
    C. ASOM   D. Adenoids

26. All the features are found in Cockayne syndrome *except:*
    A. Sensorineural deafness
    B. Goiter
    C. Dwarfism
    D. Retinal atropy

27. **Cardioauditory syndrome of Jervell and Lange-Nielsen is characterized by all the following features *except:***
   A. Prolonged P-R interval in ECG
   B. Deafness
   C. Fainting attacks
   D. Arrhythmia

28. **Collet-Siccard syndrome is characterized by all the following features *except:***
   A. Hoarsness of voice
   B. Difficulty in speech
   C. Reduced taste sensation
   D. Contralateral paralysis of soft palate

29. **The group of cranial nerves involved in the external jugular syndrome or Collet-Siccard syndrome is:**
   A. IX and X
   B. X and XI
   C. IX, X and XI
   D. IX, X, XI, XII

30. **Crouzon's syndrome is characterized by all the following features *except:***
   A. Craniofacial dystosis
   B. Sensorineural deafness
   C. Parrot beak nose
   D. Proptosis

31. **Costen syndrome or TMJ arthritis is characterized by all following features *except:***
   A. Referred otalgia
   B. Tinnitus
   C. Sensorineural hearing loss
   D. Malocclusion of TMJ

32. **Di–George syndrome is due to defective embryogenesis of pharyngeal pouches in:**
   A. 1st and 2nd
   B. 2nd and 3rd
   C. 3rd and 4th
   D. 4th and 6th

33. **The chromosomal defect found in Down's syndrome or Mongolism is:**
   A. Trisomy – 18
   B. Trisomy – 19
   C. Trisomy – 20
   D. Trisomy – 21.

34. **All the following features may be found in Down's syndrome *except:***
   A. Prominent malformed ears
   B. Hypertonia
   C. Flat nasal bridge
   D. Simian crease

35. **The brachial arch anomaly found in Duane's syndrome is due to the involvement of:**
   A. 1st arch
   B. 2nd arch
   C. 3rd arch
   D. 2nd and 3rd

36. **The cranial nerves affected in Dysmelia's syndrome is due to the paralysis of:**
   A. 3rd and 4th
   B. 4th and 5th
   C. 6th and 7th
   D. 8th and 9th

37. **All the following statements regarding DOOR syndrome are true *except:***
   A. It is autosomal recessive in nature
   B. Presence of congenital deafness
   C. Patient is mentally retarded
   D. Onycho-osteo dystrophy is also a feature

38. **All the following statements regarding Duane's syndrome are true *except:***
   A. It is otherwise know as cervical-oculo-acoustic dysplasia
   B. It is autosomal dominant in nature
   C. Congenital paralysis of 6th cranial nerve is found
   D. Presence of sensorineural deafness

39. **The chromosomal defect found in Edward's syndrome is:**
   A. Trisomy – 18
   B. Trisomy – 19
   C. Trisomy – 20
   D. Trisomy – 21

40. **All the following features may be found in Edward's syndrome except:**
   A. Mental retardation
   B. Micrognathia
   C. Hypotonicity
   D. Low set ears

41. **All the following features may be found in Ehlers-Danlos syndrome *except:***
   A. Hypoelasticity of vocal cords
   B. Hyperelasticity of joints
   C. Fragility of skins
   D. Poor wound healing

42. **The synonym of Franceshetti-Zwahlen syndrome is:**

    A. DPPK syndrome
    B. Paterson-Brown-Kelly syndrome
    C. Treacher collins syndrome
    D. Crocodile tear syndrome

43. **All the following features may be found in Fanconi's syndrome *except*:**

    A. Low frequency conductive hearing loss
    B. Mental retardation
    C. Skeletal deformity
    D. Skin pigmentation

44. **The cranial nerve paralyzed in Fobille's syndromes is:**

    A. Abducent nerve
    B. Facial nerve
    C. Auditory nerve
    D. Hypoglossal nerve

45. **Frey's syndrome is otherwise known as:**

    A. Baillarger's syndrome
    B. Fobille's syndrome
    C. Foix's syndrome
    D. None of the above

46. **Auricular temporal syndrome is otherwise know as:**

    A. Gustatory sweating
    B. Resturant syndrome
    C. Frey's syndrome
    D. All of the above

47. **The treatment of choice in Frey's syndrome is resection of:**

    A. Auriculotemporal nerve
    B. Tympanic nerve
    C. Greater superficial petrosal nerve
    D. Lesser superficial petrosal nerve

48. **The cranial nerves involved in Foix syndrome are:**

    A. III, IV and V   B. VI, VII and IX
    C. X, XI and XII   D. IX, X and XI

49. **All the features may be found in Foster-kenedy syndrome *except*:**

    A. Contralateral anosmia
    B. Contralateral papilledema
    C. Junctional scotoma
    D. Unilateral blindness

50. **The cranial nerves involvement in Foix syndrome is due to involvement of tumors or aneurysms at:**

    A. Superior orbital fissure
    B. Inferior orbital fissure
    C. Pterygomaxillary fissure
    D. Fissures of santorini

51. **Adult respiratory distress syndrome (ARDS) is charecterized by all the following features *except*:**

    A. Hypoxia
    B. Pulmonary infiltrates
    C. Decreased pulmonary vascular permeability
    D. Microvascular hemorrhage

52. **Alagille syndrome is characterized by all the following features *except*:**

    A. Temporal bone anomalies
    B. Cardiovascular anomalies
    C. Chronic cholestasis
    D. Renal anomalies

53. **All the following statements regarding Almalric syndrome are true *except*:**

    A. It may be a genetic disorder
    B. Presence of foveal dystrophy
    C. It is associated with conductive deafness
    D. Visual acuity is usually normal

54. **All the features may be present on Babinski-Nageotte syndrome *except*:**

    A. Multiple (or) scattered lesion on the distribution of vertebral artery
    B. Ipsilateral paralysis of soft palate
    C. Contralateral paralysis of pharynx and larynx
    D. Contralateral spastic hemiplegia

55. **Barre-Lieou syndrome or cervical migraine is characterised by all the following features *except*:**

    A. Frontal headache
    B. Vertigo and tinnitus
    C. Vasomotor discoress
    D. Facial spasm

56. **All the following statements regarding Barsony-palgar syndrome are ture *except*:**

    A. It is due to oesophageal spasm
    B. Caused by disruption of peristaltic waves
    C. Results in dysphagia and regurgitation
    D. Commonly affects excitable young adults

57. All following features may be present in Beckwith syndrome *except:*
    A. Macroglossia
    B. Hyperglycemia
    C. Renal hyperplasia
    D. Omphalocele

58. All the following statements regarding basal cell nevoid syndrome are false *except:*
    A. It is a sex linked familial disorder
    B. Autosomal recessive in nature
    C. Manifests late in life
    D. Bony cysts are found in maxilla and mandible

59. All the following statements regarding Bloom's syndrome are true *except:*
    A. It is an autosomal dominant disorder
    B. Associated with very high rate of cancer
    C. Presence of facial erythema and immuno deficiency
    D. Diagnosis is confirmed by chromosome analysis

60. All the following findings may be present in Bouneville Syndrome *except:*
    A. Nasal polyps
    B. Hare lip
    C. Spinal bifida
    D. Microcephaly

61. The Branchial arches involved in the branchio otorenal syndrome are:
    A. 1st and 2nd
    B. 2nd and 3rd
    C. 3rd and 4rd
    D. 4th and 5th

62. Camptomelic syndrome may be characterized by all the following features *except:*
    A. Gigantism
    B. Respiratory distress
    C. Craniofacial anomalies
    D. Prominent forehead with flat face and broad nasal bridge

63. Charcot-Weiss-Barker syndrome is other wise known as:
    A. Brown syndrome
    B. Carotid sinus syndrome
    C. Carcinoid syndrome
    D. Cavernous sinus syndrome

64. Cestan-Chenais syndrome is caused by the occlusion of:
    A. Internal carotid artery
    B. Internal auditory artery
    C. Vertebral artery
    D. Basillar artery

65. Chamion-Cregah-Klein syndrome is characterized by all the following features *except:*
    A. Cleft lip and palate
    B. Upper lip fistula
    C. Syndactaly
    D. Pesequinovarus

66. All the following features may be present in Cowden's syndrome *except:*
    A. Adenoid facies
    B. Papillomatosis of the lips and pharynx
    C. Macrostomia
    D. Serotal tongue

67. The diseases associated with Besnier-Boeck Schaumann syndrome is:
    A. Histoplasmosis
    B. Sarcoidosis
    C. Tuberculosis
    D. Cryptococcosis

68. Cri du chat syndrome is characterized by all the following features *except:*
    A. Anomaly in the long-arm of B group chromosome
    B. Mental retardation and microcephally
    C. Respiratory stridor
    D. Mid line oral cleft

69. Congenital hemifacial atrophy is otherwise known as:
    A. Chappel syndrome
    B. Chediak-Higashi syndrome
    C. Curtius syndrome
    D. Conradi-Hunerman syndrome

70. De' Jean syndrome is characterized by all the following features *except:*
    A. Diplopia
    B. Exopthalmous
    C. Otalgia
    D. Numbness over the route of trigeminal nerve

71. Dermaronay richet syndrome is charecterized by:
    A. Cleft lip and palate
    B. Upper lip fistula
    C. progeria facies
    D. Defective dentition

72. All the following statements regarding Diamond syndrome are true *except*:
    A. It is an autosomal dominant disorder
    B. Associated with diabetes mellitus and Inspidus
    C. Presence of optic atropy
    D. Deafness is hightone sensorineural type

73. The cranial nerves which may be irritated in Eagle's syndrome are:
    A. 9th and 10th
    B. 5th and 7th
    C. 5th , 7th , 9th, and 10th
    D. 11th and 12th

74. The most common theory for empty sella syndrome is:
    A. Rupture of intrasellar or parasellar cyst
    B. Infarction of pituitary adenoma
    C. Pitutary hypertrophy and subsequent involution
    D. Congenitaly deficient sella diaphragm

75. Hemifacial microsomia or lateral facial dysplasia is otherwise known as:
    A. Eisenlohr syndrome
    B. Elschnig syndrome
    C. First and second branchial arch syndromes
    D. Dandy syndrome

76. Gardner's syndrome is characterized by all the following features *except*:
    A. Chronic sinusitis
    B. Osteoma
    C. Sebaceous cysts
    D. Intestinal polyposis

77. Gargoylism is otherwise known as:
    A. Garcin syndrome
    B. Hurler's syndrome
    C. Fish syndrome
    D. Dejerine anterior bulbar syndrome

78. Goldenhar syndrome is otherwise known as:
    A. Otomandibular dysplasia
    B. Lateralfacial dysplasia
    C. Oculoauriculovertebral dysplasia
    D. All of the above

79. The cranial nerves involved in Gradenigo syndrome are:
    A. 4th and 5th   B. 5th and 6th
    C. 6th and 7th   D. 7th and 9th

80. Hadenius syndrome is otherwise known as:
    A. Goodhill and Morrison syndrome
    B. Hand foot Mouth syndrome
    C. Hydrocephalus and cocktail party syndrome
    D. Face Hand syndrome

81. Uveoparotid fever in sarcoidosis is otherwise known as:
    A. Sjogren syndrome
    B. Han harts syndrome
    C. Mickulicz syndrome
    D. Heerfordt's syndrome

82. The cranial nerve paralysis in Garcin's syndrome are nerves:
    A. III to VI   B. III to VII
    C. III to VII   D. III to X

83. The cranial nerves paralysed in Garel Gignoux syndrome are:
    A. IX and X   B. X and XI
    C. IX and XI   D. XI and XII

84. Grisel syndrome may be associated with:
    A. Nasopharyngitis
    B. Adenotonsillitis
    C. Parotitis
    D. All of the above

85. Nasopharyngeal torticoilis is otherwise known as:
    A. Gilles de latourette syndrome
    B. Giant apical air cell syndrome
    C. Grisel syndrome
    D. Hallerman streiff syndrome

86. All the following features may be associated with Hallerman streiff syndrome *except*:
    A. Hypertrichosis of scalp
    B. Dyscephally
    C. Parrot Nose
    D. Mandibular hypoplasia

87. Hanhart's syndrome is characterized by all the following features *except*:
    A. Bird like face   B. Opisthodontia
    C. Peromelia   D. Low intelligence

88. **All the following features may be found in Horner's syndrome** *except:*
    A. Ptosis
    B. Miosis
    C. Hyperhydrosis
    D. Enophthalmos

89. **The cranial nerve involved in Hugling Jacksons syndrome are:**
    A. IX and X
    B. IX, X and XI
    C. X, XI and XII
    D. IX, X, XI, and XII

90. **Mucopolysaccharide disorder is found in:**
    A. Hurler syndrome
    B. Hortons syndrome
    C. Hick syndrome
    D. Hollander syndrome

91. **An incurable, hereditary and sex linked disorder involving multiorgan system through mucopoly sacharidosis is known as:**
    A. Hunt's syndrome
    B. Hurler's syndrome
    C. Hunter's syndrome
    D. Hermann syndrome

92. **All the following features may be associated with Hallgren syndrome** *except:*
    A. Retinitis pigmentosa
    B. Progressive ataxia
    C. Mental retardation
    D. Conductive hearing loss

93. **All the following features may be associated with Immotile cilia syndrome** *except:*
    A. Bronchiectasis
    B. Sinusitis
    C. Situs inversus
    D. Female sterility

94. **Inversed jaw winking syndrome is found in supranuclear lesion of cranial nerve:**
    A. V
    B. VI
    C. VII
    D. IX

95. **All the following features may be present in Hurler's syndrome:**
    A. Hereditary sensorineural deafness
    B. Hepatosplenomegaly
    C. Cutaneous lesion
    D. Visual disturbance

96. **Large foamy PAS positive gargoyle cells in middle ear mucosa and alderbodies in neutrophils are found in:**
    A. Von-Hippel lindau syndrome
    B. Hutuchinsons syndrome
    C. Hurler's syndrome
    D. Grisches syndrome

97. **The cranial nerves involve in the Jacod syndrome or Negri Jacod syndrome are:**
    A. II and III
    B. II, III, and IV
    C. II, III, IV and V
    D. II, III, IV, V, and VI

98. **Young's syndrome may be characterized by:**
    A. Obstructive azoospermia
    B. Bronchiectasis
    C. Chronic sinusitis
    D. All of the above

99. **The cranial nerves paralyzed in Jackson syndrome are:**
    A. IX and X
    B. II, III and IV
    C. II, III, IV and V
    D. II, III, IV, V and VI

100. **Lazy leucocyte syndrome is otherwise known as:**
     A. Job's syndrome
     B. Jaccourds syndrome
     C. Leopard syndrome
     D. Larsen syndrome

101. **Cardioauditory syndrome is otherwise known as:**
     A. Norne syndrome
     B. Noonun syndrome
     C. jaruel lange Neelsen syndrome
     D. Kallmans syndrome

102. **The cranial nerves involved in jugular foramen syndrome or Vernet syndrome are:**
     A. IX and X
     B. X and XI
     C. IX, X and XI
     D. X, XI and XII

103. **All the statements regarding kallman's syndrome are true** *except:*
     A. It's transmitted by an autosomal recessive gene
     B. Loss of sense of smell
     C. Presence of hypogonadism
     D. Presence of eunuchoidism

104. All the following statements regarding Kartagener's syndrome are true *except*:

A. It's an autosomal dominant inherited disease
B. Abnormality of respiratory cilia
C. Complete or partial absence of dyncin
D. Both sex sterility may be present

105. All the following regarding klinkert's syndrome are true *except*:

A. There is paralysis of recurrent laryngeal nerve and phrenic nerve
B. It may be associated with sympathetic paralysis
C. It may be due to pancoast tumor
D. Most often occurs due to neoplastic lesions in posterior mediastinum

106. Brencolli's syndrome is otherwise known as:

A. Klippel-Feil syndrome
B. Kecrens-Sayre syndrome
C. Kleinschmidt syndrome
D. HRA syndrome

107. Angio-osteo-hypertrophy syndrome is otherwise known as:

A. Klipel-Trenaunay-Weber syndrome
B. Rendu-Weber-oslor syndrome
C. Richard-Rundel syndrome
D. Klipel-Feil syndrome

108. The karyotype in klinefelters syndrome is:

A. XXY
B. XYY
C. XXX
D. None of the above

109. Koerber-Salus-Elschng syndrome is otherwise known as:

A. Cerebral aqueduct syndrome
B. Nystagmus retraction syndrome
C. Sylvian syndrome
D. All of the above

110. Konigsmark-Gorlin syndrome is characterized by all the following features *except*:

A. Malleo-incudal fixation
B. Folding of pinna
C. Thin external nose
D. micrognathia

111. Otomandibular syndrome is otherwise known as:

A. Mandibulofacial dysostosis
B. Taylor syndrome
C. Well syndrome
D. Konigsmark-gorlin syndrome

112. The anomalies in lacrimo-auriculo –dento-digi-tal syndrome or LADD syndrome. May include all the following features *except*:

A. Facial palsy
B. Cup shaped ear
C. Sensorineural hearing loss
D. Ossicular anomaly

113. Lawrence-moon-Biedl syndrome is characterized by all of the following *except*:

A. Always familial but never hereditary
B. Pigmentary degeneration of retina
C. Syndactaly
D. Mental retardation

114. The order of symptomatology in lermoyez syn-drome or reverse meniere's is:

A. Deafness preceding tinnitus and vertigo
B. Tinnitus preceding deafness and vertigo
C. Vertigo preceding deafness and tinnitus
D. Deafness and tinnitus preceding vertigo

115. Laundry-Guillian-Barre's syndrome is character-ized by all the following *except*:

A. Rapid successions of multiple cranial nerve injuries
B. Multiple sensory nerve paralysis
C. Followed by viral infection
D. Abnormanl CSF

116. Landau-Kleffner syndrome is characterized by all the following feaures *except*:

A. Congenital aplasia
B. Epilepsy
C. Abnormal EEG
D. Severe language comprehension Problems

117. Marfans syndrome is characterized by all of the following *except*:

A. High arched palate
B. Conductive deafness
C. Convergent squint
D. Long tapering fingers

118. All the following are included in the lethal mid-line granuloma syndrome *except*:

A. Wegner's granuloma
B. Stewart granuloma
C. Polymorphic reticulosis
D. Giant cell granuloma

119. **Marcus Gunn syndrome is otherwise known as:**
   A. Louis-bar syndrome
   B. Larsen syndrome
   C. Loose wire syndrome
   D. Jan-winking syndrome

120. **Recurrent facial palsy is found commonly in:**
   A. Ramsay hunt syndrome
   B. Melkerson-Rosenthal syndrome
   C. Gradenigo syndrome
   D. Landry-guillian-barre's syndrome

121. **Polyostotic fibrous dysplasia is otherwise known as:**
   A. Mc Cune-Albright syndrome
   B. Morgagni-Stewart-Morel syndrome
   C. Mafucci syndrome
   D. Myenburg syndrome

122. **Meniere's syndrome may be found in all the following conditions *except*:**
   A. Labyrinthitis
   B. Cogan's diseases
   C. Otosclerosis
   D. Vestibular neuronitis

123. **Moecius syndrome is characterized by all the following features *except*:**
   A. Preceptive deafness
   B. Diplopia
   C. Atresia of ear
   D. Unilateral abducent palsy

124. **Cardiovocal syndrome is otherwise known as:**
   A. Morgagni syndrome
   B. Miehlke's syndrome
   C. Ortner's syndrome
   D. Myenburg syndrome

125. **Miehlke's syndrome is characterized by all the following *except*:**
   A. 7th cranial nerve palsy
   B. Phocomelia
   C. Arrested ear development
   D. Thalidomide embryopathy

126. **The cranial nerve paralysis in Millardgubblar syndrome is:**
   A. Ipsilateral 6th cranial nerve
   B. Ipsilateral 7th cranial nerve
   C. Contralateral 6th cranial nerve
   D. Ipsilateral 6th & 7th cranial nerve

127. **Progressive hemifacial atrophy is otherwise known as:**
   A. Parry-Romberg syndrome
   B. Muckle-Wells syndrome
   C. Nelson's syndrome
   D. Mezelof's syndrome

128. **Maffucci's syndrome is otherwise known as:**
   A. Klippel-Trenaunay syndrome
   B. Struge-Weber syndrome
   C. Vonhippel –Lindau syndrome
   D. None of the above

129. **Munchausen syndrome is otherwise known as:**
   A. Mobins syndrome
   B. Occulo-Dento-Digital syndrome
   C. Opthalmo-Mandibulo-Melic syndrome
   D. None of the above

130. **The cranial nerve paralyzed in Nothangel's syndrome is:**
   A. 3rd cranial nerve   B. 5th cranial nerve
   C. 7th cranial nerve   D. 9th cranial nerve

131. **The genetic anomaly in Patau syndrome is:**
   A. Trisonomy 13 to 15
   B. Trisonomy 15 to 17
   C. Trisonomy 17 to 19
   D. Trisonomy 19 to 21

132. **Plummer-Vinson syndrome or Paterson-Brown-kelly syndrome is characterized by all the following *except*:**
   A. Siderophenic anemia
   B. Pharyngeal web
   C. Koilonychia
   D. Decreased iron binding capacity

133. **Bilateral profound childhood deafness with diffuse or nodular goiter is found in:**
   A. Perinaud's syndrome
   B. Pendred's syndrome
   C. Pfeiffer's syndrome
   D. Potter's syndrome

134. **Pickwickian's syndrome may associate all the following factors *except*:**
   A. Obesity
   B. Short face and neck
   C. Heavy Snoring
   D. Pruder-willi syndrome

135. **Acrofacial Dystosis is otherwise known as:**
    A. Nager's syndrome
    B. Nager-de regnier syndrome
    C. Potter's syndrome
    D. Pruder-willi syndrome

136. **Pierre-Robbin syndrome is characterized by all the following *except:***
    A. Micrognathia
    B. Perceptive deafness
    C. Glossoptosis
    D. Cleft palate

137. **Pruder-Willi syndrome is characterized by all the following *except:***
    A. Bird like face
    B. Obesity
    C. Hypogonadism
    D. IDDM

138. **The cranial nerves involved in orbital apex syndrome are:**
    A. II, III and IV
    B. III, IV and V
    C. IIII, IV and VI
    D. II, III and IV

139. **OPD syndrome is otherwise known as:**
    A. Occulopalatodigital syndrome
    B. Oropalatodigital syndrome
    C. Otopalatodigital syndrome
    D. Odonto-palato-digital syndrome

140. **Hereditary hemorrhagic telangiectasia is otherwise known as:**
    A. Struge-Weber syndrome
    B. Rendu-Osler-Weber syndrome
    C. Peutz-Jeghers syndrome
    D. Von hippel-lindau syndrome

141. **Horner's syndrome is associated with:**
    A. Oro-Facial-digital syndrome
    B. Raeder's syndrome
    C. Refsum's syndrome
    D. Pancoast's syndrome

142. **Phonatological syntactic syndrome is otherwise known as:**
    A. Suethre-Chotzens syndrome
    B. Rapin Allen's syndrome
    C. Reicher syndrome
    D. Rutherford syndrome

143. **Reiter's syndrome may follow after any of the following infections *except:***
    A. Campylobacter
    B. Salmonella
    C. Shigella
    D. Yersinia

144. **Benign intracranial hypertension is otherwise known as:**
    A. SCID syndrome
    B. Samter syndrome
    C. Pseudotumor syndrome
    D. Arnold-Chiari syndrome

145. **Orbital Apex-sphenoidal syndrome is otherwise known as:**
    A. Orbital Apex syndrome
    B. Rollet syndrome
    C. Reye syndrome
    D. Hunt's syndrome

146. **The cranial nerves involved in Schmidt's syndrome are:**
    A. 9th and 10th
    B. 10th and 11th
    C. 9th, 10th and 11th
    D. 10th, 11th and 12th

147. **The symptoms in scalenus anticus syndrome are due to pressure or compression are:**
    A. Brachial plexus
    B. Subclavian artery
    C. Sympathetic nerves
    D. All of the above

148. **The clinical symptoms in cervical syndrome are identical with:**
    A. Eagle's syndrome
    B. Pancoast's syndrome
    C. Horner's syndrome
    D. Scalenus anticus syndrome

149. **The clinical test for diagnosis of scalenus anticus syndrome is known as:**
    A. Adson's test
    B. Corradi's test
    C. Teuber test
    D. Wallastrom's test

150. **Schafer syndrome is characterized by all the following *except:***
    A. Photogenic epilepsy
    B. Conductive hearing loss
    C. Mental retardation
    D. Prolinemia

151. **Schafer syndrome is due to the deficiency of:**
    A. Iron
    B. Vitamin B12
    C. Pyridoxine
    D. Proline oxidase

152. Shy- Drager syndrome is a degenerating disease of:
A. Central nervous system
B. Peripheral nervous system
C. Autonomic nervous system
D. None of the above

153. All of the following features may be found in Sjogren's syndrome except:
A. Hypergammaglobulinemia
B. Cryoglobulinemia
C. Primary biliary cirrhosis
D. Kerratoconjuctivitis sicca

154. Acute erythema multiforme is otherwise known as:
A. Sprengel's syndrome
B. Stevens-Johnson syndrome
C. Scimitar syndrome
D. Seckel syndrome

155. The cranial nerve involved in Steele-Richardson-Olszewski syndrome is:
A. 5th cranial nerve
B. 7th cranial nerve
C. 9th cranial nerve
D. 11th cranial nerve

156. All the following features may be found in Struge-Weber syndrome expect:
A. Unilateral congenital cutaneous capillary angioma in face with port-wine stain
B. Leptomeningeal angiomatosis
C. Ipsilateral homonymous hemianopia
D. Ipsilateral glaucoma

157. The compression in subclavian steal syndrome may be due to:
A. Scalenus anticus muscles
B. Osteoarthritic spur
C. Disc herniation
D. All of the above

158. Sphenoid fissure syndrome is otherwise known as:
A. Superior orbital fissure syndrome
B. Orbital apex syndrome
C. Optic foramen syndrome
D. All of the above

159. Earpits deafness syndrome is otherwise known as:
A. Sleck-Phelps syndrome
B. Tietze syndrome
C. Trotters syndrome
D. None of the above

160. Superior vena cava syndrome may be caused by:
A. Bronchogenic carcinoma
B. Mediastinal neoplasm
C. Substernal goitre
D. All of the above

161. The cranial nerves involved in Tapia's syndrome are:
A. IX and X   B. X and XI
C. XI and XII   D. X and XII

162. The cranial nerves involved in Tolosa-Hunt syndrome are:
A. II, III, IV and V   B. III, IV, V and VI
C. IV, V, VI and VII   D. V, VI, VII and VIII

163. Mandibulofacial dysostosis is otherwise known as:
A. Berry syndrome
B. Treacher Collins syndrome
C. Tranceschtti-zwahlen-klien syndrome
D. All of the above

164. The incidence of turners syndrome is:
A. 1:1000 live births   B. 1:2000 live births
C. 1:3000 live birth   D. 1:4000 live birth

165. Turner's syndrome or gonadal dysgenesis is characterized by all the following except:
A. Small ear lobes
B. Poorly developed mastoid air cell system
C. Low set external ears
D. XO: with 80% sex chromatic negative

166. The race usually affected by Tay-Sachs syndrome is:
A. Jews   B. Africans
C. Mongoloids   D. Caucasians

167. Trotter's syndrome is characterized by all the following except:
A. Neuralgia of the inferior maxillary nerve
B. Conductive hearing loss
C. Contralateral akinesia of soft palate
D. Pre auricular edema

168. **Sinus of Morgagni syndrome is otherwise known as:**
    A. Morgagni syndrome
    B. Morgagni-Stewart-Morrel syndrome
    C. Trotter's syndrome
    D. Sprengel's syndrome

169. **Turpin's syndrome is characterized by all the following except:**
    A. Congenital bronchiectasis
    B. Situs inversus
    C. Mega esophagus
    D. Tracheo oesophageal fistula

170. **Among the entire congenital deafness syndrome which of the following is most likely to include vestibular symptoms:**
    A. Usher's syndrome
    B. Wardenburg's syndrome
    C. Pendred's syndrome
    D. Alport's syndrome

171. **As per the Gorlin and coworker classification 90% of the Usher's syndrome belong to:**
    A. Type I
    B. Type II
    C. Type III
    D. Type IV

172. **Among all the hereditary deafness the incidence of Usher's syndrome is around:**
    A. 5%
    B. 10%
    C. 20%
    D. 25%

173. **The neuralgia associated with vail syndrome is:**
    A. Trigeminal neuralgia
    B. Vidian neuralgia
    C. Sphenopalatine neuralgia
    D. None of the above

174. **The syndrome which is often confused with VATER syndrome is:**
    A. Van der Hoeve syndrome
    B. Vogt-Kouanagi-Harada syndrome
    C. Hold-Oram syndrome
    D. Van-Buchem's syndrome

175. **VATER syndrome is a nonrandom association of:**
    A. Vertebral defects and anal atresia
    B. TOF with esophageal atresia
    C. Renal defects and radial limb dysplasia
    D. All of the above

176. **Vander-hoeve syndrome is otherwise known as:**
    A. De-Klegn's syndrome
    B. Frigilitis osseum
    C. Osteogenis is imperfecta
    D. All of the above

177. **All the following may be associated with Van-der-Hoeve syndrome except:**
    A. Blue sclera
    B. Brittle bones
    C. Thick skin
    D. Otosclerotic deafness

178. **The cranial nerve paralysis in Vernet's syndrome includes:**
    A. IX and X
    B. X and XI
    C. IX, X and XI
    D. X, XI and XII

179. **Posterior retropharyngeal syndrome is otherwise known as:**
    A. Vernet's syndrome
    B. Villaret's syndrome
    C. Vail syndrome
    D. None of the above

180. **Horner's syndrome may be associated with:**
    A. Schmidt's syndrome
    B. Tapia syndrome
    C. Vernet's syndrome
    D. Villaret's syndrome

181. **The cranial nerves involved in Villaret's syndrome are:**
    A. IX and X
    B. IX, X and XI
    C. IX, X, XI and XII
    D. None of the above

182. **Van-Buchem's syndrome is characterized by all the following features except:**
    A. Bilateral progressive sensorineural hearing loss
    B. Skull thickening & narrowing of foramens
    C. Facial palsy
    D. Vertigo

183. **Uveomenigoencephalitis syndrome is otherwise known as:**
    A. Weber syndrome
    B. Werdning-Hoffman syndrome
    C. Wildervac syndrome
    D. Vogt-Koyanagi-Harada syndrome

184. **All the following features maybe associated with Vogt-Koyanagi-Harada syndrome** *except:*
    A. Conductive deafness
    B. Vitiligo
    C. Bilateral uveitis
    D. Pseudobulbar palsy

185. **von Willebrand's syndrome is associated with deficiency of factor:**
    A. VI
    B. VII
    C. VIII
    D. IX

186. **von Willebrand's syndrome or hereditary telangectasia is associated with prolonged:**
    A. Bleeding time
    B. Clotting time
    C. Prothrombin time
    D. None of the above

187. **Von-Hippel-Lindau disease may be associated with:**
    A. Cerebellar hemangioblastoma
    B. Medullary hemangioblastoma
    C. Spinal hemangioblastoma
    D. All of the above

188. **Wallenberg's syndrome is due to the occlusion of:**
    A. Anterior inferior cerebellar artery
    B. Posterior inferior cerebellar artery
    C. Anterior cerebral artery
    D. Posterior cerebral artery

189. **Lateral medullary syndrome is otherwise known as:**
    A. Dorsolateral-medullary infarction
    B. Wallenberg's syndrome
    C. Syndrome of PICA thrombosis
    D. All of the above

190. **The cranial nerves involved in the lateral medullary syndrome are:**
    A. IX and X
    B. X and XI
    C. IX, X and XI
    D. X, XI and XII

191. **Poland syndrome is the congenital absence of:**
    A. Pectoralis minor
    B. Pectoralis major
    C. Latismus dorsi
    D. None of the above

192. **Horner's syndrome may be associated with all the following syndrome** *except:*
    A. Pancoast's syndrome
    B. Villaret's syndrome
    C. Vernet's syndrome
    D. Wallenberg's syndrome

193. **Wardenberg's syndrome is characterized by all the following features** *except:*
    A. White forelock
    B. Hetochromia ididia
    C. Perceptive deafness
    D. Medial displacement of lateral canthus

194. **Weber syndrome is characterized by all the following features** *except:*
    A. Ipsilateral ocular palsy
    B. Ipsilateral facial palsy
    C. Contralateral hemiplegia
    D. Contralateral hypoglossal palsy

195. **Craniocarpotarsal dysplasia is otherwise known as:**
    A. Wildervank's syndrome
    B. Whistling Face syndrome
    C. Wiskott-Aldrich syndrome
    D. Werding-Hoffman syndrome

196. **Wildervank's syndrome is associated with:**
    A. Bilateral facial palsy
    B. Bilateral abducen'se palsy
    C. Unilateral facial palsy
    D. Unilateral abducen'se palsy

197. **Wernicke's syndrome is associated with the deficiency of vitamin:**
    A. B_1
    B. B_2
    C. B_6
    D. B_{12}

198. **The synonym of cervico-occulo-acoustic syndrome is:**
    A. Werdning-Hoffman syndrome
    B. Wildervac syndrome
    C. Well syndrome
    D. None of the above

199. **Wiskott-Aldrich syndrome is associated with:**
    A. B cells defect
    B. T cells defect
    C. Combined B and T cells defect
    D. None of the above

ANSWERS

1 C	2 A	3 D	4 D	5 B	6 D	7 D	8 D
9 A	10 B	11 A	12 A	13 B	14 B	15 C	16 D
17 D	18 B	19 A	20 D	21 A	22 D	23 B	24 A
25 D	26 B	27 A	28 D	29 D	30 B	31 C	32 C
33 D	34 B	35 A	36 C	37 A	38 D	39 A	40 C
41 A	42 C	43 A	44 A	45 A	46 D	47 B	48 A
49 A	50 A	51 C	52 D	53 C	54 C	55 A	56 D
57 B	58 D	59 D	60 A	61 A	62 A	63 B	64 C
65 B	66 C	67 B	68 A	69 C	70 C	71 B	72 A
73 C	74 D	75 C	76 A	77 B	78 D	79 B	80 C
81 D	82 D	83 B	84 D	85 C	86 A	87 D	88 C
89 C	90 A	91 C	92 A	93 D	94 A	95 B	96 C
97 D	98 D	99 D	100 A	101 C	102 C	103 A	104 A
105 D	106 A	107 A	108 A	109 D	110 A	111 D	112 A
113 C	114 D	115 B	116 A	117 D	118 D	119 D	120 B
121 A	122 C	123 D	124 C	125 A	126 B	127 A	128 D
129 D	130 A	131 A	132 D	133 B	134 D	135 A	136 B
137 D	138 C	139 C	140 B	141 D	142 B	143 C	144 C
145 B	146 B	147 D	148 D	149 A	150 B	151 D	152 C
153 A	154 B	155 B	156 C	157 D	158 D	159 A	160 D
161 D	162 B	163 D	164 D	165 A	166 A	167 C	168 C
169 B	170 A	171 A	172 B	173 B	174 C	175 D	176 D
177 C	178 C	179 B	180 D	181 C	182 D	183 D	184 A
185 C	186 A	187 D	188 B	189 D	190 D	191 B	192 C
193 D	194 B	195 B	196 B	197 A	198 B	199 C	

Foramen, Fossa and Fissure

1. **The bones taking part in the formation of anterior ethmoidal foramen are:**
   A. Ethmoid and vomer
   B. Ethmoid and frontal
   C. Ethmoid and maxilla
   D. Ethmoid and temporal

2. **The location of anterior ethmoidal foramen is on the:**
   A. Medial wall of orbit
   B. Lateral wall of orbit
   C. Floor of orbit
   D. Root of orbit

3. **Foramen cacum is present in the:**
   A. Anterior cranial fossa
   B. Middle cranial fossa
   C. Posterior cranial fossa
   D. None of the above

4. **The contents of foramen ceacum are:**
   A. Greater petrosal nerve
   B. Lesser petrosal nerve
   C. Emissary veins
   D. All of the above

5. **Condyloid foramen is present on the:**
   A. Temporal bone
   B. Parietal bone
   C. Sphenoid bone
   D. Occipital bone

6. **The bones taking part in the formation of greater palatine foramen are:**
   A. Palatine and vomer
   B. Palatine and maxilla
   C. Palatine and ethmoid
   D. None of the above

7. **Incisive foramen contains:**
   A. Emissary vein
   B. Ascending septal artery
   C. Descending palatine artery
   D. Nasopalatine nerve

8. **All the following bones take part in the formation of inferior orbital fissure *except*:**
   A. Sphenoid
   B. Maxilla
   C. Ethmoid
   D. Palatine

9. **All the following structures are contents of the inferior orbital fissure *except*:**
   A. Opthalmic division of 5th cranial nerve (V1)
   B. Maxillary division of 5th cranial nerve (V2)
   C. Zygomatic nerve
   D. Pterygoid plexus

10. **Infraorbital foramen is present on the:**
    A. Lacrimal bone
    B. Zygoma
    C. Maxilla
    D. None of the above

11. **The bones taking part in the formation of Jugular foramen are:**
    A. Temporal and sphenoid
    B. Occipital and temporal
    C. Temporal, occipital and sphenoid
    D. Parietal, temporal and occipital

12. **All the following structures are contents of Jugular foramen *except*:**
    A. Inferior petrosal sinus
    B. Superior petrosal sinus
    C. Transverse sinus
    D. Meningeal arteries

13. **All the following cranial nerves are contents of jugular foramen *except:***

    A. IX
    B. X
    C. XI
    D. XII

14. **All the following statements regarding foramen lacerum are correct *except:***

    A. Present in posterior cranial fossa
    B. Formed by temporal, occipital, sphenoid bones
    C. Lies lateral to basilar part of occipital
    D. Covered by cartilaginous plate

15. **All the following structures are contents of foramen magnum *except:***

    A. Medulla oblongata
    B. Spinal root of XI cranial nerve
    C. Vertebral arteries
    D. Preganglionic sympathetic fibers

16. **Mandibular foramen is present on the:**

    A. Medial surface of ramus of mandible
    B. Lateral surface of ramus of mandible
    C. External surface of body of mandible
    D. Internal surface of body of mandible

17. **All the following statements regarding mastoid foramen are true *except:***

    A. It's location is on the posterior external surface of skull
    B. It lies below and behind the mastoid process
    C. It is near the temparo occipital suture
    D. It's content is emissary vein

18. **Optic foramen is present on the:**

    A. Lacrimal bone
    B. Frontal process of maxilla bone
    C. Maxillary process frontal bone
    D. Sphenoid bone

19. **All the following structures are contents of the optic foramen *except:***

    A. Opthalmic artery
    B. Central artery of retina
    C. Emissary veins
    D. Postganglionic sympathetic fibers

20. **The location of the optic foramen is on the:**

    A. Apex of orbit
    B. Floor of orbit
    C. Medial wall of orbit
    D. Lateral wall of orbit

21. **The optic foramen lies between the two root of:**

    A. Greater wing of sphenoid
    B. Lesser wing of sphenoid
    C. Pterygoid hamulus
    D. None of the above

22. **Foramen ovale is present on the:**

    A. Greater wing of sphenoid
    B. Lesser wing of sphenoid
    C. Medial Pterygoid plate
    D. Lateral Pterygoid plate

23. **All the following structures are contents of the foramen ovale *except:***

    A. Mandibular division of 5th cranial nerve
    B. Maxillary division of 5th cranial nerve
    C. Accessory meningeal artery
    D. Lesser petrosal nerve

24. **Which of the following nerve passes through foramen rotandum?**

    A. Abducent
    B. Trochlear
    C. Mandibular division of 5th cranial nerve
    D. Maxillary division of 5th cranial nerve

25. **All the following statements regarding sphenopalatine foramen are true *except:***

    A. It opens to the nasal cavity
    B. It lies between the sphenoidal and orbital processes
    C. It is located on the lateral wall of pterygopalatine fossa
    D. It's contents are pterygopalatine nerves and vessels.

26. **All the following structures are contents of the foramen spinosum *except:***

    A. Middle meningeal artery
    B. Recurrent meningeal nerve
    C. Middle meningeal vein
    D. Lesser superficial petrosal nerve

27. **Stylomastoid foramen lies:**

    A. Anterior to the base of styloid process
    B. Posterior to the styloid process
    C. Medial to the styloid process
    D. Lateral to the styloid process

28. All the following foramens are located on the zygoma *except*:

- A. Zygomaticofacial
- B. Zygomatico orbital
- C. Zygomatic frontal
- D. Zygomatic temporal

29. The supraorbital foramen lies:

- A. Above the supercilliary arch
- B. Below the supercilliary arch
- C. Medial to supercilliary arch
- D. Lateral to supercilliary arch

30. Foramen of luschka is otherwise known as:

- A. Foramen of Key and Retzius
- B. Huschke's foramen
- C. Hyrtl's foramen
- D. Morrand's foramen

31. Foramen of luschka communicate between:

- A. Third and fourth ventricle
- B. Lateral and third ventricle
- C. Fourth and lateral ventricle
- D. Fourth ventricle and subarachnoid space

32. CSF passes from lateral to third ventrical through:

- A. Foramen of megendie
- B. Foramen of monro
- C. Foramen of Retzius
- D. None of the above

33. Foramen of megendie is otherwise known as:

- A. Apertura mediana
- B. Ventriculi quarti
- C. All of the above
- D. None of the above

34. Foramen of morgagni is otherwise known as:

- A. Foramen of Retzius
- B. Foramen singulare
- C. Interventricular foramen
- D. Appertura lateralis ventricularis Quarti

35. Foramen of morgani transmits:

- A. Auditory nerve
- B. Facial nerve
- C. Posterior ampullary nerve
- D. None of the above

36. All the following statement's regarding Huschke's foramen are correct *except*:

- A. It is caused by arrest of development
- B. It is found near the inner extremity of tympanic plate
- C. It lies between the tympanic and Jugular fossa
- D. Chordatympani nerve passes through the foramen

37. Hyrtl's foramen is found on:

- A. Petrous part of temporal bone
- B. Squamous part of temporal bone
- C. Sphenoid bone
- D. Ethmoid bone

38. The relation of Hyrtl's foramen to foramen ovale is that the former is:

- A. Below and lateral
- B. Above and lateral
- C. Below and medial
- D. Above and medial

39. Foramen of Rivinus is found on:

- A. Tectorial membrane
- B. Sharpnell's membrane
- C. Secondary tympanic membrane
- D. Reissner's membrane

40. Foramen of vessalium is a minute inconsistent opening found on:

- A. Ethmoid
- B. Sphenoid
- C. Petrous part of temporal
- D. Squamous part of temporal

41. The relationship of foramen vessalium to foramen ovale is that the former is:

- A. Anteromedial
- B. Anterolateral
- C. Posteromedial
- D. Posterolateral

42. Foraman of vessalium transmits emissary vein from:

- A. Superior sagital sinus
- B. Inferior sagital sinus
- C. Cavernous sinus
- D. Sigmoid sinus

43. Morrand's foramen is otherwise known as:
A. Fallopian foramen
B. Farrien's foramen
C. All of the above
D. None of the above

44. Fallopian foramen transmits:
A. Facial nerve
B. Singular nerve
C. Lesser petrosal nerve
D. Greater petrosal nerve

45. Scarpas foramen is found in the:
A. Inter maxillary suture
B. Sphenoparietal suture
C. Occipitomastoid suture
D. Sagittal suture

46. Foramen of Huschke, an embryologic remnant, if persists, may allow the spread of tumor or infection to:
A. Preauricular area   B. Glenoid fossa
C. Parotid   D. All of the above

47. The posterior compartment of Jugular foramen contains all the following structure's except:
A. Internal Jugular vein
B. Meningeal branch of ascending pharyngeal artery
C. X cranial nerve
D. Nodes of Kause

48. The anterior compartment of jugular foramen contains:
A. Inferior petrosal sinus
B. Internal jugular vein
C. XI cranial nerve
D. IX cranial nerve

49. Internal carotid artery is a content of:
A. Foramen magnum
B. Jugular foramen
C. Foramen lacerum
D. None of the above

50. All the following statements regarding foramen caecum are true except:
A. It's a shallow pit like depression on tongue
B. Lies just posterior to sulcus terminalis
C. Indicates the opening of embryological thyroglossal duct
D. Hypoglossal nerve passes through the foramen

51. The facial fossa lodges all the following structure except:
A. Facial nerve
B. Intermediate nerve of wrisburg
C. Internal auditory artery
D. Stylomastoid artery

52. Fossa of Rossenmuller is otherwise known as:
A. Fossa of malgaign
B. Pyramidal fossa
C. Facial recess
D. Pharyngeal recess

53. Fossa of Rossenmuller opens to the nasopharynx:
A. Above the foramen lacerum
B. Below the foramen lacerum
C. Medial to foramen lacerum
D. Lateral to the foramen lacerum

54. Fossa of Rossenmuller is present:
A. Behind the posterior margin of torus tubaris
B. Behind the anterior margin of torus tubaris
C. Below the posterior margin of torus tubaris
D. Below the anterior margin of torus tubaris

55. Fossa of malgogin is otherwise known as:
A. Gerdy's hyoid fossa
B. Carotid trigone
C. Carotid triangle
D. All of the above

56. Mastoid fossa is otherwise known as:
A. Mac-Ewen's triangle
B. Suprameatal triangle
C. All of the above
D. None of the above

57. Meckel's fossa contains:
A. Semilunar ganglion
B. Otic ganglion
C. Geniculate ganglion
D. Scarpas ganglion

58. Pyramidal fossa is present in the jugular foramen in:
A. Anterior compartment
B. Middle compartment
C. Posterior compartment
D. None of the above

59. Cochlear aqueduct empties into:
A. Pyramidal fossa   B. Cerebellar fossa
C. Meckel's fossa   D. Mastoid fossa

60. Cochlear fossa corresponds to:
A. Base of cochlea
B. Apex of cochlea
C. Cochlear acqueduct
D. None of the above

61. Pterygopalatine fossa is enclosed by all the following bones *except*:
A. Maxilla   B. Palatine
C. Ethmoid   D. Pterygoid

62. Pterygopalatine fossa communicates with:
A. Intracranial cavity
B. Nasal cavity
C. Orbit
D. All the above

63. Mandibular fossa is otherwise known as:
A. Glenoid fossa
B. Pyramidal fossa
C. Retromolar fossa
D. None of the above

64. Scaphoid fossa is a small depression at the:
A. Base of medial pterygoid plate
B. Base of lateral pterygoid plate
C. Apex of medial pterygoid plate
D. Apex of lateral pterygoid plate

65. The deepest portion of sella turica is known as:
A. Subarcuate fossa
B. Hypophyseal fossa
C. Tuberculum Sellae
D. Dorsum Sellae

66. All the following boundaries of canine fossa are correct *except*:
A. Anteriorly canine ridge
B. Posteriorly posterior border of maxillary tuberosity
C. Superiorly infraorbital ridge
D. Inferiorly alveolar margin

67. All the fossae are present on the mandible *except*:
A. Digastric   B. Sublingual
C. Submandibular   D. Glenoid

68. All the following boundaries of infratemporal fossa are correct *except*:
A. Anterior wall by body and tuberosity of maxilla
B. Medial wall by medial pterygoid plate
C. Lateral wall by ramus of mandible
D. Root by greater wing of sphenoid and squamous temporal

69. Jugular fossa lies between the following two bones:
A. Occipital and parietal
B. Occipital and sphenoid
C. Temporal and occipital
D. Temporal and sphenoid

70. The pitutary fossa is otherwise known as:
A. Sellae turcila
B. Hypophyseal fossa
C. Tuberculum sellae
D. Dorsum Sellae

71. All the following structures are contents of Infratemporal fossa *except*:
A. Lateral pterygoid muscle
B. Medial pterygoid muscle
C. Maxillary artery
D. Maxillary nerve

72. The key orientation structure for the contents of infratemporal fossa is:
A. Temporalis muscle
B. Medial pterygoid muscle
C. Lateral pterygoid muscle
D. Pterygoid venous plexus

73. The middle cranial fossa is associated with cranial nerves:
A. II – V   B. III – VI
C. II – VII   D. III – VIII

74. Which of the following boundaries of epitympanum is formed by fossa incudis?
A. Medial   B. Lateral
C. Superior   D. Inferior

75. 2/3rd of the floor of middle cranial fossa is formed by:
A. Sphenoid   B. Temporal
C. Occipital   D. Parietal

76. **Triangular fossa is present in:**
    A. External auditory meatus
    B. Internal auditory meatus
    C. Auricle
    D. None of the above

77. **Subarcuate fossa, present on the temporal bone is in:**
    A. Squamous part   B. Mastoid part
    C. Petrous part   D. Tympanic part

78. **Vermion fossa is present in the:**
    A. Anterior cranial fossa
    B. Middle cranial fossa
    C. Posterior cranial fossa
    D. None of the above

79. **Pterygomaxillary fossa contains all the following structures *except*:**
    A. Maxillary nerve
    B. Sphenopalatine ganglion
    C. Pterygoid venous Plexus
    D. Internal maxillary artery

80. **The lateral boundary of the pterygopalatine fossa is formed:**
    A. Lateral pterygoid muscle
    B. Medial pterygoid muscle
    C. Temporalis muscle
    D. Masseter muscle

81. **The fissure through which the chorda tympani nerve leaves the middle ear is known as:**
    A. Squamotympanic fissure
    B. Petrotympanic fissure
    C. Petrosquamous fissure
    D. None of the above

82. **The fissure which transmits the anterior tympanic branch of the maxillary artery is:**
    A. Tympanosquamous
    B. Petrosquamous
    C. Petrotympanic
    D. Pterygomaxillaru

83. **The petrosquamous suture overlies the auditory tube in it's:**
    A. Medial aspect   B. Lateral aspect
    C. Superior aspect   D. Inferior aspect

84. **Petrosquamous suture in relation to Petrotympanic suture lies:**
    A. Medially   B. Laterally
    C. Anteriorly   D. Posteriorly

85. **The medial extension of tympanosquamous suture is known as:**
    A. Petrotympanic suture
    B. Petrosquamous suture
    C. Tympanomatoid suture
    D. None of the above

86. **The pterygomaxillary fissure opens into the:**
    A. Temporal fossa
    B. Infratemporal fossa
    C. Pterygopalative fossa
    D. None of the above

87. **In relation to the Infratemporal fossa the pterygomaxillary fissure is in the:**
    A. Medial aspect of the anterior wall
    B. Medial aspect of the medial wall
    C. Lateral aspect of anterior wall
    D. Lateral aspect of medial wall

88. **The superior orbital fissure lies between the:**
    A. Greater wing of sphenoid and maxilla
    B. Lesser wing of sphenoid and maxilla
    C. Lesser and greater wings of sphenoid
    D. None of the above

89. **The inferior orbital fissure lies between the:**
    A. Greater wing of sphenoid and maxilla
    B. Lesser wing of sphenoid and maxilla
    C. Greater wing of the sphenoid and lacrima bone
    D. Lesser wing of sphenoid and lacrima bone

90. **The inferior orbital fissure transmits all the following structure's *except*:**
    A. Infraorbital vessels
    B. Inferior ophthalmic veins
    C. Lacrimal branch of ophthalmic nerve
    D. Infraorbital branch of maxillary nerve

91. **The remnant of the postembryonic fussion between the right and left half of frontal bone is known as:**
    A. Coronal suture   B. Sagittal suture
    C. Metopic suture   D. None of the above

92. The longitudinal fissure separates:
   A. Frontal parietal lobes
   B. Occipital and temporal lobes
   C. Frontal and temporal lobes
   D. Both cerebral hemispheres

93. The floor of the longitudinal fissure is formed by:
   A. Septum pellucidum
   B. Corpora quadrigemina
   C. Corpus callosum
   D. Hypothalamus

94. The spread of tumor or infection from the parotid can passthrough the:
   A. Hyrtle's fissure
   B. Fissure of Santorini
   C. All of the above
   D. None of the above

95. All the following statements regarding Hyrtle's fissure are true *except*:
   A. It is an embryological remnant that normally obliterates
   B. It may persists as epitympanic connection

   C. The connection is to the subarachnoid space
   D. It allow transmission of middle ear/mastoid infection to the CSF

96. Which of the following statement regarding petrotympanic fissure is true?
   A. It is otherwise known as Glaserian fissure
   B. It open s anteriorly just above the attachment of the tympanic membrane on the bone of the medial surface of the lateral wall of the
   C. The chorda tympani enter s the medial surface of the fissure through a separate anterior canaliculus (canal of Huguier)
   D. All of the above

97. The following statements regarding squamosal foramen are true *except*:
   A. Very rarely present just above the anterior root of the zygomatic process
   B. When present transmits petrosquamous sinus
   C. Present on the medial wall of temporal fossa
   D. Present just above the posterior root of the zygomatic process

ANSWERS

1 B	2 A	3 A	4 C	5 D	6 B	7 D	8 C
9 A	10 C	11 B	12 B	13 D	14 A	15 D	16 A
17 B	18 D	19 C	20 A	21 B	22 A	23 B	24 D
25 C	26 D	27 B	28 C	29 B	30 A	31 D	32 B
33 B	34 B	35 C	36 D	37 C	38 A	39 B	40 B
41 A	42 C	43 C	44 D	45 A	46 D	47 C	48 A
49 C	50 D	51 C	52 D	53 B	54 A	55 D	56 D
57 A	58 A	59 B	60 A	61 C	62 D	63 A	64 A
65 B	66 B	67 D	68 B	69 C	70 B	71 D	72 C
73 C	74 D	75 B	76 C	77 C	78 C	79 C	80 C
81 B	82 C	83 A	84 C	85 A	86 C	87 A	88 C
89 A	90 C	91 C	92 D	93 C	94 B	95 B	96 D
97 D							

History

1. **Sir Charles Bell was born in:**
   - A. Dublin (1574)
   - B. London (1674)
   - C. Edinburg (1774)
   - D. Glasgow (1874)

2. **Wilhelm Freidrich von Ludwig who first described Ludwigs angina was:**
   - A. French
   - B. British
   - C. German
   - D. Dutch

3. **Prosper meniere died of:**
   - A. Influenzal Pneumonia (1867)
   - B. Tuberculosis (1861)
   - C. Pneumonic Plague (1762)
   - D. Cancer Stomach (1761)

4. **Alfred Higginson closely resembles:**
   - A. Hippocrates
   - B. Soccrates
   - C. Charles Darwin
   - D. Galen

5. **The father of otology is:**
   - A. George Shambaugh
   - B. Adam Politzer
   - C. Prosper Menier
   - D. Charles Bell

6. **Alfonso Corti first described the organ of corti in:**
   - A. 1841
   - B. 1851
   - C. 1861
   - D. 1871

7. **The first description of ankylosis of stapes is attributed to:**
   - A. Antonio Valsalva
   - B. Joseph Toynbee
   - C. Adam Politzer
   - D. Michale Portman

8. **The clinical diagnosis of otosclerosis was first clarified by:**
   - A. Freidrich Bezold
   - B. Jullius Lempert
   - C. Adam Politzer
   - D. Terence Cawthrone

9. **The modern operation of stapedectomy was first described by:**
   - A. Lempert
   - B. Shambaugh
   - C. Rosel
   - D. John Shea

10. **The foremost advocate of endaural approach is:**
    - A. George Portman
    - B. Jullius Lempert
    - C. Michale Portman
    - D. George Shambaug Jr.

11. **The endolymphatic hypertension hypothesis of Meniere's disease was first proposed in 1890 by:**
    - A. Terence Cawthrone
    - B. George Portman
    - C. Gabriel Follopius
    - D. Prosper Menier

12. **Gabriel fallopius, who first described the intra-temporal position of 7th cranial nerve in Fallopian Canal is:**
    - A. Italian anatomist
    - B. British anatomist
    - C. French surgeon
    - D. British surgeon

13. **The concept of tympanoplasty was first developed by:**
    - A. Rutherford and Helmholtz
    - B. Wullstein and Zollener
    - C. Ballantyne and Shambaug
    - D. None of the above

14. The Otomicroscope for ear surgery was introduced in 1921 by:
A. George Shambaugh
B. John Ballantyne
C. Charles Hallpike
D. Carl Olaf Nylen

15. Charles Skimmer Hallpike was born (1900) in:
A. London   B. India
C. New York   D. Paris

16. The nobel prize winner Robert Barany worked at University hospital of:
A. London   B. Dublin
C. Uppasala   D. Stockholm

17. The rare fortune of achieving immortality in the medical world for a single case report goes to:
A. Neils Stenson   B. von Ludwig
C. Prosper Meniere D. Charles Bell

18. The name of a famous otologist and a contemporary of victor Hugo who became director of Paris Institute of Deaf-mute is:
A. Alfonso Corti
B. Prosper Meniere
C. Alfred Higginson
D. Charles Bell

19. The doctor who worked as a curator in Guy's hospital but subsequently abandoned the practice of medicine after discovering a disease is:
A. Robert Koch   B. Henery Koplik
C. Thomas Hodgkin D. Victor Hosley

20. Nobel prize in medicine for his work on vestibular physiology was awarded in 1914 to:
A. Charles Hallpike B. Robert Barany
C. Rutherford   D. Helmholtz

21. Nobel prize in medicine was awarded to a Hungarian scientist in 1961 for his work on physical transmission of sound in cochlea to:
A. von Bekesy   B. Wever
C. Rutherford   D. Helmholtz

22. The famous Quote "As to diseases, make a habit of two things – to help or at least do no harm" is associated with:
A. Galen   B. Hippocrates
C. Paracelsus   D. Louis Pasture

23. The aphorism "Life is short but the art is long experiment risky, the crisis fleeting and decision difficult" is told by:
A. Hippocrates   B. Paracelsus
C. Robert Koch   D. Louis Pasture

24. Hippocrates lived between:
A. 460 to 370 BC   B. 370 to 220 BC
C. 220 to 170 BC   D. 170 to 80 BC

25. The first physician to describe cranial nerve was:
A. Galen   B. Paracelsus
C. Hippocrates   D. None of the above

26. Thomas Wharton, who published the first description of submandibular duct, obtained his MD degree from the University of:
A. Oxford
B. Cambridge
C. Both of the above
D. None of the above

27. Neil Stensen, who described the parotid duct at the age of 22 years only died aged:
A. 28 years   B. 38 years
C. 48 years   D. 58 years

28. Neil Stensen was born in:
A. Netherland   B. Denmark
C. Italy   D. England

29. A famous work titled "The Anatomy of Expression" was written by:
A. Alfred Higginson
B. Adam Politzer
C. Gabriel Fallopius
D. Sir Charles Bell

30. John Cheyne (1777-1836) who described cheyne – stokes breathing while working in the hospital at:
A. Dublin   B. Belfast
C. Edinburg   D. London

31. The father of nasal endoscopy is:
A. Wigand   B. Messerklinger
C. Killian   D. Hirschmann

32. The first successful laryngectomy was done in the year:
A. 1854   B. 1864
C. 1874   D. 1884

33. The first successful laryngectomy was done by:
    A. Hyesmartine   B. Schodinger
    C. Macfee   D. Billorth

34. Radium was discovered by Marie and pierre curie in the year:
    A. 1868   B. 1878
    C. 1888   D. 1898

35. The father of bronchoscopy is:
    A. Sutave Killian   B. Chevalier Jackson
    C. Ambroise Parre   D. Friedrich Bezold

36. The father of endoscopy is:
    A. Messerklinger
    B. Chevalier Jackson
    C. Antonio Valsalva
    D. Johannes Kessel

37. Which of the following personality is regarded as the father of surgery?
    A. Billorth
    B. Nylen
    C. Ambroise Parre
    D. None of the above

38. Which of the following personality is regarded as the father of neurotology?
    A. William F House
    B. Jullius Lempert
    C. John J. Shea
    D. Carl Olef Nylen

39. Which of the following personality is regarded as the father of mediastinoscopy?
    A. Rufus Guild   B. Theodor Bast
    C. William Wild   D. Eric Carlens

40. Which of the following otologists first performed endaural radical mastoidectomy?
    A. WF House   B. Jullius Lempert
    C. Johannes Kessel   D. George Portman

41. Who among the following was credited with for first discovery of glomus Jugulare?
    A. SR Guild   B. WF House
    C. DW Kennedy   D. JJ Shea

42. Who among the following, first coined the term FESS?
    A. DW Kennedy   B. Maurice Cottle
    C. Wigand   D. Messerklinger

43. Which of the following name is credited with for doing the first tracheostomy?
    A. Aclepiades   B. Bozzini
    C. Kayser   D. None of the above

44. Who among the following is credited with, for first using a mirror to visualise his own larynx?
    A. Kustner   B. Bozzini
    C. Kyser   D. Politzer

45. Who among the following performed the first rigid oesophagoscopy?
    A. Kyser   B. Kussmaul
    C. Wullstein   D. Schuknecht

46. Who and When first coined the term otosclerosis?
    A. Harrold Schuknechet in 1850
    B. Horst Wublstein in 1855
    C. Adam politzer in 1894
    D. Siebenmann in 1812

47. Who and when first described acoustic neuroma?
    A. Sandifort (1777)   B. Valentin (1848)
    C. Boeck (1905)   D. Willis (1666)

48. Who and when recorded the first case of CSF rhinorrhea?
    A. Friedmann (1966)   B. Sindifort (1777)
    C. Willis (1666)   D. Pilz (1868)

49. Who among the following ancient Indian is credited with for performing the rhinoplasty?
    A. Susrutha   B. Charak
    C. Dhanvantri   D. Aswinikumar

50. Who among the following, first observed fluid within the labyrinth?
    A. Antonio Maria Valsalva
    B. Sterling Bunnell
    C. Sir Terence Caw throne
    D. Harry Rosen Wasse

ANSWERS

1 C		2 C		3 A		4 C		5 B		6 B		7 A		8 A
9 D		10 B		11 B		12 A		13 B		14 D		15 B		16 C
17 B		18 B		19 C		20 B		21 A		22 B		23 A		24 A
25 A		26 C		27 C		28 B		29 D		30 A		31 D		32 C
33 D		34 D		35 B		36 B		37 C		38 A		39 D		40 C
41 A		42 A		43 A		44 B		45 B		46 C		47 A		48 C
49 A		50 A												

Skull Base Surgery

1. **Cerebrospinal fluid is produced in:**
   A. Choroid plexus of lateral ventricle
   B. Ependyma of 3rd & 4th ventricles
   C. Both the above
   D. None of the above

2. **Spontaneous CSF leaks occur in:**
   A. Mondini's dysplasia
   B. Large vestibular aqueduct
   C. Widely patent cochlear aqueduct
   D. All of the above

3. **Fisch type I lateral skull base approach is used for:**
   A. Glomus tumours
   B. Nasopharyngeal angiofibromas
   C. Schwannoma of vagus nerve
   D. squamous cell ca of temporal bone

4. **Pathognomonic test for confirmation of CSF is:**
   A. Handkerchief test
   B. Flourescein dye test
   C. Betaz transferrin
   D. Biochemical analysis.

5. **Routes of intracranial spread of CSOM are:**
   A. Trautmann's triangle
   B. Periarteriolar spaces of virchow-Robin
   C. Dural dehiscence.
   D. Dural venous sinus thrombosis.
   E. All of the above.

6. **Battle's sign is seen in:**
   A. # anterior cranial fossa
   B. # middle cranial fossa.
   C. # posterior cranial fossa.
   D. None of the above.

7. **Post-traumatic profound hearing loss occurs in:**
   A. Transverse # of temporal bone.
   B. Longitudinal # of temporal bone.
   C. Lefort's type III #
   D. Rupture of tympanic membrane.

8. **Bilateral facial palsy is seen in:**
   A. Lyme's disease.
   B. Guillain-Barré syndrome.
   C. Merkleson-Rosenthal syndrome.
   D. Congenital facial agenesis
   E. All of the above.

9. **Fisch described facial nerve decompression:**
   A. From internal acoustic meatus till its exit
   B. Horizontal segment till its exit
   C. Second genu to its exit
   D. At the stylomastoid foramen

10. **Stereotactic radiosurgery is a treatment modality for:**
    A. Olfactory meningioma
    B. Acoustic neuroma
    C. Craniopharyngeoma
    D. Retinoblastoma

11. **Facial nerve monitoring by House-Brackmann included all *except*:**
    A. Synkinesis
    B. Forehead creases
    C. Eye closure
    D. Clenching of teeth

12. **Anaesthesia over the posterior superior conchal-skin in CP angle tumours is called:**
    A. Hitselberger's sign
    B. Hennebert's sign
    C. Hurtle's sign
    D. Holman Miller sign

13. **Facial nerve grafting is done using:**
    - A. Ansa cervicalis.
    - B. Sural nerve.
    - C. Common peroneal nerve .
    - D. None of the above.

14. **Structures passing through foramen spinosum:**
    - A. Middle meningeal artery.
    - B. Nerve of Wrisberg.
    - C. Accesory meningeal vein.
    - D. Lesser petrosal nerve.
    - E. None of the above.

15. **Approches to Petrous apex are *all except:***
    - A. Thornwaldt's
    - B. Eagleton's.
    - C. Almoor's
    - D. Ramadier-Lempert's
    - E. Cushing's

16. **CSF leak repair is done with:**
    - A. Gel foam.
    - B. Muscle.
    - C. Fat.
    - D. Fascia lata.
    - E. Surgicel
    - F. All the above.

17. **Botulinum toxin is used in the treatment of:**
    - A. Blepharospasm.
    - B. Spasmodic dysphonia.
    - C. Tic dolourex.
    - D. All the above.

18. **Superior vestibular schwannoma is best diagnosed by:**
    - A. Contrast pnuemoencephalogram.
    - B. Technicium - 99 radionucleide scan.
    - C. Gadollinium enhanced MRI.
    - D. High resolution CT of temporal bone.

19. **Structure in superior relation to foramen lacerum:**
    - A. Maxillary nerve.
    - B. Ascending pharyngeal artery
    - C. Dorello's canal
    - D. Spine of sphenoid

20. **Steps in surgery for glomus jugulare include *all except:***
    - A. Anterior transposition of facial nerve
    - B. Blind sac closure
    - C. Sigmoid sinus obliteration
    - D. Radical mastoidectomy
    - E. Labyrinthectomy.

21. **Congenital cholesteatoma is classified by:**
    - A. House-Brackmann
    - B. Janssen-Claussen
    - C. Perry-Smith
    - D. Derlake-Clemis

22. **A 6-month-old child presenting with trans-illuminant swelling arising from roof of the nasal cavity:**
    - A. Meningoencephalocele
    - B. Rathke's bursitis
    - C. Thornwald's cyst
    - D. Olfactory neuroblastoma

23. **Erosion of clivus is pathagnomonic of:**
    - A. Nasopharyngeal carcinoma
    - B. Juvenile nasopharyngeal angiofibroma
    - C. Cavernous sinus thrombosis
    - D. Craniopharyngeoma
    - E. None of the above

24. **Pterygopalatine fossa is approached for which surgery:**
    - A. Vidian neurectomy
    - B. Internal maxillary artery
    - C. Juvenile nasopharyngeal angiofibroma
    - D. Sphenopalatine ganglion block
    - E. All of the above

25. **Lateral sinus thrombosis is diagnosed by:**
    - A. Toynbee's test
    - B. Queckenstedt's test
    - C. Mueller's test
    - D. Frenckner's test

26. **Bitemporal hemianopia seen in:**
    - A. Hypophsial tumour
    - B. Cavernous sinus thrombosis
    - C. Cerebellar abscess
    - D. Retinitis pigmentosa

27. **Nerve involved in Frey's syndrome is:**
    - A. Vidian nerve
    - B. Singular nerve
    - C. Auriculotemporal nerve
    - D. Jacobson's nerve
    - E. Arnold's nerve

28. **Optic canal dehiscence within the sphenoid sinus is seen in:**
    - A. 24% cases.
    - B. 0.5% cases.
    - C. 12% cases.
    - D. 6% cases.
    - E. 48% cases.

29. Phelp's sign is the pathagnomonic radiographic sign showing erosion of:

A. Korner's septum
B. Lateral attic wall
C. Petrotympanic fissure
D. Caroticojugular spine

30. Approches to the internal acoustic meatus include *all except*:

A. Translabrynthine
B. Middle cranial fossa
C. Retrosigmoid
D. Transcochlear
E. Extended facial recess

ANSWERS

1 C	2 D	3 A	4 C	5 E	6 C	7 A	8 E
9 A	10 B	11 D	12 A	13 B	14 A	15 E	16 F
17 D	18 C	19 C	20 E	21 D	22 A	23 D	24 E
25 B	26 A	27 C	28 D	29 D	30 E		

Section 3
Allied Subjects

Radiology

1. **For thorough noninvasive evaluation of nasal cavity and paranasal sinuses the following provides the maximum detail:**
   - A. Direct observation
   - B. Radiography
   - C. Both
   - D. None

2. **Superior and lateral extent of frontal sinuses are best evaluated by the following view:**
   - A. Water's view
   - B. Caldwell view
   - C. Skull lateral view
   - D. Both Caldwell and Water's view

3. **Ethmoid sinuses are best evaluated in:**
   - A. Caldwell view
   - B. Water's view
   - C. Skull lateral view
   - D. Both

4. **If Anterior ethmoid sinuses are of specific interest which view will be most useful?**
   - A. Caldwell view
   - B. Waters' view
   - C. Skull Towne's view
   - D. Skull lateral view

5. **Maxillary sinuses are best evaluated by:**
   - A. Water's view
   - B. Caldwell view
   - C. Skull lateral view
   - D. Skull Towne's view

6. **The following pair of sinuses are quite symmetric in size and configuration:**
   - A. Frontal sinus
   - B. Sphenoid sinuses
   - C. Maxillary sinuses
   - D. Both frontal and sphenoidal sinuses

7. **For the best evaluation of sphenomaxillary (pterygomaxillary) fissure, following view is most useful:**
   - A. Lateral view
   - B. Basal view of skull
   - C. Towne's view of skull
   - D. Neither of the above

8. **Canal like lucency seen in lateral maxillary sinus wall as seen in Water's view is due to:**
   - A. Posterior superior alveolar canal
   - B. Fracture line
   - C. Lipoma
   - D. Neither of the above

9. **For sphenoidal sinuses, the following radiography is most useful:**
   - A. Basal view of skull
   - B. Lateral view of skull
   - C. Open mouth view of skull
   - D. All of the above

10. **Lack of sphenoidal sinus pneumatization beyond the age of 10 years strongly suggests the presence of:**
    - A. Occult sphenoid sinus pathology
    - B. Nil pathology
    - C. 67% to 75% of associated maxillary sinuses inflammatory pathology
    - D. Both A and C

11. **The following sinus is the most commonly affected by mucocoele:**
    - A. Ethmoid sinus.
    - B. Maxillary sinus
    - C. Frontal sinus
    - D. Sphenoid sinus

12. **The nasolacrimal duct opens into:**
    - A. Middle Meatus
    - B. Superior Meatus
    - C. Inferior meatus
    - D. Neither of the above

13. **Nasal atrium is the:**
    A. Space between superior and middle turbinate
    B. Space above the inferior turbinate and anterior to the middle turbinate
    C. Space below the inferior turbinate
    D. Neither of the above

14. **Lateral margin of nasal cavity is formed by:**
    A. Frontal processes of maxillary bone
    B. Maxillary process of frontal bone
    C. Zygomatic process of frontal bone
    D. Neither of the above

15. **Agger nasi or nasal ridge is the:**
    A. Soft tissue thickening
    B. Small bony thickening along the upper lateral nasal wall
    C. Soft tissue and bony thickening
    D. Neither of the two

16. **The ethmoid sinuses are clearly delineated in the CT in:**
    A. Axial projection
    B. Coronal projection
    C. Both
    D. Neither

17. **CT scan image of paranasal sinuses should be reviewed:**
    A. Only in soft tissue window setting (200 to 400HU)
    B. Only in bony windows setting (1000HU or more)
    C. Both soft tissue and bony window setting
    D. Neither

18. **Cribriform plates are identified as very thin horizontal densities located:**
    A. To medial side of nasal septum
    B. To lateral side of nasal septum
    C. To either side of the nasal septum
    D. Neither of the above

19. **Axial CT scan of ethmoid sinus reveals lamina papyracea on the lateral aspect of:**
    A. Nasal cavity   B. Orbital cavity
    C. Neither   D. Both

20. **Air fluid levels are commonly seen in:**
    A. Chronic bacterial sinusitis
    B. Acute bacterial sinusitis
    C. Pan sinusitis
    D. Allergic sinusitis

21. **True polypoid hypertrophy seen radiographically as hypertrophic polypoid mucosal thickening when present, it is suggestive of:**
    A. Bacterial sinusitis   B. Allergic sinusitis
    C. Neither   D. Both

22. **Presence of nasal polyp in the first few years of life should suggest the possibility of:**
    A. Myelococle
    B. Encephalocoele
    C. Encephalomyelocole
    D. Neither

23. **Persistent opacification or recurrent episode of sinusitis by the age of 1 year may indicate the presence of:**
    A. Allergic rhinitis
    B. Cystic fibrosis (mucoviscoidosis)
    C. Acute sinusitis
    D. Neither

24. **Most sinus pathology is readily diagnosable by:**
    A. Plain X-ray   B. CT
    C. MRI   D. CT and MRI

25. **In allergic rhinitis, when plain X-ray are negative?**
    A. Further imaging is necessary
    B. Further imaging is unnecessary
    C. Contrast investigation needed
    D. None

26. **In acute infection of the sinuses such as maxillary antritis the following will confirm the diagnosis and monitor the effects of treatment without further imaging:**
    A. Plain X-ray   B. CT scan
    C. MRI   D. None of the above

27. **Frontal lobe abscess is common following spread of infection in one of the sinuses given below, resulting in intracranial, subdural or extra dural abscess:**
    A. Ethmoid sinuses   B. Maxillary sinuses
    C. Frontal sinuses   D. Sphenoidal sinuses

28. **After intravenous contrast, abscess will show the characteristic of the following:**
    A. No enhancement
    B. Ring enhancement
    C. Thick irregular ring enhancement
    D. None of the above

29. **Orbital cellulitis follows one of the following and results in abscess formation, often situated outside periorbital region:**
    A. Maxillary antritis
    B. Ethmoiditis
    C. Frontal sinusitis
    D. None of above

30. **Inward collapse of the antral walls is the characteristic finding of CT in:**
    A. Osteomyelitis
    B. Neoplastic bone destruction
    C. Polypoid mass
    D. None of the above

31. **Bony expansion and soft tissue mass of the sinus is characteristic CT finding in:**
    A. Neoplastic bone destruction
    B. Osteomyelitis
    C. Polypoid mass
    D. None of the above

32. **Identification of the following is essential to treat the primary infection by endoscopic surgery:**
    A. Osteomeatal complex
    B. Middle meatus of the nose
    C. Frontal recess
    D. Anterior ethmoid cells and infundibulam

33. **Identification of important anatomic landmarks by one of the following avoids the known hazards of endoscopic surgery such as blindness, ocular motility dysfunction, orbital hematoma, CSF leak and carotid cavernous fistula:**
    A. Plain X-ray   B. CT
    C. MRI   D. Neither

34. **In MRI signal hypointensity is the distinctive feature of:**
    A. Aspergillosis
    B. Mucocoele
    C. Neoplastic mass lesion
    D. None of the above

35. **The following tumor show areas of calcification or produce sclerotic changes in the walls of sinus involved:**
    A. Inverted papilloma
    B. Osteoma
    C. Ossifying fibroma
    D. Neither

36. **One of the following tumors takes origin within the sphenopalatine foramen and if it is expansile will enlarge the foramen:**
    A. Antrochoanal polyp
    B. Ossifying fibroma
    C. Inverted papilloma
    D. Infantile angiofibroma

37. **Angiofibroma could be differentiated from antrochoanal polyp by:**
    A. Identifying the extent of tumor
    B. Plain X-ray
    C. By MRI studies
    D. Neither

38. **The more constant and characteristic demonstration of a deformity of the base of the medial pterygoid plate seen on coronal section is being seen in:**
    A. Juvenile angiofibroma
    B. Ossifying fibroma
    C. Antrochoanal polyp
    D. Inverted papillona

39. **Early stage of development of sinus malignancy, the tumor:**
    A. Accessible by clinical methods of examination
    B. Initial diagnosis made by radiologist
    C. Diagnosis made by pathologist
    D. Neither of the above

40. **Best method to establish the extent of disease prior to treatment is by:**
    A. Clinical evaluation
    B. Imaging (gadolinium enhanced MRI)
    C. Surgical procedure
    D. Neither of the above

41. **Extension of malignancy through the cribriform plate into anterior cranial fossa is best demonstrated by:**
    A. Gd MRI
    B. Contrast CT
    C. Plain X-ray
    D. Neither of the above

42. **Invasion of pterygopalatine and Infratemporal fossa best demonstrated by:**
    A. MRI   B. CT
    C. Plain X-ray   D. Neither of the above

43. **Extension of malignancy into orbit is best shown by:**
    A. CT
    B. MRI
    C. CT or MRI
    D. Plain X-ray

44. **Many tumor recurrence in the accessible areas are best diagnosed by:**
    A. Clinical inspection by endoscopy
    B. Contrast CT
    C. Gadolinium MRI
    D. Neither of the above

45. **Tumor recurrences occurring in inaccessible areas are best diagnosed by:**
    A. Contrast CT
    B. MRI
    C. Subtraction Gd MRI
    D. Neither of the above

46. **The whole length of petrous bone is best demonstrated by:**
    A. Stenvers' view
    B. Basal view of skull
    C. Townes view
    D. Lateral view

47. **Middle and inner ears are best studied by:**
    A. High resolution CT of 1 or 2 mm thick
    B. Contrast CT
    C. Plain CT of 5 mm thickness
    D. Neither of the above

48. **Glomus jugulare tumors are best assessed by full assessment of their vascular nature by:**
    A. Angiography
    B. CT examination
    C. MRI
    D. Neither of the above

49. **The mastoid is unpneumatized and the attic and antrum are absent or slit like , being replaced in varying degrees by solid bone in:**
    A. Mandibulofacial dysostosis(Treacher-Collin syndrome)
    B. Michel and Mondini deformities
    C. Cholesteatoma
    D. Neither of the above

50. **Labryinth capsule is affected only in late stage in one of the following condition:**
    A. Cholesteatoma
    B. Infective and neoplastic process
    C. Neither of the above
    D. Either of the above

51. **Cholesterol granulomas give:**
    A. Strong signal on all protocols
    B. Hypo in TI and Hyper in T2
    C. Hypo in T2 and Hyper in T1
    D. Neither of the above

52. **For demonstration of small cholesteatoma in the attic and antrum, the optimum method to diagnose:**
    A. Computed tomography in coronal plate
    B. CT in axial plane
    C. Plain X-ray lateral view skull
    D. Towne's view

53. **One of the following well defined usually single bony mass of high density, may arise in any bony surface of petrous temporal bone, will cause conductive deafness, if it blocks the external meatus or middle ear:**
    A. Osteoma
    B. Glomus tumor
    C. Neuromas
    D. Neither of the above

54. **Presence of rugged erosion, usually extensive in the external auditory meatus, middle ear cleft or in a mastoid cavity suggests:**
    A. Carcinoma
    B. Bone dysplasia
    C. Osteoma
    D. Fibrous dysplasia

55. **To diagnose patchy or ring rarefaction around the cochlear coils or adjacent to oval window in otospongiosis is by:**
    A. Axial CT
    B. Axial CT with densitometry
    C. Contrast CT
    D. Plain X-ray.

56. **Congenital cholesteatoma originating from ectodermal cell rests, may arise:**
    A. Only in middle ear cleft
    B. Only in attic
    C. Only in petrous temporal bone
    D. Any of the cranial bone, the petrous temporal bone being the most commonly affected

57. **Acquired cholesteatoma arise in:**
    A. Posteroinferior part of middle ear
    B. Posterosuperior part of middle ear
    C. Rest of tympanic cavity
    D. From mastoid antrum

58. **Which of the following condition give rise to extensive ragged destruction?**
    A. Tuberculosis otitis media
    B. Adhesive otitis media
    C. Benign lesion
    D. Neither of the above

59. Intracranial complications of suppurative ear disease, particularly abscess in the temporal lobe and cerebellum are best detected by:
- A. Contrast CT
- B. Plain CT
- C. Lateral view of skull
- D. Neither of the above

60. Fractures of petrous temporal bone, ossicular dislocation and foreign bodies could be well demonstrated by:
- A. Contrast CT
- B. Axial CT
- C. High resolution CT
- D. MRI

61. Localized mid-facial destruction resulting in severe mutilation and bone necrosis, is Characteristic of:
- A. Wegener's granulamatosis
- B. Stewarts' granulamatosis
- C. Fibrous dysplasia
- D. Inverted papilloma

62. The bone destruction in the nose and sinuses is obvious in plain X-rays in:
- A. Stewart's granulamotosis
- B. Wegener's granulamotosis
- C. Osteoma
- D. Fibrous dysplasia

63. Multisystem disease characterized by necrotizing granulomas of upper and lower respiratory tract, together with glomerulonephritis and systemic vasculitis is seen in:
- A. Stewart's granulamatosis
- B. Wegner's granulamatosis
- C. Allergic rhinitis
- D. Fibrous dysplasia

64. Both on Plain X-ray and CT, generalized opacity in the sinuses, accompanied by thinning of the sinus walls and nasal and ethmoid septa is characteristic of:
- A. Multiple polyps
- B. Mucocoele
- C. Fungal disease
- D. Neither of the above

65. Prior to endoscopic surgery, to avoid complication such as blindness, CSF leaf, cavernous sinus fistula etc:
- A. CT is essential
- B. Plain X- ray needed
- C. Contrast (CT) to be done
- D. Neither of the above

66. Osteomyelitis leading to bone involvement is common following:
- A. Empyema of the sinus
- B. Mucocoele
- C. Allergic rhinitis
- D. Fungal infection

67. Loss of out line of sinus wall, followed by frank osteolysis and bone sequestration is characteristic of:
- A. Osteomyelitis
- B. Orbital cellulitis
- C. Frontal lobe abscess
- D. Mucocoele

68. Increased bone density in a sinus cavity and in some cases partial obliteration of sinus cavity is seen in:
- A. Acute sinusitis
- B. Chronic sinusitis of long standing
- C. Orbital cellulitis.
- D. Neither of the above

69. Opaque sinus on a plain X-ray is characteristic of:
- A. Chronic sinusitis
- B. Acute sinusitis
- C. Mucocoele
- D. Osteomyelitis

70. Expansion of maxillary antrum with formation of mucocoele is due to:
- A. Odontogenic cyst
- B. Fungal disease
- C. Inverted papilloma
- D. Acute sinusitis

71. The following is misdiagnozed as tumor on plain X-ray:
- A. Nasopharyngeal tumor invading sphenoid
- B. Pituitary tumor
- C. Sphenoid mucocoele
- D. Neither of the above

72. Rounded or partially rounded expansion of sinus is the characteristic CT finding:
- A. Sphenoid mucocoele
- B. Malignancy
- C. Fungal disease
- D. Neither of the above

73. Fluid content of sphenoid mucocoele is better demonstrated by:
- A. MRI
- B. CT
- C. Plain X-ray
- D. Neither of the above

74. Destruction of sphenoid bone *in situ* is by:
    A. Sphenoid mucocoele
    B. Malignancy
    C. Sphenoid sinusitis
    D. Neither of the above

75. Following sinuses are rudimentary at birth, appear at about the age of 2 years continuing to enlarge until the end of puberty:
    A. Maxillary sinuses
    B. Ethmoid sinuses.
    C. Sphenoid sinuses
    D. Frontal sinuses

76. The following sinuses appear at about the age of 3 years and reach adult size at puberty:
    A. Maxillary sinuses
    B. Ethmoid sinuses
    C. Sphenoid sinuses
    D. Frontal sinuses

77. Anatomic detail of ENT is well shown in:
    A. T-2 weighted images
    B. T1 weighted images
    C. T1 weighted images after Gd-DTPA contrast
    D. Neither of the above

78. Tumor is more readily seen in:
    A. T2 weighted images
    B. T1 weighted images
    C. T1 weighted images after Gd-DTPA
    D. Neither of the above

79. Detection of tumor spread is best done by:
    A. T1 weighted images
    B. T2 weighted images
    C. T1 weighted images after Gd-DTPA. contrast enhancement
    D. Neither of the above

80. Hypoplastic sinuses are seen in:
    A. Kartagener's syndrome
    B. Parry-Romberg's syndrome
    C. Steiner's syndrome
    D. Grouzon's syndrome

81. Localized enlargement of paranasal sinus is termed as:
    A. Pneumocephaly
    B. Aerocoele
    C. Pneumo sinus dilatans
    D. Neither of the above

82. Simultaneous involvement of two or more sinuses and presence of mucosal swelling is a feature of:
    A. Chronic sinusitis
    B. Acute sinusitis
    C. Fungal infection
    D. Complicated allergy

83. Persistent antral fluid level with the presence of oro antral fistula is common following:
    A. Sinus drainage
    B. Chronic sinusitis
    C. Dental extraction
    D. Neither of the above

84. Cavernous sinus thrombosis is best evaluated non invasively by:
    A. Orbital phlebography
    B. Contrast CT
    C. MR
    D. None of the above

85. Difficulties in distinguishing tumors from mucocoele, and in detecting tumors underlying secondary mucocoele may be resolved by use of:
    A. Contrast CT
    B. Phlebography
    C. Gd-DTPA T1 weighted MR
    D. T2 weighted MR

86. Upward expansion of sphenoid mucocoele is into:
    A. Planum sphenoid ale
    B. Pituitary fossa
    C. Cavernous sinus
    D. Middle cranial fossa

87. Polyps are most often found in:
    A. Maxillary sinus
    B. Sphenoid sinus
    C. Ethmoid air cell complex and nasal cavity
    D. Frontal sinus

88. Bilateral ethmoidal involvement is common in:
    A. Polyps   B. Malignancy
    C. Neither of the above   D. Inflammation

89. Multiple sinus osteomas are seen in:
    A. Gardner's syndrome
    B. Inverted papilloma
    C. Fibrous dysplasia
    D. Neither of the above

90. Nodular plaque like calcification seen on CT in the nasal and paranasal sinus region is suggestive of:
    A. Lymphoma
    B. Chondrosarcoma
    C. Plasmacytoma
    D. Olfactory neuroblastorna

91. Perineural tumor extension best detected by MR in:
    A. Adenoid cystic carcinoma
    B. Squamous cell carcinoma
    C. Olfactory neuroblastoma
    D. Plasmacytoma

92. Lobulated sessile mucosal lesions with local bone erosion is seen in:
    A. Adenoid cystic carcinoma
    B. Squamous cell carcinoma
    C. Plasmacytoma
    D. Chondrosarcoma

93. Radiologically, a soft tissue mass without calcification with local bone expansion or destruction is seen in:
    A. Chondrosarcoma
    B. Olfactory neuroblastoma
    C. Plasmacytoma
    D. Lymphoma (Non- Hodgkin's type)

94. 7th and 8th nerves in their intracanalicular and CP angle segments are best shown by:
    A. T1 weighted images
    B. T2 weighted images
    C. Modern fast spin echo T2 weighted images
    D. Neither of the above

95. The cochlea, vestibule and semicircular canals are show with great clarity on:
    A. T1 weighted images
    B. T2 weighted images
    C. CT scan
    D. Neither of the above

96. In malignant otitis externa, soft tissue and bony components of the disease process are best demonstrated by:
    A. CT   B. MRI
    C. CT and MRI D. Neither of the above

97. In uncomplicated acute otitis media or mastoiditis, the following to be done immediately:
    A. CT
    B. MRI
    C. Plain X-ray
    D. Radiological investigation rarely undertaken

98. Osteomyelitis of petrous temporalal bone, causing pain of trigeminal distribution with 6th nerve cranial palsy is seen:
    A. Gardners' syndrome
    B. Gradenigo's syndrome
    C. Bezold's abscess
    D. Neither of the above

99. Cholesterol granuloma can be distinguished from congenital cholesteatoma by:
    A. High signal intensity in T1 weighted image
    B. High signal intensity in T2 weighted image
    C. High signal intensity in both T1 and T2 weighted images
    D. Gd-DTPA, T1 weighted MR

100. In the absence of MRI, the diagnosis of intrameatal tumors and extrameatal tumours less than 1 cm in diameter must be made by:
    A. Plain X- ray
    B. CT
    C. Contrast CT
    D. Air CT meatography

101. Meningiomas of cerebellopontine angle, could be best differentiated from acoustic neuroma by:
    A. Plain X-ray
    B. Contrast enhanced CT
    C. MRI
    D. Contrast enhanced CT or MRI

Bibliography

1. Thomas Bergeon: Head and Neck Imaging Excl Brain; Q.Nos. 1 to 23.
2. David Sutton-sixth: Text book of Radiology and Imaging - edition; Vol- II.Q.Nos. 24 to 74.
3. Grainger and Allison's: Diagnostic Radiology; IIIrd Edition Vol- 3.Q.Nos. 75 to 101.

ANSWERS

1 B	2 D	3 A	4 B	5 A	6 C	7 A	8 A
9 D	10 C	11 C	12 C	13 B	14 A	15 B	16 A
17 C	18 C	19 A	20 B	21 B	22 B	23 B	24 A
25 B	26 A	27 C	28 B	29 B	30 A	31 A	32 A
33 B	34 A	35 A	36 D	37 C	38 A	39 B	40 B
41 A	42 B	43 C	44 A	45 C	46 A	47 A	48 A
49 A	50 B	51 A	52 A	53 A	54 A	55 B	56 D
57 B	58 A	59 A	60 B	61 B	62 A	63 B	64 A
65 A	66 A	67 A	68 B	69 B	70 A	71 C	72 A
73 A	74 B	75 D	76 C	77 B	78 A	79 C	80 A
81 C	82 D	83 C	84 C	85 C	86 B	87 C	88 A
89 A	90 B	91 A	92 C	93 D	94 C	95 B	96 C
97 D	98 B	99 C	100 D	101 D			

Radiation Oncology

HEAD AND NECK—GENERAL

1. Adenoid cystic variety mainly found in:
- A. Thyroid gland
- B. Salivary gland
- C. Oral cavity
- D. Tongue

2. AJCC staging system of stage IV B represents:
- A. Distant metastasis locally advanced
- B. Resectable disease locally advanced
- C. Nonresectable disease locally advanced
- D. Vascular invasion locally advanced

3. The main prevention of head and neck cancer are the following *except one*:
- A. Sharp tooth removal
- B. Tobacco-non use
- C. Isoretinin
- D. Facial creams

4. Exclusive RT management in head and neck cancer require the following dose:
- A. 4500 to 5000 CGY
- B. 6500 to 7500 CGY
- C. 5000 to 5500 CGY
- D. 3500 to 4500 CGY

5. Indication for postoperative RT include the following *except one*:
- A. Close margin
- B. Inadequate resection
- C. Poorly differentiated growth
- D. One node involvement

6. Incidence of clinical metastasis percentage in true vocal cord tumor is:
- A. 3%
- B. 6%
- C. 1%
- D. Nil

7. RT is treatment of choice to one of the following area of tumor involvement:
- A. Nasopharynx
- B. Anterior part of tongue
- C. Cheek
- D. Tonsil

8. Most effective drug used in head and neck cancer concomitantly with RT and surgery:
- A. VCR
- B. Bleomycin
- C. Paclitaxol
- D. CDDP

9. Lehrmitte's syndrome is seen mostly in head and neck cancer after:
- A. Radical surgery
- B. Radiotherapy
- C. Chemotherapy
- D. Hormone therapy

10. Match the possible etiology (head & neck) cancer:
- A. NPC- Beetal nut
- B. Ca Buccal mucosa – EBV
- C. Postcricoid – HPV 16
- D. Cancer larynx- Irondeficiency

11. Stage B in Kadish system for esthesioneuro-blastoma represent:
- A. Disease confined to nasal cavity
- B. Disease confined to one or more paranasal sinus
- C. Extension beyond nasal cavity or paranasal sinus
- D. *In situ*

12. Nasopharyngeal angiofibroma stage II in chandler management:

A. Confined to nasopharynx
B. Extend to nasal cavity/sphenoid Sinus
C. Extend to one or more antrum, ethmoid, etc
D. Intracranial extension

RADIOTHERAPY—GENERAL

13. X-rays were discovered by:

A. Henri Coutard
B. Wilhelm Konrad Roentgen
C. Henri Becquerel
D. Marie Curie

14. Radioactivity was discovered by:

A. Wilhem Konrad Roentgen
B. Henri Coutard
C. Pierrie Curie
D. Henri Becquerel

15. Radium was discovered by:

A. Wilhem conrad Roentgen and Henri Becquerel
B. Marie and Pierrie Curie
C. Henri Coutard and Claude Regad
D. Fetcher

16. Artificial radioactivity was discovered in:

A. 1936
B. 1953
C. 1934
D. 1928

17. Which one of the following statements is not true:

A. Becquerel was awarded Nobel Prize in Physics for the discovery of radioactivity
B. Roentgen was awarded the first Nobel prize in physics
C. Marie and Pierrie Curie were awarded a Nobel prize in physics for their work on radioactivity
D. Holzknecht was awarded the Nobel prize for his work on his chromoradiometer

18. Radiation therapy units operating at approximately 50 to 120 kVp are referred to as:

A. Linear accelerators
B. Orthovoltage units
C. Superficial units
D. Betatrons

19. Insertion of aluminium, copper and tin filters into the X-ray beam causes:

A. Low-energy X-rays to be absorbed
B. The kVp to increase
C. An unnecessary dose on the skin surface
D. The dose to increase

20. Orthovoltage X-ray units usually operate at:

A. 15 to 20 cm of source-surface distance (SSD)
B. 20 to 40 cm of source –surface distance (SSD)
C. 50 to 70 cm of source – surface distance (SSD)
D. 80 to 100 cm of source – surface distance (SSD)

21. Orthovoltage X-ray units usually operate in the range of:

A. 20 to 150 kVp
B. 150 to 500 kVp
C. 200 to 1200 kVp
D. Any kVp below 200 kVp

22. Linear accelerators produce high energy beams:

A. By accelerating charged particles in a linear tube
B. By accelerating photons in a circular orbit
C. By accelerating charged particles in a circular orbit
D. None of the above is correct

23. The half life of a cobalt^{60} source is:

A. 30.3 years
B. 1600 years
C. 5.26 years
D. 74 days

24. 1 GY is the same as:

A. 1 rad
B. 10 CGY
C. 100 CGY
D. 1 erg

25. A HVT (Half Value Thickness) is a way of expressing:

A. The filtration of beam
B. The dose
C. The quality of the beam
D. The TAR

26. Simulators are primarily used to:

A. Localize the target
B. Duplicate the geometry of therapy machines
C. Duplicate the mechanical movements of the therapy machine
D. All of the above

EAR

27. Inner ear-lymphatic drains into:

A. Superficial parotid lymph nodes
B. Retroauricular lymph node
C. Superficial cervical node
D. No lymphatics drainage

28. Commonest pathology – external earmalignacy:

A. Basal cell   B. Squamous cell
C. Lymphoma   D. Melanoma

29. The 7th nerve palsy indicates:

A. Excellent local control
B. Partial local control
C. Poor local control
D. No significance

30. Type of RT for early external ear tumor:

A. Megavoltage
B. Orthovoltage
C. Electron beam
D. Either ortho. or electron beam

31. Good cosmesis obtained in < 4 cm tumor by:

A. Wide excision
B. Chemotherapy
C. I^{192} afterloading (Interstitial)
D. Cryotherapy

32. Best RT dosage for lesions of upto 2 cm in pinna:

A. 65 GY   B. 70 GY
C. 50 GY   D. 80 GY

33. Doses in the range of 70 GY in ear lesions results in:

A. Good control of tumor
B. No control of tumor
C. Osteoradio necrosis
D. None of them is true

34. Type of field preferred for pinna tumors is usually (Ext.RT):

A. Oval   B. Round
C. Rectangular   D. Polygonal

35. 5 yr survival match:

A. Middle ear – 90%
B. Ext. auditory canal – 40%
C. Inner ear – 60%
D. Pinna – 10%

NASOPHARYNX

36. RT sequelae – majority of them:

A. Cartilage necrosis
B. Bone necrosis
C. Neural damage
D. Bleeding sequelae

37. Tumor of nasopharynx frequency order:

A. Roof of nasopharynx
B. Fossa of rosenmuller
C. Lateral wall
D. Posterior wall

38. Distant metastasis in nasopharyx primarily:

A. Lung   B. Liver
C. Bone   D. Brain

39. Distant metastasis influenced by:

A. Size of tumor
B. Stage of tumor
C. Lymph node involvement
D. None of the above

40. Ominous prognostic factor:

A. Cranial nerve involvement
B. Bilateral cervical node involvement
C. RT failure
D. Pathological entity (histologic subtype)

41. Advanced nasopharynx tumours treated mainly by:

A. Chemotherapy
B. RT
C. Surgery
D. Chemoradiotherapy

42. Normal RT field covers over the following area *except:*

A. Posterior ethmoid cells
B. Posterior 3rd of maxillary antrum
C. Nasal cavity
D. Orbit

43. RT field used mainly:

A. Unilateral
B. Opposing lateral
C. Straight facial
D. Wedge fields

44. Correct angulation in treating posterior wall of nasopharynx:
    A. 10°
    B. 12°
    C. 7°
    D. 5°

45. Spinal cord dosage is important after:
    A. 45 GY
    B. 50 GY
    C. 60 Gy
    D. Not necessary

46. Postneck lymph node is boosted by:
    A. 9 Mev electrons
    B. 15 Mev electrons
    C. Co^{60}
    D. 4 Mev - photon

47. Area to be careful in nasopharynx tumor with RT:
    A. Base of skull
    B. Ear
    C. Orbit
    D. Temporomandibular joint

48. Nasopharynx boost can be done by:
    A. Co^{60}
    B. Cs^{137}
    C. Electron – 9 Mev
    D. Photon – 18 Mev

49. The following treatment modalities have a role in nasopharynx tumors except:
    A. Conformal therapy
    B. IMRT
    C. Proton therapy
    D. 250 KV

50. Major chemotherapeutic agent in the nasopharynx tumor is:
    A. CDDP
    B. 5 Fu
    C. Endoxan
    D. Mitomycin

51. Complications of RT in nasopharynx tumor are true except one:
    A. Symphathetic nerve palsy
    B. Spine mylopathy
    C. Hypopituitarism
    D. Hypothyroidism

52. Average dose for nasopharynx tumor:
    A. 50 to 55 GY
    B. 60 to 70 GY
    C. 40 to 45 GY
    D. 80 > GY

53. For patients 30 yrs and below RT dose range is for nasopharyngeal lesion is:
    A. 30 to 40 GY
    B. 45 to 50 GY
    C. 50 to 60 GY
    D. 60 to 70 GY

54. Lymph node metastasis in nasopharynx regions most common is:
    A. Upper cervical
    B. Lower cervical
    C. Preauricular
    D. Submandibular

55. Most common pathologic entity:
    A. Salivary gland tumor
    B. Malignant melanoma
    C. Squamous cell carcinoma
    D. Sarcoma

56. Nasal cavity radiotherapy postoperative dose is:
    A. 68 GY
    B. 50 GY
    C. 70 GY
    D. 60 GY

57. Preoperative RT preferred in:
    A. Nasal cavity tumor
    B. Ethmoid tumor
    C. Maxillary tumor
    D. Sphenoid tumors

58. Treatment with wedges are necessary except in one area:
    A. Orbit
    B. Nasal cavity
    C. Ethmoid
    D. Maxillary cavity

59. Primary interstitial radiotherapy is favored among the:
    A. Maxillary tumours
    B. Ethmoid tumours
    C. Paranasal tumours
    D. Nasal vestibule tumours

60. Head and neck accessible area the preferred isotope for brachy therapy is:
    A. Co^{60}
    B. Cs^{137} pellet
    C. I^{192} wire
    D. Radium needle

61. Bolus mainly needed in Ext. RT for the below mentioned area:
    A. Nasal vestibule area
    B. Paranasal sinus area
    C. Maxillary antrum
    D. Pinna

62. Known RT complications in the dose range of > 60 GY *except* one is:
A. Otitis media
B. Chronic sinusitis
C. Vision loss
D. Brain tumours

SALIVARY GLAND

63. Acinic cell tumor occurs only in:
A. Submandibullar
B. Lacrimal gland
C. Parotid gland
D. Sublingual gland

64. Mucoepidermoid variety commonly found in:
A. Adult patient male
B. Adult patient female
C. Children
D. Patient older than 60 years

65. Percentage of facial nerve involvement in parotid gland tumor is:
A. 25%
B. 50%
C. 10%
D. 60%

66. Diagnostic assistant test best in salivary gland tumor by:
A. Contrast examination
B. CT
C. MRI
D. Plain X-ray

67. Adenoidcystic cancer mainly found in:
A. Parotid
B. Sublingual
C. Submaxillary
D. Palatal gland

68. In salivary gland tumors all are correct for prognostic indices *except*:
A. Grade
B. Residual disease
C. Age
D. Facial nerve involvement

69. One of the particulate radiation tried in parotid tumor is:
A. Proton
B. Electron
C. Neutron
D. Negative p meson

70. Wedge pair in RT to parotid gland is:
A. Not necessary
B. Necessary
C. Used in a single field
D. Partly used

71. Inferior angulation of beam in parotid tumor treatment is done to protect:
A. Contralateral parotid
B. Preventing mucositis
C. Contralateral eye
D. To reduce skin reaction

72. Adenoid cystic carcinoma and radiation field covering to one of the area is important:
A. Postcervical lymph node group
B. Preauricular node
C. Subdigastric
D. Base of skull region

73. Usual dose for elective neck irradiation:
A. 35 GY
B. 50 GY
C. 60 GY
D. 45 GY

74. Preferred modality for elective neck irradiation is:
A. Co^{60}
B. 9 MeV photon
C. 10 MeV electron
D. Proton

75. Irradiation for submandibular gland tumor involves the following area only:
A. Gland with 2 cm margin
B. Gland with subdigastric node
C. Gland with base of skull region
D. Gland with ipsilateral neck

76. Notable complication of parotid tumor treatment (surgery +RT):
A. Facial nerve paralysis
B. Neuromas greater auricular nerve
C. Fistula
D. Xerostomia

MINOR SALIVARY GLAND

77. Put in order the adenoidcystic carcinoma – as per the commonality:
A. Nasal cavity
B. Tongue
C. Paranasal sinuses
D. Palate

78. RT not generally indicated for minor salivary gland tumor in one of the following:

A. Surgical inaccessible site
B. Incomplete excision
C. Locally aggressive tumors
D. Early stage hard palate lesion

79. Advanced/residual disease – total RT dose recommended is:

A. 70 GY   B. 80 GY
C. 66 GY   D. 58 GY

80. 5 yrs survival for adenoidcysticcarcinoma approximately is:

A. 45%   B. 60%
C. 70%   D. 80%

ORAL CAVITY

81. Majority of bilateral positive lymph node found in:

A. Tongue   B. Check
C. Tonsil   D. Floor of mouth

82. Preferred treatment for post 3rd of tongue:

A. Surgery alone
B. External RT alone
C. External RT and interstitial therapy
D. Chemotherapy

83. Irradiation to neck node not recommended in one of the following presentation:

A. One neck node no extracapsular extension
B. Multiple neck node
C. One neck node with extracapsular extension
D. More than one nodal station

84. Nodal involvement in CT scan evaluation requires:

A. Ipsilateral nodal clearance
B. Bilateral nodal clearance
C. Ipsilateral clearance and bilateral neck RT
D. Bilateral neck RT

85. Time interval required after dental extraction for RT to oral cavity usually is:

A. 5 days
B. 15 days
C. 10 days
D. 3 weeks

86. For oral cavity tumors, preferred irradiation dose to neck node is:

A. 60 GY   B. 50 to 60 GY
C. 45 to 50 GY   D. 50 GY

87. RT to mobile tongue requires primarily:

A. Wedge field
B. Tongue bite block
C. Bolus
D. Closed mouth position

88. Posterior chain node irradiation requires dose adjustment for cord after:

A. 50 GY   B. 60 GY
C. 30 GY   D. 45 GY

89. T_1,T_2 tumour dose for oral cavity is:

A. 40 to 45 GY   B. 65 to 70 GY
C. 60 to 65 GY   D. 55 to 60 GY

90. In oral cavity tumor irradiation, importance should be given to:

A. Mandible   B. Tempromandible joint
C. Lips   D. Neck

TONGUE

91. Most commonly used isotope for interstitial implant:

A. Co^{60} B. Cs^{137}
C. Tantulam wires D. I_R^{192}

92. Classic dose rate for interstitial implant as follows:

A. 7 to 7.5 Gy/hr   B. 6 to 7 Gy/hr
C. 4.5 to 5.0 Gy/hr D. 3.5 to 4 Gy/hr

93. Intraoral cone largely used in:

A. Pharyngeal wall tumor
B. Base of tongue
C. Anterior tongue
D. Tonsilar growth

94. The following beam energy is ideal for Intraoral irradiation:

A. Cs^{137} - 0.62 MeV
B. Strontium 89 – 1.4 β Max
C. Electron – 6 MeV
D. 250 KeV (orthovoltage)

LIP

95. Treatment of choice for lesion (carcinoma) 2- 4 cm in lip is:

A. Surgery
B. Radiotherapy
C. Chemotherapy
D. Cryotherapy

96. RT is not advised in one of the following presentation:

A. Positive margin
B. Perineural invasion
C. Node presentation
D. Commisural involvement

97. Which of alternative energy used in lip malignancy?

A. Co^{60} / CS^{137}
B. 200 KeV / electron 6 MeV
C. Proton / X-ray photon
D. p meson / neutron

98. Equate the given radiation doses below for the stages $T_1 - T_4$ lesion in tongue:

A. 50-60 Gy - T_1
B. 60-65 Gy - T_2
C. 70-75 Gy - T_3
D. 65-70 Gy - T_4

99. Edentulous patient and anterior lesion suitable for:

A. External RT
B. Intraoral cone
C. Surgery
D. Chemotherapy

FLOOR OF MOUTH

100. Tempered dose of irradiation for small superficial lesion is:

A. Interstitial implant – 60 to 65 GY
B. Ext. RT – 50 to 55 GY
C. Mould – 60 GY
D. Strontium 90 (SR 90 Y 90) plaque 40 GY

101. One of the newer modality practiced for advanced $T_3 - T_4$ lesion is:

A. Hypo #
B. Hyper #
C. Hyper thermia
D. Hyperbaric O_2

BUCCAL MUCOSA

102. The best combination of approach to T_1, T_2 lesion, negative node is:

A. Photon + surgery
B. Photon + implant
C. Implant + surgery
D. Intraoral cone therapy

103. Important structure to be taken care for Ext. RT and advanced lesion (buccal area):

A. Tongue
B. Palate
C. Neck
D. Mandible

GINGIVA

104. Best form of investigative approach in gingival lesion is facilitated by:

A. Biopsy
B. Panorex
C. CT
D. MRI

105. Choice of treatment for positive neck node with advanced gingival lesion:

A. Surgery
B. Ipsilateral RT
C. Interstitial implant
D. Chemotherapy

TONSILLAR FOSSA (OROPHARYNX)

106. Lymph node metastasis and tonsillar fossa lesion has less propensity *except* for one group:

A. Postcervical chain
B. Mid jugular chain
C. Subdigastric
D. Submaxillary

107. Trismus manifestation seen in tonsillar fossa lesion as:

A. Early manifestation
B. Late manifestation
C. No manifestation
D. Typical manifestation

108. **Least common tumor pathology in tonsil:**
    A. Non Hodgkin lymphoma
    B. Squamous cell carcinoma
    C. Lymphoepithelioma
    D. Melanoma

109. **Survival decreases with following presentation in tonsil:**
    A. Ulceroproliferative presentation
    B. Base of tongue involvement
    C. Faucial arch extention
    D. Regional node involvement

110. **RT dosage for T$_2$ lesion of tonsil is:**
    A. 40 to 50 GY   B. 55 to 60 GY
    C. 60 to 75 GY   D. 80 > GY

111. **Dose interstitial boost to tonsillar tumor:**
    A. 25 to 30 GY   B. 40 to 45 GY
    C. 10 to 15 GY   D. 45 > GY

112. **Nodal dose for lymph node of tonsillar tumour ranges from:**
    A. 30 to 40 GY   B. 40 to 50 GY
    C. 50 to 70 GY   D. 75 to 85 GY

113. **Lymph node dissection in faucial arch lesion indicated when:**
    A. Prophylactic   B. Fixed node
    C. Palpable node   D. Radiation failure

114. **For T$_1$ No faucial arch tumor, RT includes the following area (field) _except:_**
    A. Subdigastric   B. Midjugular
    C. Submaxillary   D. Postcervical

115. **One of the following radiation modality has a role in oropharynx tumor:**
    A. IORT (intraoperative radiotherapy)
    B. IMRT
    C. Photodynamic therapy
    D. pimession therapy

116. **Primary faucial arch tumor and preoperative RT dose is:**
    A. 40 to 45 GY   B. 55 to 60 GY
    C. 30 to 45 GY   D. 70 to 75 GY

117. **Except one, all other structures limit the RT dosage to oropharynx:**
    A. Mandible
    B. Salivary gland
    C. Subcutaneous tissue
    D. Nerve trunks

118. **One of the fractionation schedule has a role in oropharynx tumors:**
    A. Hyper #   B. Hypo #
    C. Split course   D. Accelerated #

119. **One of the optimal beam energy used in faucial arch tumor:**
    A. 6 MV photon
    B. 6 MeV Electron
    C. Fast neutron
    D. Protons

120. **Xerostomia not experienced in one of the radiation modality:**
    A. 6 MV photon
    B. 18 MV photon
    C. IMRT
    D. p Meson

121. **Important complication of surgery in post RT failure of oropharynx lesion:**
    A. Wound healing delay
    B. Carotid rupture
    C. Fistula
    D. Necrosis

122. **Percentage of lymph node presentation in base of tongue lesion is:**
    A. 40%   B. 50%
    C. 30%   D. 80%

123. **Prognosis influenced greatly by one of the following factors:**
    A. Greater size at diagnosis
    B. Spread to adjacent structures
    C. Lymphatic spread
    D. Difficulty in swallowing

124. **Radiotherapy indicated in the following presentation:**
    A. Exophytic
    B. Ulcerative
    C. Endophytic
    D. Fixed

125. **Postoperative irradiation indicated in:**
    A. N$_1$
    B. N$_2$
    C. N$_3$
    D. All the above + extra capsular invasion

BASE OF TONGUE

126. Select best form of approach for tumor base of tongue with infiltration and partial fixation:
   A. Surgery only
   B. RT only
   C. Surgery + RT
   D. Chemotherapy only

127. The portal used in lower neck irradiation in base of tongue lesion:
   A. Anterior portal
   B. Lateral portal
   C. Oblique portal anterior
   D. Anterior oblique portal post

128. The maximum spinal cord dose during irradiation in the base of tongue lesion is:
   A. 50 GY   B. 45 GY
   C. 35 GY   D. 60 GY

129. Electron energy normally used for neck treatment in base of tongue lesion:
   A. 4 MeV   B. 6 MeV
   C. 14 MeV   D. 20 MeV

130. Dose to primary tumor and lymph node can go up to:
   A. 50 – 55 GY   B. 60 – 65 GY
   C. 65 – 75 GY   D. 75 – 80 GY

131. Subclinical lesion and RT dose base of tongue range up to:
   A. 30 GY   B. 40 GY
   C. 50 GY   D. 60 GY

132. Selective drug for nonkeratinising head and neck cancer can be:
   A. CDDP   B. 5 Fu
   C. Paclitaxal   D. Bleomycin

133. Newer RT modality tried in base of tongue lesion is:
   A. IORT
   B. IMRT
   C. Stereotactic radiosurgery
   D. Photodynamic therapy

134. One of the main complication with RT at the site is:
   A. Xerostomia
   B. Ulceration
   C. Trismus
   D. Bleeding

HYPOPHARYNX

135. Most of the malignancy commonly found in the area of:
   A. Larynx
   B. Postcricoid
   C. Pyriform fossa
   D. Hypopharyngeal wall

136. Hypopharynx lymph node metastasis mainly to:
   A. Subdigastric
   B. Submandibular
   C. Postcervical
   D. Midcervical

137. Arnold's nerve involvement is reflected as:
   A. Ipsilateral paralysis of tongue
   B. Hoarseness
   C. Headache
   D. Pain in ear

138. Ipsilateral tongue paralysis reflects the involvement of:
   A. Vagus
   B. Trigeminal
   C. Facial
   D. Hypoglossal

139. Esophageal inlet involvement require the investigation by:
   A. CT
   B. Indirect laryngoscopy
   C. Endoscopy
   D. Barium swallow

140. Major pathological entity of hypopharynx tumour is:
   A. Squamous cell carcinoma
   B. Adenocarcinoma
   C. Lymphoma
   D. Metastasis entity

141. Arrange in order the best form of cure expected in hypopharyngeal lesion:

   A. Postcricoid
   B. Pharyngeal wall
   C. Pyriform fossa
   D. Vallecula

142. Grave prognostic factor indicated in hypopharynx lesion by:

   A. Vocal cord fixation
   B. Extracapsular invasion
   C. Pyriform apex involvement
   D. Postcricoid involvement

143. Conditions contribute to contraindication for conservative surgery:

   A. Cartilage invasion
   B. Vocal cord paralysis
   C. Postcricoid
   D. All the above conditions

144. For T$_1$ (hypopharynx) pyriform sinus, total RT dose can be:

   A. 50 GY   B. 55 GY
   C. 60 GY   D. 70 GY

145. Best form of approach for pharyngeal wall tumor cure is:

   A. Surgery   B. Surgery + RT
   C. RT   D. Chemotherapy

146. Posterior neck is irradiated with:

   A. Co^{60}
   B. CS^{137}
   C. 10 MeV photons
   D. 9 MeV electrons

147. Chemo and irradiation in hyopharynx mainly use:

   A. Bleomycin   B. Adriamycin
   C. Cisplatin   D. Endoxan

LARYNX

148. Carcinoma larynx strongly related to:

   A. Smoking
   B. Alcohol
   C. Tobacco chewing
   D. Singing

149. *In situ* vocal cord cancer, the treatment is:

   A. Striping (surgery)
   B. RT
   C. Chemotherapy
   D. Laser therapy

150. One of the following is not contraindicated to hemilaryngectomy:

   A. Extension to epiglottis
   B. Extension to false cord
   C. Arytenoids involvement
   D. One full cord involvement

151. Ideal energy used for laryngeal lesion in radiotherapy:

   A. 6 MV X-ray
   B. 8 MV X-ray
   C. 10 MeV electrons
   D. 20 MeV photons

SUPRAGLOTTIC LARYNX

152. The adjuvant approach for advanced supraglottic lesion is:

   A. Neoadjuvant chemo
   B. Hyperbaric oxygen
   C. Hyperthermia
   D. Proton irradiation

153. Boost RT to clinically positive cervical node, the preferred beam is:

   A. Photon X-ray   B. Gamma ray
   C. Electron   D. Neutron

154. Compare the following doses for postoperative RT in supraglottic tumor dose:

   A. –ve margin   - 65 GY
   B. Microscopic +ve margin - 70GY
   C. Gross residual   - 66GY
   D. Minor residual   - 60GY

155. Electron energy for stoma boost is:

   A. 4 MeV   B. 6 MeV
   C. 14 MeV   D. 20 MeV

156. Voice restoration in responding tumor of laryngeal lesion is expected in:

   A. 3 months   B. 6 months
   C. 12 months   D. 4 weeks

NONEPITHELIAL TUMOR

157. Middle cranial fossa glomus tumor can cause all the following *except*:

A. Retroorbital pain

B. Perisis of cranial nerves

C. Ataxia

D. Proptosis

158. Chemodectoma and metastasis seen in:

A. 90% of cases   B. 80% of cases

C. 2% of cases   D. 40% of cases

159. RT mainly indicated for glomus tumor in the following area *except*:

A. Carotid body chemodectomas

B. Small jugular bulk tumors

C. Tympanicum jugular tumors

D. Occipital bone jugular tumors

160. Wedge with the following specification used in RT with localized glomus tumor:

A. 35° wedge   B. 45° wedge

C. 15° wedge   D. 25° wedge

161. Following beam energy preferred for glomus tumor treatment:

A. 6 MeV   B. 4 MeV

C. 15 MeV   D. 10 MeV

162. The normal RT dose given to glomus tumor is:

A. 60 GY   B. 30 GY

C. 55 GY   D. 70 GY

HEMANGIOPERICYTOMA

163. Characteristic angiographic feature of hemangio pericytoma is:

A. Radial projection B. Spiral projection

C. Tortus projection D. Stellate projection

164. Role of radiation in hemangiopericytoma can be described as:

A. Radioresistant

B. Relatively radioresistant

C. Radiosensitive

D. Radiation no role

165. Tumor dose of hemangiopericytoma:

A. 50 to 55 GY   B. 40 to 45 GY

C. 60 to 70 GY   D. 30 to 40 GY

CHORDOMA

166. MRI is good in helping to investigate:

A. Delineation of tumor extent

B. Bony destruction

C. Calcification

D. Pathology

167. Irradiation type most useful is:

A. Photon beam

B. Electron beam

C. Proton beam

D. Interstitial therapy

168. Proton therapy in clivus tumor can result in:

A. Brain damage

B. Soft tissue necrosis

C. Cranial nerve damage

D. Hypothyroidism

169. Etiology of lethal midline granuloma may be due to:

A. HPV virus   B. Streptococcal virudance

C. EB virus   D. HIV

170. LMG (Lethal Midline Granuloma) treated mainly by:

A. Surgery   B. Chemotherapy

C. RT   D. Antibiotics

171. RT dose for LMG (lethal midline granuloma):

A. 45 to 50 GY   B. 35 to 45 GY

C. 35 to 40 GY   D. 60 to 70 GY

CHLOROMA

172. Chloroma usually associated with:

A. AML

B. ALL

C. CLL

D. CML

173. One of the isotope scintigraphy useful in chloromas:

A. I^{131} B. Tec^{99}M
C. I^{125} D. Gallium ^{67}

174. RT as emergency in one of the nonepithelial head and neck lesion:

A. Orbital chloroma
B. Cervical chordoma
C. Choroidal melanoma
D. Midline granuloma

ESTHESIONEUROBLASTOMA

175. Kadish staging system for stage B Esthesioneuroblastoma indicates:

A. Nasal cavity involvement
B. Paranasal sinus involvement
C. Orbit involvement
D. Cervical lymph node involvement

176. Intracranial extention of esthesioneuroblastoma mainly through perineural invasion of:

A. Facial nerve
B. Trigeminal nerve
C. Glossopharyngeal
D. Olfactory nerve

177. Radiotherapy for esthesioneuroblastoma is indicated mainly by:

A. Grade
B. Nodal secondaries
C. Distant metastasis
D. Size

178. 5 years acturial survival in esthesioneuroblastoma:

A. 40%   B. 50%
C. 70%   D. 60%

179. High inhomogenous dose in esthesioneuroblastoma by RT can be prevented by:

A. Anterior field
B. Lateral field with wedges
C. Vertex field
D. Reducing field

180. Dose of irradiation selected for inoperable disease is:

A. 45 to 50 GY   B. 65 to 70 GY
C. 35 to 40 GY   D. 50 to 60 GY

EXTRAMEDULLARY PLASMACYTOMA

181. Usually Extramedullary plasmacytoma is presented in nasopharynx as:

A. Sessile   B. Pedunculated
C. Circumscribed   D. Ulcerated

182. The choice of therapy for pedunculated type is:

A. Radiation   B. Surgery
C. Chemotherapy   D. Laser therapy

183. Radiation dose for sessile variety is:

A. 55 GY   B. 40 GY
C. 70 GY   D. 35 GY

NASOPHARYNGEAL ANGIOFIBROMA

184. Age group of presentation of nasopharyngeal angiofibroma:

A. Pediatric age group
B. Adult age
C. Old age
D. Pubertal age

185. Anomolous sexual development can be noted in:

A. Esthesioneuroblastoma
B. Chloroma
C. Chordoma
D. Nasopharyngeal angiofibroma

186. One of them is contra indicated in nasopharyngeal angiofibroma:

A. CT Plain
B. CT Contrast
C. Biopsy
D. Angiogram

187. The role of RT is to be appreciated in the light of:

A. Intracranial extension
B. Extracranial advanced lesion
C. Embolisation failure
D. Risk of secondary malignancy

188. Important region to be protected in radiation is:

A. Ear
B. Vocal cord
C. Eye
D. Parotid

189. Dose max ranges to:

A. 30 to 35 GY
B. 40 to 45 GY
C. 50 to 55 GY
D. 60 to 65 GY

190. Dose in the range of 60 GY and above the most noted risk to be:

A. Cataract
B. Hypopitutarism
C. Sarcoma
D. Carcinoma

NON-LENTIGINOUS MELANOMA

191. One of the adjuvant modality tried in melanoma (recurrent) is:

A. Photodynamic theory
B. Hyperthermia
C. p mesons
D. Brachy therapy

192. Metastatic potential of nodular type (Melanoma):

A. 10%
B. 15%
C. 50%
D. 40%

193. Raidotherapeutic dose in case of melanoma ranges from:

A. 45 – 50 GY
B. 50 –55 GY
C. 60 – 65 GY
D. 70 GY

194. Preferred radiation in RT management of melanoma is:

A. Photon
B. Protons
C. p mesons
D. Electrons

195. Clinically nodal negative presentation in LMM requires:

A. Surgery
B. Radiotherapy
C. Chemotherapy
D. Observation

SARCOMA OF HEAD AND NECK

196. Most common type in head and neck region is:

A. Liposarcoma
B. Myosarcoma
C. Rhabdomyosarcoma
D. Synovil sarcoma

197. Clinical presentation of sarcoma match:

A. Scalp or face – 27%
B. Orbit/Paranasal sinus – 14%
C. Upper aero digestive tract 26%
D. Neck – 33%

198. Supplimentation of diagnostic work utilizes the help of:

A. Plain X-ray
B. CT
C. MRI
D. Ultra sonogram

199. Preoperative RT dose preferred in sarcoma is:

A. 50 GY
B. 40 GY
C. 70 GY
D. 60 GY

200. Newer modality approach for sarcoma in RT includes:

A. IORT
B. Hyperthermia
C. 3D conformal therapy
D. Ir^{192} implantation

THYROID

201. Diagnostic work not necessary in thyroid nodule evaluation:

A. Angiography
B. Plain X-ray
C. Nuclide imaging
D. FNAC

202. Follicular cancer of thyroid mainly seen in:

A. 50 – 60 yrs of age
B. 40 –50 yrs of age
C. 25 – 30 yrs of age
D. < 10 yrs

203. Indication of isotope of Iodine in thyroid cancer *except* in one pathology:

A. Medullary
B. Follicular
C. Anaplastic
D. Papillary

204. Emperical dose of I ^{131} in thyroid cancer is:

A. 60 to 70 MCi
B. 70 to 80 MCi
C. 80 to 90 MCi
D. 100 to 150 MCi

205. Dose of EXRT in anaplastic thyroid carcinoma:

A. 60 GY
B. 70 GY
C. 50 GY
D. 45 GY

206. Side effects of I ^{131} administration are the following *except* one:

A. Sialadenitis
B. Hyperthyroidism (transient)
C. Pneumonitis
D. Dysphagia

HEAD AND NECK ASSOCIATED NODES

207. Diagram (i)   Diagram (ii)

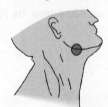 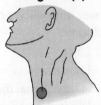

Name the nodal region in both:

Diagram (i)	Diagram (ii)
A. Preauricular	(a) Low jugular
B. Submental	(b) Mid jugular
C. Submaxillary triangle	(c) Supraclavicular
D. Supraclavicular	(d) Low posterior cervical

208. Diagram (i)   Diagram (ii)

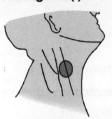 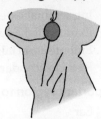

Identify the nodal region in both:

Diagram (i)	Diagram (ii)
A. Subdigastric	1. Preauricular
B. Mid jugular	2. Upper posterior cervical
C. Low jugular	3. Subdigastric
D. Mid posterior cervical	4. Submental

209. Diagram (i)   Diagram (ii)

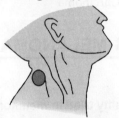 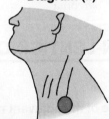

Identify the nodal region in both:

Diagram (i)	Diagram (ii)
A. Low posterior cervical	1. Supraclavicular
B. Mid posterior cervical	2. Preauricular
C. Supraclavicular	3. Lower posterior cervical
D. Mid jugular	4. Low jugular

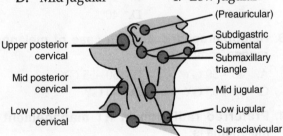

ANSWERS

1 B	2 C	3 D	4 B	5 D	6 D	7 A	8 D
9 B	10 BADC	11 B	12 B	13 B	14 D	15 B	16 C
17 D	18 C	19 A	20 C	21 B	22 A	23 C	24 C
25 C	26 B	27 D	28 A	29 C	30 D	31 C	32 A
33 C	34 D	35 BCDA	36 A	37 BACD	38 C	39 C	40 B
41 D	42 D	43 B	44 D	45 A	46 A	47 D	48 D
49 D	50 A	51 D	52 B	53 C	54 A	55 C	56 D
57 C	58 A	59 D	60 C	61 A	62 D	63 C	64 C
65 A	66 C	67 C	68 C	69 C	70 B	71 C	72 D
73 B	74 C	75 D	76 A	77 DCBA	78 D	79 A	80 D
81 D	82 C	83 A	84 C	85 C	86 C	87 B	88 D
89 B	90 A	91 D	92 C	93 C	94 C	95 B	96 C
97 B	98 BDCA	99 B	100 A	101 B	102 B	103 D	104 C
105 B	106 A	107 B	108 C	109 B	110 C	111 A	112 C
113 C	114 D	115 B	116 A	117 D	118 A	119 A	120 C
121 B	122 C	123 A	124 A	125 D	126 C	127 A	128 B
129 B	130 C	131 C	132 A	133 B	134 A	135 C	136 D
137 D	138 D	139 D	140 A	141 DBAC	142 A	143 D	144 D
145 C	146 D	147 C	148 A	149 B	150 D	151 A	152 A
153 C	154 DCBA	155 C	156 A	157 C	158 B	159 B	160 B
161 C	162 C	163 A	164 B	165 C	166 A	167 C	168 D
169 C	170 C	171 A	172 A	173 D	174 A	175 B	176 D
177 A	178 C	179 C	180 B	181 B	182 B	183 A	184 D
185 D	186 C	187 D	188 C	189 A	190 C	191 B	192 C
193 B	194 D	195 D	196 C	197 DCBA	198 C	199 A	200 C
201 A	202 A	203 C	204 D	205 A	206 D	207 (I)C (II)A	208 (I)B (II)C
209 (I)B (II)A							

Anesthesiology

1. **Identify the true statement regarding lower oesophageal tone:**
   A. It is increased by sympathetic beta stimulation and alpha block
   B. It is reduced by suxamethonium
   C. It is increased with vagal stimulation
   D. It is increased with opiates
   E. It is reduced with ranitidine

2. **All the statements regarding laryngeal and tracheal anatomy are true *except*:**
   A. The adult trachea is normally 10-12 cm long
   B. The vocal cords lie just below the notch of the thyroid cartilage
   C. In bilateral partial recurrent laryngeal nerve paralysis there is loss of voice but no respiratory impairment
   D. The right main bronchus lies more vertically, and is shorter than the left main bronchus
   E. In the desperate situation of a patient with complete respiratory obstruction, cricothyroid puncture is one of the safest ways of providing an airway

3. **Which one statement is true regarding the nerve supply of larynx?**
   A. The recurrent laryngeal nerve supplies the mucous membrane below the true vocal cords
   B. The recurrent laryngeal nerve supplies the cricothyroid muscle
   C. The external laryngeal nerve is entirely sensory
   D. The larynx has no sympathetic nerve supply

4. **Which is the most efficient breathing system during controlled ventilation?**
   A. Mapleson A.
   B. Mapleson B.
   C. Mapleson C.
   D. Mapleson D.
   E. Mapleson E.

5. **Difficult intubation may be anticipated in all these conditions *except*:**
   A. Treacher-Collins syndrome
   B. Pierre-Robin syndrome
   C. Klippel-Feil syndrome
   D. Sturge-Weber syndrome

6. **All the undermentioned areas are supplied by trigeminal nerve *except*:**
   A. The mucosa of the soft palate
   B. The tympanic membrane
   C. The skin over the angle of the mandible
   D. The ala nasae

7. **The pressor response to laryngoscopy and intubation can be attenuated by all of these measures *except*:**
   A. Intravenous fentanyl in dose of 1 mcg / kg
   B. Lignocaine surface spray to the larynx and trachea
   C. Nasal nitroglycerine
   D. Diltiazem

8. **Identify the false statement when conducting a pre-use check of an anesthetic machine:**
   A. When nitrous oxide supply is disconnected there should be a reduction in the flow of oxygen
   B. There should be no flow of nitrous oxide when oxygen supply is disconnected
   C. The standard check gives no indication as to which gas flows through which flowmeter
   D. The pressure relief valve should operate only if the common outlet is completely occluded
   E. The gas hose probes should not fit into an outlet for another gas

9. **Identify the false statement with regard to antistatic precautions in operating theatres:**
   A. An electrically conductive floor is necessary
   B. Cotton clothing should have conductive strips
   C. Foot wear with a leather sole is acceptable
   D. The zone of risk is 25 cm from the patient breathing system

10. **Identify the false statement regarding larynx:**
    A. Lies at level with cervical vertebrae 3-6
    B. The vestibule lies between the false cords and the aryepiglottic folds
    C. The saccule is between false cords and vocal cords
    D. The vocal cords are covered with ciliated epithelium

11. **Granuloma after short-term intubation most commonly occurs:**
    A. At the carina
    B. In the trachea
    C. On the arytenoids
    D. Anterior two-thirds of the cords
    E. Posterior third of the cords

12. **Identify the false statement regarding adult trachea:**
    A. It extends from vertebral levels C6 to T5
    B. Has sensory supply from the vagus nerve
    C. Has squamous epithelium
    D. Is supplied by the inferior thyroid artery
    E. Is crossed by the aorta

13. **Identify the false statement:**
    A. The lungs biodegrade fentanyl
    B. The lungs are a site of action of angiotensin converting enzyme
    C. The lungs produce interleukin-1
    D. The lungs are rich in macrophages
    E. The lungs are a source of catecholamines

14. **All the statements regarding smoking are true except:**
    A. Smoking causes carboxyhemoglobinemia
    B. Smoking causes postoperative chest complications
    C. Smoking reduces ciliary activity
    D. Smoking reduces sputum
    E. Smoking reduces wound healing

15. **Identify the true statement regarding sterilization:**
    A. Boiling for 15 minutes destroys spores
    B. Gluteraldehyde can destroy spores
    C. Tubercle bacilli are destroyed by ethyl alcohol
    D. Phenol destroys spores

16. **Identify the true statement regarding total intravenous anesthesia:**
    A. Does not require resuscitation equipment
    B. Can be monitored by esophageal contractions
    C. The airway is secure
    D. Oxygen is not required

17. **Identify the correct statement with respect to the cuff of a tracheal tube:**
    A. The cuff deflates with time
    B. Intracuff pressure should not exceed 100 mmHg
    C. Its filling tube has a longer intramural length in a nasal tube
    D. Causes a fall of IPPV pressure when herniated

18. **All the statements below, when intubating children, are true except:**
    A. The epiglottis is shorter and flatter than in adults
    B. The narrowest part of the upper airway is the cricoid
    C. Length of trachea is, age divided by 4, plus 4 cm
    D. The rima glottidis is in level with C3/4

19. **All the statements below are true except:**
    A. Bleeding during surgery is reduced by elevating the operative site
    B. Bleeding during surgery is reduced by local vasopressin
    C. Bleeding during surgery is reduced by bradycardia
    D. Bleeding during surgery is reduced by hypertension
    E. Bleeding during surgery is reduced by hypocapnia

20. **In clinical doses, glyceryl trinitrate causes all except:**
    A. Reduces preload
    B. Reduces afterload
    C. Reduces intracranial pressure
    D. Reduces intraocular pressure
    E. Reduces intracranial blood volume

21. All the statements below regarding upper airway obstruction are true *except*:

    A. Stridor implies that the adult airway is reduced to less than 6 mm diameter
    B. May be caused by epiglottitis
    C. It is solved by using a relaxant
    D. Causes paradoxical respiration

22. A patient who becomes cyanosed in the postoperative ward:

    A. May need laying on his/her side
    B. May be hypervolamic
    C. Will always need oxygen
    D. May need neostigmine
    E. All of the above

23. All the situations below can indicate respiratory failure in the adult *except*:

    A. Ten words per breath
    B. Cyanosis
    C. Tachypnea greater than 30 per minute
    D. Grimacing and alar flaring

24. All the statements regarding the complications of tracheostomy are true *except:*

    A. Tracheal dilation
    B. Tracheal stenosis
    C. Carotid hemorrhage
    D. Increased dead space
    E. Pneumothorax

25. Acute inflammatory epiglottitis:

    A. Is caused by *Hemophilus influenzae* type B
    B. Is often accompanied by drooling in children
    C. Is helped by breathing 21% oxygen in helium
    D. May be visible on X-ray
    E. All of the above

26. Identify the true statement regarding acute laryngotracheitis in children:

    A. Has an insidious onset
    B. The child drools
    C. Pulmonary edema may occur
    D. Tracheostomy is indicated

27. With regard to accidental esophageal intubation, the negative pressure test is more reliable than chest auscultation in determining tracheal intubation (True/False)

28. esophagitis is a premalignant condition for carcinoma of esophagus (True/Flase)

29. Incidence of laryngospasm is not increased by upper respiratory tract infections (TRUE/FALSE)

30. Laryngeal edema is more prone to develop in the supraglottic region than in the subglottic area (TRUE/FALSE)

31. Epiglottitis is usually caused by a viral infection (TRUE/FALSE)

32. If intubation is deemed necessary in a 4-yr old child with epiglottitis, a 5.5 mm diameter tube should be used (TRUE/FALSE)

33. Surgery for carcinoma of the bronchus is usually contraindicated by left recurrent laryngeal nerve palsy (TRUE/FALSE)

34. The VII cranial nerve (facial nerve) has no branches before its exit from the stylomastoid foramen (TRUE/FALSE)

35. The glottis is closed by the extrinsic muscles (TRUE/FALSE)

36. The vocal cords are covered by ciliated epithelium (TRUE/FALSE)

37. The trachea is surrounded by cartilages (TRUE/FALSE)

38. Pulmonary shunt is increased by anesthesia (TRUE/FALSE)

39. Hypoxia causes pulmonary vascular constriction (TRUE/FALSE)

40. The oxygen dissociation curve of hemoglobin is moved to the right by hypercapnia (TRUE/FALSE)

41. Autoclaving destroys rubber and plastics (TRUE/FALSE)

42. Total intravenous anesthesia can be monitored by esophageal contractions (TRUE/FALSE)

43. In children, the RAE tube cannot enter the right main bronchus (TRUE/FALSE)

44. Upper airway obstruction can be solved by use of a laryngeal mask (TRUE/FALSE)

45. Hypotensive anesthesia is the anesthetic technique of choice for middle ear surgery (TRUE/FALSE)

46. Nitrous oxide should be avoided in operations on middle ear (TRUE/FALSE)

47. A pharyngeal pack is not necessary while using cuffed endotracheal tube for adult tonsillectomy surgery (TRUE/FALSE)

48. Placing a wet swab in the larynx prevents tracheal damage while doing laser surgery (TRUE/FALSE)

49. PVC endotracheal tubes can be used for laser surgery of the larynx (TRUE/FALSE)

50. Patients can be allowed to recover in the supine position in the immediate post-tonsillectomy period (TRUE/FALSE)

51. Extubation should be preferably done in the post-tonsillar position after tonsillectomy (TRUE/FALSE)

52. Injury to the superior laryngeal nerve can be suspected if there is a change in voice (TRUE/FALSE)

53. Eedema of larynx is seen in the immediate post-operative period after thyroidectomy (TRUE/FALSE)

54. In which of the following situations associated with cardiac arrest is the use of sodium bicarbonate acceptable. A: 1,2,3 Correct B: 1,3 Correct C: 2,4 Correct D: 4 Correct E: All Correct
    A. Hyperkalemia.
    B. Tricyclic antidepressant overdose.
    C. Pre-existing metabolic acidosis.
    D. Hypoxic lactic acidosis subsequent to prolonged period of circulatory arrest.

55. To operate on the ear, one would have to block which of the following nerves A: 1,2,3 Correct B: 1,3 Correct C: 2,4 Correct D: 4 Correct E: All Correct
    A. Auriculotemporal.
    B. Great auricular nerve.
    C. Auricular branch of the vagus.
    D. Greater occipital.

56. Which of the following are methods of measuring the content of oxygen in a gas mixture? A: 1,2,3 Correct B: 1,3 Correct C: 2,4 Correct D: 4 Correct E: All Correct
    A. Paramagnetic analysis
    B. Mass spectrometry.
    C. Fuel cell analysis
    D. Katharometry.

57. Which of the following materials are flammable in air? A: 1,2,3 Correct B: 1,3 Correct C: 2,4 Correct D: 4 Correct E: All Correct
    A. Polyethylene.
    B. Polyvinylchloride (PVC).
    C. Polymethylmethacrylate.
    D. Polytetrafluoroethylene (Teflon)

58. The following techniques should be given particular attention while administering anesthesia for middle ear surgery A: 1,2,3 Correct B: 1,3 Correct C: 2,4 Correct D: 4 Correct E: All Correct
    A. To provide clear airways
    B. To position the patient carefully
    C. To avoid hypercarbia
    D. Small quantities of a local vasoconstrictor are indicated

59. Moffet's solution contains the following drugs A: 1,2,3 Correct B: 1,3 Correct C: 2,4 Correct D: 4 Correct E: All Correct
    A. Cocaine   B. Procaine
    C. Adrenaline   D. Felypressin

60. In Mackintosh and Ostlere modification, the Moffet's solution is deposited in the ethmoidal recess to block A: 1,2,3 Correct B: 1,3 Correct C: 2,4 Correct D: 4 Correct E: All Correct
    A. Greater palatine nerve
    B. Anterior ethmoidal nerve
    C. Ciliary ganglion
    D. Sphenopalatine ganglion

61. Regarding tonsillectomy A: 1,2,3 Correct B: 1,3 Correct C: 2,4 Correct D: 4 Correct E: All Correct
    A. Surgical ligation of post-tonsillectomy bleeding is required in 1-2 % of cases
    B. Insufflation method of anesthesia without intubation is suitable
    C. Early return of reflex activity is important
    D. Patients can be allowed to recover in the supine position

62. The following conditions must be ruled out before diagnosing collapse of trachea after thyroidectomy A: 1,2,3 Correct B: 1,3 Correct C: 2,4 Correct D: 4 Correct E: All Correct
   A. Edema of the larynx
   B. Recurrent laryngeal nerve injury
   C. Hemorrhage under the strap muscles
   D. None of the above

63. The methods used to provide topical analgesia of the nasal cavities include A: 1,2,3 Correct B: 1,3 Correct C: 2,4 Correct D: 4 Correct E: All Correct
   A. Sluder's method   B. Moffet's method
   C. Curtiss method   D. Bodman's method

64. Bilateral vagus nerve blockade produces A: 1,2,3 Correct B: 1,3 Correct C: 2,4 Correct D: 4 Correct E: All Correct
   A. Tachycardia
   B. Aphonia
   C. Abolition of cough reflex
   D. Hypotension

65. Features of Horner's syndrome include A: 1,2,3 Correct B: 1,3 Correct C: 2,4 Correct D: 4 Correct E: All Correct
   A. Mydriasis   B. Miosis
   C. Exophthalmos   D. Enophthalmos

66. The Moffet's solution consists of 2 ml of ____ % Cocaine , 2 ml of 1% sodium bicarbonate and 1ml of 1:1000 adrenaline

67. In the Bodman's method ____ ml of 1.25 % lignocaine with adrenaline are used for the topical analgesia of the nasal cavities

68. The concentration of cocaine in the cocaine paste used for topical analgesia of the nasal cavities is ____ %

69. Cocaine is a powerful _____ (vasoconstrictor/vasodilator)

70. The vagus nerve emerges from the skull through the _____ foramen

71. The _____ nerve is the only sensory nerve supplying the floor of the mouth between the alveolar margin and the midline

72. The vagus nerve contains _____ , _____ and _____ fibres

73. The anatomical landmark for the lingual nerve block is _____ of the mandible

74. Superior laryngeal nerve block causes analgesia of the larynx _____ (above the vocal cords/below the vocal cords)

75. Stuffiness of nostril is known as _____ sign

76. Mueller's syndrome consists of injection of tympanic membrane and _____

77. Chassaignac tubercle is at the level of _____ cervical transverse process

78. Moore's method of stellate ganglion block uses the _____ approach

79. The nerve plexus supplying the tonsil is known as _____

ANSWERS

1 C	2 C	3 A	4 D	5 D	6 C	7 A	8 A
9 B	10 D	11 E	12 C	13 E	14 D	15 B	16 B
17 C	18 A	19 D	20 E	21 C	22 E	23 A	24 D
25 E	26 C	27 TRUE	28 FALSE	29 FALSE	30 FALSE	31 FALSE	32 FALSE
33 TRUE	34 FALSE	35 FALSE	36 FALSE	37 FALSE	38 TRUE	39 TRUE	40 TRUE
41 TRUE	42 TRUE	43 FALSE	44 FALSE	45 TRUE	46 TRUE	47 TRUE	48 TRUE
49 FALSE	50 FALSE	51 TRUE	52 TRUE	53 FALSE	54 A	55 A	56 A
57 B	58 E	59 B	60 C	61 B	62 A	63 E	64 A
65 C	66 8%	67 40 ML	68 25%				

69 VASOCONSTRICTOR
70 JUGULAR FORAMEN
71 LINGUAL NERVE
72 MOTOR, SECRETORY AND SENSORY
73 RETROMOLAR FOSSA
74 ABOVE THE VOCAL CORDS
75 GUTTMANN'S SIGN
76 WARMTH OF FACE
77 SIXTH
78 THE PARATRACHEAL APPROACH
79 CIRCULUS TONSILLARIS

Medicine

EAR

1. Wardenburg's syndrome characterized by the followings *except*:

A. It is due to an abnormal migration of melanoblast.

B. Type II is associated with vestibular dysfunctions.

C. Due to mutation in endothelin β receptor and SOX-10 gene.

D. Congenital sensory neural hearing loss.

2. Digeorge syndrome is include all *except*:

A. Abnormal ears

B. Shortened philtrum

C. Micrognathia

D. Hypotelorism

3. Following features are correct about Alport syndrome *except*:

A. More common in male.

B. X-linked recessive

C. X-linked dominant

D. Defects in Type IV collagen molecule.

E. Sensory neural deafness develop earlier to nephritis.

4. These are the features of craniometaphyseal dysplasia *except*:

A. An autosomal recessive condition.

B. Presents with conductive hearing loss.

C. Fixation of the malleus head.

D. Sensorineural deafness may be present.

5. Which is *not* correct about the hearing loss in Osteogenesis Imperfecta (OI)?

A. Usually begins in the second decade.

B. Hearing loss can be conductive, sensorineural or mixed type.

C. Hearing loss mostly present in Type II of OI.

D. Middle ear exhibit maldevelopment and deficient ossification

6. Deafness is the feature of which of the following muscular dystrophy:

A. Duchenne.

B. Becker

C. Limb-girdle

D. Facios-capulohumeral .

7. In refsum disease which is *not* correct.

A. Cochlear hearing loss present in 80% of cases.

B. High phytanate diet may arrest hearing deterioration.

C. Plasmapheresis may also arrest hearing loss.

D. Onset is in 1st or 2nd decade.

8. Following type of mucopolysaccarodosis can have deafness *except*:

A. Type II   B. Type IV

C. Type V   D. Type VI

9. In X-linked hypophosphotamic rickets which is *not* correct

A. Due to decrease in renal tubular phosphate reabsorption

B. It is a X-linked recessive disorder

C. Causes low frequency cochlear hearing loss

D. Hearing loss due to hydropic pattern or from occlusion of the endolymphatic duct.

10. Sensorineural deafness is a feature of:

A. Klinfelter syndrome

B. Turner's syndrome

C. Mixed gonadal dysgenesis

D. True hermaphrodite

11. Features of Turner's syndrome are:

A. Otitis media

B. Sensorineural deafness

C. Auricular deformity

D. Commonly seen in male population

12. Which of the following feature(s) are / is *not* correct about the hearing loss in typhoid fever?

A. Due to cochleovestibular lesion

B. Occurred between second and third week of the disease

C. More often seen in males

D. Occurred in first week of the disease

E. May be reversible

13. Which of the following mitochondria myopathies is *not* associated with hearing loss:

A. Progressive external ophthalmoplegia syndrome with ragged red fiber.

B. Kearns-sayre syndrome

C. Autosomal dominant progressive external ophthalmoplegia

D. Myoclonic epilepsy with ragged red fiber(MERRF)

14. Following features are correct about Wegener's granulomatosis *except*:

A. Severe crusting and pain over the nose

B. Type-I is widely disseminated disease

C. Hearing loss and otitis media are not seen

D. Also viewed as vasculitis and an autoimmune disease

15. About Melkersson-Rosenthal syndrome following are correct *except*:

A. Edema in periorbital skin

B. Bilateral facial palsy

C. Fissured tongue

D. Papillary projections of tongue

16. Which of the following statements best represents Bell's palsy:

A. Hemi paresis and cotralateral facial N. palsy.

B. Combined paralysis of facial, trigeminal and abducent N.

C. Idiopathic ipsilateral paralysis of facial N

D. Facial nerve paralysis with a dry eye.

17. Rheumatological disorder(s) associated with relapsing polychondritis is/ are:

A. Systemic vasculitis

B. Rheumatoid arthritis

C. Systemic lupus erythmatosus

D. Sjögren syndrome

E. All of the above

18. Nonrheumatic disorder(s) associated with relapsing polychondritis is/are:

A. Behcet's syndrome

B. Inflammatory bowel disease

C. Primary biliary cirrhosis

D. Mylodysplastic syndrome

E. All of the above.

19. Most often involve cranial nerves in relapsing polychondritis are:

A. III, VI, VII, VIII   B. II, III, VI, VII

C. V, VI, VIII, IX   D. IX, X, XI, XII

20. Most common valvular lesion in relapsing polychondritis is:

A. Mitral stenosis

B. Aortic regurgitation

C. Pulmonary regurgitation

D. Tricuspid regurgitation

21. Drugs are used for the treatment of relapsing polychondritis:

A. Dapsone   B. Prednisolone

C. Methotrexate   D. Cyclosporine

E. Lamivodine   F. Clotrimoxazole

G. Metronidazole

22. The following features are correct about Gout *except*:

A. Tophi are commonly seen in the external ear

B. Heberden's node or Bouchard's node may be first manifestation

C. Tyrosinase enzyme deficiency results in this disease

D. Martel's sign or G–sign present

E. Cyclosporin is the drug of choice

23. **Following are the features of polyarteritis nodusa** *except:*
    A. It is a necrotising vasculitis of small and medium sized arteries
    B. Incidence of pulmonary arteries involvement same as bronchial arteries
    C. There may be complete disappearance of organ of corti and atrophy of stria vascularis
    D. Favorable therapeutic agents are cyclophosphamide and prednisolone

24. **About Cogan's syndrome which is *not* correct:**
    A. Vestibuloauditory symptoms
    B. Syphilitic interstitial keratitis
    C. Associated with systemic vasculitis
    D. Glucocorticoids are the mainstay of treatment

25. **Molluscum contagiosum caused by:**
    A. Herpes virus-1
    B. Human herpes virus Type 8
    C. Pox virus
    D. Human herpes virus Type 2

26. **"Cauliflower" ear and deformed nose seen in:**
    A. Sarcoidosis
    B. Amyloidosis
    C. Relapsing polychondritis
    D. Leprosy

27. **The most common virus implicated in etiopathogenesis of Bell's palsy:**
    A. Herpes zoster virus (HZV)
    B. Herpes simplex virus (HSV-1)
    C. Human herpes virus Type 8
    D. CMV

28. **Facial nerve degree of damage in Bell's palsy is generally:**
    A. Neuropraxic
    B. Axnonotemesis
    C. Neurotemesis
    D. Non of the above

29. **Functional outcome of Bell's probably improve when treated with:**
    A. Prednisolone alone
    B. Acyclovir alone
    C. Prednisolone plus acyclovir
    D. None of the above

30. **Which of the following diagnostic test indicated in Heerfordt's syndrome?**
    A. Serum ANA
    B. Serum angiotensin-converting enzyme level
    C. Rheumatoid factor
    D. Serum C-ANCA

31. **Fluctuating hearing loss is a feature of following disease** *except:*
    A. Cogan syndrome
    B. SLE
    C. Scleroderma
    D. All of the above

32. **Pulsatile tinitus may be present in:**
    A. Arterial aneurysm
    B. Stenotic arterial lesion
    C. Glomus jugulare tumor
    D. Suppurative otitis media
    E. A-V fistula
    F. All of the above

33. **Chronic suppurative otitis media can lead to the following** *except:*
    A. Paralysis of VIIth Cr N
    B. Paralysis of VIIIth Cr N
    C. Brain abscess
    D. Meningitis

34. **Which of the following is *not* correct about" Swimmer's ear":**
    A. It can not develop in the absence of swimming
    B. Heat and humidity are predisposing factor
    C. Elevation of the pH of the ear canal
    D. Superadded predominant pathogen is *P. aeruginosa*

35. **Chronic otitis externa can caused by the following pathogen** *except:*
    A. Syphilis   B. Tuberculosis
    C. Typhoid fever   D. Leprosy

36. **The close differential diagnosis for chronic otitis external are following** *except:*
    A. Atopic dermatitis
    B. Psoriasis
    C. Dermatomycosis
    D. Dermatomycosis

37. The most common causative pathogen for necrotising (malignant) otitis externa is:

A. *P. aeruginosa*
B. *S. aureus*
C. *S. epidermidis*
D. Actinomycosis

38. The cranial N. usually affected first and most often in C.S.O.M is:

A. VIth
B. VIIth
C. VIIIth
D. IXth

39. Congenital deafness associated with the following *except*:

A. Pendred syndrome
B. Congenital rubella syndrome
C. Wardenburg syndrome
D. Ramsay hunt syndrome

40. In DIDMOAD syndrome "A" stands for:

A. Autosomal
B. Atrophy
C. Abnormal
D. Absence

NOSE

41. Noninfectious causes of acute sinusitis is/are:

A. Barotrauma
B. Wegener's granulomatosis
C. Cystic fibrosis
D. All of the above

42. Rhinocerebral mucor mycosis can occur in following conditions *except*:

A. Diabetes ketoacidosis
B. Deferoxamine therapy
C. Transplant recipient
D. Diabetes insipidus

43. Followings are complication of Pott's puffy tumor *except*:

A. Epidural abscess
B. Cerebral abscess
C. Myocarditis
D. Meningitis

44. Postanginal septicemia (Lemierr's disease) predominantly caused by:

A. Fusobacterium *necrophurum*
B. *H. influenzae*
C. Group A *Streptococcus*
D. *H. parainfluenza*

45. Nasopharyngeal carcinoma associated with which viral infection:

A. Human herpes virus-8
B. Human herpes virus-6
C. Epstein barr virus
D. Cytomegalo virus

46. Nasalmucosa involvement in in sarcoidosis is up to:

A. 10 %
B. 20 %
C. 30 %
D. 40 %

47. Lupus pernio is a form of:

A. SLE
B. Leprosy
C. Nasal tuberculosis
D. Nasal sarcoidosis

48. Following are the cutaneous manifestations of SLE *except*:

A. Lupus vulgaris
B. Discoid lupus erythmatosus (DLE)
C. Subacute cutaneous lupus erythmatosus
D. Lupus pernio

49. Following are correct about Churg –Strauss syndrome *except*:

A. Classified under a granulomatous vasculitis
B. Histopathological feature is coagulative or liquifactive necrotizing epitheloid granuloma
C. Allergic rhinitis and sinusitis developed up to 61 % of patients.
D. Associated with eosinophilic gastroenteritis
E. Usually have the diffuse nasal mucosa destruction

50. Rhinoscleroma following are correct *except*:

A. Caused by *Klebsiella rhinoscleromatis*
B. It involves the nose only but not larynx, trachea or bronchi.
C. Mikulie's cell is definitely pathognomomic of the disease.
D. Streptomycin and tetracycline are recommended for treatment
E. In stage – IV disease stent not useful

51. Lupus vulgaris is a form of:

A. Nasal sarcoidosis
B. Nasal tuberculosis
C. SLE
D. Leprosy

52. Drugs of choice to histoplasmosis:

A. Itraconazole
B. Metronidazole
C. Clotrimazole
D. Clotrimoxazole
E. Amphotericin B

53. Following are correct about von Willebrand's disease except:

A. It is an autosomal recessive disorder
B. It is one of the most common congenital bleeding disorder
C. Epistaxis is most common presentation
D. There is no aquired form the disease
E. Increase factor VIII activity

54. Followings are correct about Osler-Weber-Rendu disease except:

A. Recurrent epistaxis is the most common manifestation
B. It is an autosomal recessive disease
C. Produce pulmonary A-V fistula
D. Genetic defects are HHT-1 and HHT-2 gene

55. The term phantosmia refers to:

A. Perceptionof an odorant where none is present
B. Absence of smell in a prosthetic nose
C. A decrease ability to smell
D. Distortion in the perception of an odor.

56. Anosmia associated with following conditions except:

A. Kallmann's syndrome
B. Turner's syndrome
C. Schizophrenia
D. Cogan syndrome

57. Kaposi's sarcoma of nose is caused by:

A. Herpes simplex virus 2
B. Human herpes virus Type 8
C. Human herpes virus 1
D. CMV

THROAT

58. Phagophobia may occur in following conditions except:

A. Hysteria
B. Rabies
C. Tetanus
D. Tuberculosis

59. Unilateral paratracheal lymphadenopathy can occur in following conditions except:

A. Histoplasmosis
B. Primary amyloidosis
C. Sarcoidosis
D. Tuberculosis

60. About Plummer-Vinson syndrome which is not correct:

A. Presence of hypopharyngeal web
B. Commonly in middle aged women
C. Presence of glositis
D. Presence of megaloblastic anemia

61. Vascular compression producing dysphagia is/are:

A. Aberrant right subclavian artery
B. Right sided aorta
C. Left atrial enlargement
D. Aortic aneurysm
E. All of the above

62. Drugs causing xerostomia are the following except:

A. Benzhexol
B. Clonidine
C. Phenothiazine
D. Pilocarpine

63. A double lip with colloid goiter known as:

A. Pendred's syndrome
B. Ascher's syndrome
C. Albright' syndrome
D. Pemberten's syndrome

64. Brownish green teeth seen in:

A. Congenital hemolytic anemia
B. Hemochromatosis
C. Congenital billiary atresia
D. Iron deficiency anemia

65. Following features are correct about acanthosis nigricans except:

A. It is appears as dark, velvety, skin lesion in corner of mouth and tongue
B. It is a reflection of GI malignancy
C. It occurs primarily in extensor surface
D. It also seen in obesity and insulin resistance

66. Drugs producing gingival hyperplasia are the following except:

A. Phenytoin
B. Nifedipine
C. Cyclosporine
D. Azathioprine

67. Premature tooth loss resulting from periodontitis seen in following conditions *except:*

A. Papillon-lefevre syndrome
B. Chediac-Higashi syndrome
C. Leukemia
D. Churg-Strauss syndrome

68. Strawberry gum is a feature of:

A. Wegener's granulomatosis
B. Churg –Strauss syndrome
C. Sarcoidosis
D. Scarlet fever

69. Aphthous ulcers seen in following conditions *except:*

A. Behcet's syndrome
B. Reiter's syndrome
C. Systemic lupus erythmatosus
D. Rheumatoid arthritis

70. Which type of AML more prone to have gingival bleeding, ulceration and enlargement:

A. Promylocytic leukemia
B. Myelomonocytic leukemia
C. Megakaryoblastic leukemia
D. Erythroleukemia

71. Following features are correct about scurvy *except:*

A. Bleeding gums   B. Ulcer gums
C. Atrophic gums   D. Loosening of the teeth

72. Fordyce "spots" is due to:

A. Hyperplasia of sebaceous gland
B. Mucous gland
C. Taste buds
D. Minor salivary gland

73. Bilateral nontender parotid enlargement occur in following conditions *except:*

A. Diabetes mellitus   B. Cirrhosis
C. Bulimia   D. AIDS
E. Hepatitis   F. Anorexia nervosa

74. Enlarged tongue found in:

A. Down's syndrome
B. Klinfelter' syndrome
C. Primary amyloidosis
D. Hemangioma of tongue
E. Acromegaly
F. Diabetes mellitus

75. Pigmented oral lesion associated with HIV infection present in:

A. Kaposi's sarcoma
B. Bacillary angiomatosis
C. Addison's disease
D. Burkitt's lymphoma
E. Angiosarcoma

76. In *Helicobacter* pylori gastritis odor of the breath is:

A. Ammoniacal   B. Fishy
C. Fruity   D. Garlic

77. The diagnosis of subclinical hypothyroidism is mainly based on:

A. Clinical criteria
B. Biochemical criteria
C. Autoantibody positive
D. None of the above

78. In hypothyroidism all following can be seen *except:*

A. Hypernatremia
B. Precocious puberty
C. Hyperprolactimia
D. Goiter

79. Subclinical hypothyroidism must be treated if there is:

A. Antithyroid antibody positive
B. Constipation and cold intolerance
C. Goiter
D. All of the above

80. Primary hypothyroidism can be associated with:

A. Pituitary hyperplasia
B. Anovulation
C. Menorrhagia
D. All of the above

81. Following are correct about the tracheal involvement in Wegener granulomatosis (WG) *except:*

A. Tracheal stenosis resulting from granulomatus involvement
B. It has been noted 10 to 30 % patient of WG
C. More than 90% of patients with tracheal stenosis complicating WG are male
D. Results in hoarseness, dyspnoea,strider and progressive airway obstruction

82. **The most important risk factor for obstructive sleep apnea (OSA) syndrome is:**
    A. Female gender
    B. Diabetes mellitus
    C. Hyperthyroidism
    D. Obesity

83 **Apnea Hypopnea Index (AHI):**
    A. Sum of apnoea and hypopnea divided by by minutes of sleep
    B. Sum of apnea and hypopnea divided by hours of sleep
    C. Sum of apnea and hypopnea multiplied by minutes of sleep
    D. Sum of apnea and hypopnea multiplied by hours of sleep

84. **The most frequent symptoms with obstructive sleep apnea syndrome is:**
    A. Day time somnolence
    B. Sleep fragmentation
    C. Habitual snoring
    D. Weight loss

85. **The treatment of choice for obstructive sleep apnea syndrome is:**
    A. Antidiabetic therapy
    B. Antiobesity therapy
    C. Sedatives
    D. Continuous positive airway pressure

86. **The most common surgical procedure indicated for OSA syndrome is:**
    A. Ovulopalatopharyngoplasty
    B. Uvuloplasty
    C. Tonsillectomy
    D. Reconstruction of mandible

87. **In mild to moderate OSA syndrome can be managed by following measures except:**
    A. Modest weight reduction
    B. Avoidance of alcohol
    C. Sleeping in supine position
    D. Cessation of smoking

88. **The following are the consequences of OSA syndrome except:**
    A. Hypertension
    B. Neurocognitive impairment
    C. Coronary artery disease
    D. Osteoarthritis

89. **Risk factors for OSA syndrome are following except:**
    A. Alcohol intake
    B. Increased neck circumference
    C. Microglossia
    D. Adenotonsillar hypertrophy
    E. Obesity

90. **Obesity, hypersomonolence, alveolar hypoventilation and corpulmonale represent:**
    A. Pickwickian's syndrome
    B. Metabolic syndrome
    C. Syndrome X
    D. POEMS syndrome

91. **Laryngeal tuberculosis commonly involve:**
    A. Posterior portion of the true vocal cord
    B. Anterior portion of the true vocal cord
    C. Arytenoid cartilages
    D. Intra- arytenoids space

92. **The most common presenting symptoms of laryngeal TB is:**
    A. Weight loss
    B. Hoarseness
    C. Cough
    D. Hemoptysis

93. **Laryngeal involvement in patients with rheumatoid arthritis is:**
    A. 5 to 10 %   B. 15 to 20 %
    C. 25 to 30%   D. 35 to 40%

94. **Laryngeal involvement in patients with relapsing polychondritis is about:**
    A. 10%   B. 30%
    C. 50%   D. 70%

95. **Laryngeal involvement in sarcoidosis is about:**
    A. 3 to 5 %   B. 5 to 10 %
    C. 10 to 20 %   D. 25 to 30 %

96. **Rheumatoid involvement of larynx is/are:**
    A. Arthitis of the cricoarytenoid joint
    B. Laryngeal myositis
    C. Ischemic atrophy of the recurrent laryngeal nerve(s)
    D. Rheumatoid nodule of the vocal cord
    E. All of the above

97. Following features are true about the esophageal involvement in scleroderma *except*:

A. Diposition of fibrous tissue in submucousa and mascularis mucusa

B. Esophageal smooth musle hypertrophy

C. Esophageal dysmotility and atonia

D. Occur more than 50% of the patients

98. "CREST" syndrome represents:

A. Calcinosis, Raynaud's phenomenon, ECG changes, scleroderma, telangiectasia

B. Cardiomyopathy, rhematoid arthritis, eye changes, scleroderma, tracheoesophageal fistula

C. Calcinosis, Raynaud's phenomenon, esophageal dysmotility, sclerodactyli, and telangiectasia

D. Conduction block, rickets, ear deformity, sensorineural deafness, and telangiectasia.

99. The term "Tracheobronchopathia osteoplastica" refers to:

A. Sarcoidosis

B. Amyloidosis

C. Midline granuloma

D. Osteogenesis imperfecta

E. Paget's disease

100. The most common area of laryngeal involvement in amyloidosis is:

A. Aryepiglottic fold

B. Vestibulae

C. Subglottic region

D. False cord

101. All of the followings are correct about laryngeal sarcoidosis *except*:

A. Symptomatic laryngeal involvement about 5% patients of sarcoidosis

B. Dyspnoea is the most common manifestation

C. The epiglottis and area around the true vocal cord are usually involved

D. Vocal cord themselves not involved.

E. Upper airway obstruction may occur

102. Followings are correct about esophageal sarcoidosis *except*:

A. Primary involvement of esophagus < 1%

B. Serum ACE is the best useful parameter

C. Methotrexate is the drug of choice for treatment

D. There may be hypocalcaemia

ANSWERS

EAR

1	C	2	D	3	E	4	A	5	C	6	D	7	B	8	C
9	B	10	B	11	A,B,C	12	D,C	13	A	14	B,C	15	B	16	C
17	E	18	E	19	B	20	B	21	A,B,C,D	22	C,E	23	B	24	B
25	C	26	C	27	B	28	A	29	C	30	B	31	D	32	F
33	B	34	A	35	C	36	D	37	A	38	B	39	D	40	B

NOSE

41	D	42	D	43	C	44	A	45	C	46	B	47	D	48	A,D
49	B,E	50	B,C,E	51	B	52	A,E	53	A,D,E	54	B	55	A	56	D

THROAT

57	B	58	D	59	B	60	D	61	E	62	D	63	B	64	A,C
65	C	66	D	67	D	68	A	69	D	70	A	71	C	72	A
73	E,F	74	A,C,D,E	75	A,B,C	76	A	77	B	78	A	79	D	80	D
81	C	82	D	83	B	84	C	85	D	86	A	87	C	88	D
89	C	90	A	91	B	92	B	93	C	94	C	95	A	96	E
97	B	98	C	99	B	100	B	101	B,D	102	C				

Psychiatry

1. **Sudden onset of painful deviation of the tongue to one side is reported by the patient. Patient was on which of the following medicine?**
   - A. Haloperidol
   - B. Alprazolam
   - C. Olazepine
   - D. Lithium

2. **Patient complains of dryness of mouth and throat. Which of the medicine can cause these side-effects?**
   - A. Trihexyphenidyl
   - B. Carbamazepine
   - C. Lithium
   - D. Diazepam

3. **Lack of the taste is seen in:**
   - A. Anxiety disorder
   - B. Schizophrenia
   - C. Depression
   - D. Mania

4. **Paroxysmal episodes of bell-ringing noises seen in the following condition:**
   - A. Schizophrenia
   - B. Simple partial seizures
   - C. Otitis media
   - D. Depression

5. **Patient reports of a feeling of obstruction in the throat. This is seen in:**
   - A. Schizophrenia
   - B. Anorexia nervosa
   - C. Anxiety disorder
   - D. Mania

6. **Ball-rolling sensation in the throat (Globus hystericus) is seen in:**
   - A. Anxiety disorder
   - B. Mania
   - C. Dementia
   - D. Schizophrenia

7. **The child is not responding to verbal commands but the response to noises is present. This condition is seen in:**
   - A. Mental retardation
   - B. Receptive language disorder
   - C. Expressive language disorder
   - D. Selective mutism

8. **Communication deviance is seen in:**
   - A. Stammering
   - B. Social phobia
   - C. Autism
   - D. Mental retardation

9. **Which of the following is most common among head and neck malignancies?**
   - A. Schizophenia
   - B. Depression
   - C. Dementia
   - D. Hallucinations

10. **Hysterical conversion disorders can present with:**
    - A. Aphonia
    - B. Deafness
    - C. Dysphagia
    - D. All of the above

11. **Body dysmorphobia patients frequently ask for:**
    - A. Investigation of body parts
    - B. Change of facial appearance with surgery
    - C. Medicines for pain
    - D. All of the above

12. **Insects crawling into the ear is reported by:**
    - A. Elderly depressed patients
    - B. Young anxious women
    - C. Children with anxiety
    - D. All of the above

13. Grunting noises are repeatedly made by patients with:
    A. Stammering
    B. Tourette's disorder
    C. Obsessive compulsive disorder
    D. All of the above

14. Prevalence of stammering among children is:
    A. 5% - 10%
    B. 1%
    C. Males and females have equal prevalence
    D. Not clearly known

15. "Voices of 2 to 3 people talking amongst themselves about the patient in third person" – Which is not real – is a:
    A. Hallucination   B. Delusion
    C. Illusion   D. Obsession

16. 'Emiting foul odor from the self' and due to that other people are avoiding me. This phenomenon is known as:
    A. Hypochondriasis
    B. Bromosiderophobia
    C. Body dysmorphobia
    D. Obsession

17. Partial seizures can present with:
    A. Olfactory hallucinations
    B. Behavioral abnormalities
    C. Gustatory hallucinations
    D. All of the above

18. One of the following is an 'Autism Spectrum' disorder:
    A. Asperger's syndrome
    B. Cotard syndrome
    C. Tourette's syndrome
    D. All of the above

19. "Cotard Syndrome" is characterized by:
    A. Foul smelling odor emiting from internal organs
    B. Delusion of love
    C. Tinnitus
    D. All of the above

20. Central type of sleep apnea can be associated with:
    A. Depression   B. Narcolepsy
    C. Schizophernia   D. Anorexia nervosa

21. Paranoid ideation may be increased in:
    A. Stammering   B. Tinnitus
    C. Deafness   D. Vertigo

22. Sudden and spontaneous attacks of giddiness may be seen in:
    A. Social phobia   B. Panic disorder
    C. Depression   D. Schizophernia

23. Children reporting inability to speak in school 'alone' is:
    A. Selective mutism B. Autism
    C. Social phobia   D. Mental retardation

ANSWERS

1 A	2 A	3 C	4 B	5 C	6 A	7 B	8 C
9 B	10 D	11 B	12 D	13 B	14 B	15 A	16 B
17 D	18 A	19 A	20 B	21 C	22 B	23 A	

General Surgery

1. **CSF leak is commonly seen in fracture of:**
   A. Petrous temporal bone
   B. Frontal bone
   C. Parietal bone
   D. Occipital Bone

2. **The treatment for cold nodule of one lobe of thyroid gland is:**
   A. Total thyroidectomy
   B. Subtotal thyroidectomy
   C. Hemi thyroidectomy
   D. Radioactive Iodine

3. **Secondaries in the neck in an unknown primary malignancy is commonly from:**
   A. Ca bronchus   B. Ca thyroid
   C. Ca nasopharynx D. Ca larynx

4. **A cystic swelling in the midline of neck that moves on deglutition and protrusion of the tongue is:**
   A. Subhyoid bursitis
   B. Branchial cyst
   C. Thyroglossal cyst
   D. Cold abscess

5. **Medullary carcinoma of the thyroid gland arises from:**
   A. Parafollicular C cells
   B. Parathyroid glands
   C. Thyroglossal cyst
   D. Tracheal lymph nodes

6. **Complications of total thyroidectomy are:**
   A. Hemorrhage
   B. Airway obstruction
   C. Recurrent laryngeal nerve paralysis
   D. All the above

7. **Calcitonin level is raised in:**
   A. Anaplastic carcinoma of thyroid gland
   B. Medullary carcinoma of thyroid gland
   C. Reidls thyroiditis
   D. Multinodular Goiter

8. **Hashimoto's thyroiditis is treated by:**
   A. Total thyroidectomy
   B. Thyroxine
   C. Radioiodine
   D. Antibiotics

9. **Sternomastoid tumor leads to:**
   A. Wry neck
   B. Facial nerve palsy
   C. Facial disfiguration
   D. None of the above

10. **The following structures are the contents of the carotid sheath *except*:**
    A. Carotid artery
    B. Phrenic nerve
    C. Vagus nerve
    A. Internal jugular vein

11. **A cystic hygroma:**
    A. Occurs anywhere in the neck
    B. Is brilliantly transluscent
    C. Multiloculated.
    D. All of the above.

12. **Carotid body tumor:**
    A. Can be easily enucleated.
    B. Adherent to carotid artery.
    C. Adherent to external jugular vein.
    D. Treated by irradiation

13. **Sistrunk's operation is:**
    A. Block dissection of neck
    B. Enucleation of sublingual dermoid
    C. Excision of thyroglossal cyst
    D. None of the above

14. **Retrosternal goiter is:**
    A. common in females
    B. Blood supply is from neck
    C. Frequently turns malignant
    D. None of the above

15. **Branchial fistula:**
    A. Opens in the midline of the neck
    B. Opens into the trachea
    C. Excised by transverse incision
    D. Remnant of fourth branchial arch

16. **Killian's dehiscence is the site of:**
    A. Origin of laryngeal diverticulum
    B. Cold abscess
    C. Pharyngeal diverticulum
    D. Polyp

17. **Collar stud abscess is seen in:**
    A. Ludwig's angnia
    B. Alveolar abscess
    C. Tubercular infection of the deep cervical lymph nodes
    D. All the above

18. **Branchial cyst:**
    A. Is a remnant of thyroglossal tract
    B. Remant of second branchial cleft
    C. Is a dermoid
    D. Remnant of fourth branchial cleft

19. **In functional neck dissection the following structures are preserved:**
    A. A sternocleidomastoid muscle
    B. Internal jugular vein
    C. Spinal accessory nerve
    D. All the above

20. **Cervicofacial lesion is seen in:**
    A. Blastomycosis
    B. Histoplasmosis
    C. Maduramycoses
    D. Actinomycoses

21. **An open wound presenting after 8 hours is:**
    A. Debrided and sutured
    B. Debrided and left open
    C. Debrided and left open for secondary suture
    D. None of the above

22. **In maxillofacial injury, priority is to:**
    A. Arrest hemorrhage
    B. Keep airway open
    C. Diagnosis of the injuries
    D. X-ray face

23. **Melanoma is removed with a margin of:**
    A. 5 cms   B. 3 cms
    C. 6 cms   D. 10 cms

24. **Scalene node biopsy is obtained from:**
    A. Jugular group
    B. Deep cervical group
    C. Superior mediastinum
    D. Carotid sheath

25. **Chemodectoma arises from:**
    A. Carotid bodies   B. Spinal cord
    C. Left ventricle   D. Pituitay.

26. **In an unconcious patient, the better method of keeping airway open is:**
    A. Ambubag ventilation
    B. Cuffed endotracheal tube
    C. Uncuffed endotracheal tube
    D. Tracheostomy

27. **Sebaceous cyst does not occur in:**
    A. Sole   B. Scalp
    C. Scrotum   D. Back

28. **Squamous cell carcinoma arises from:**
    A. Long standing venous ulcer
    B. Basal cell carcinoma
    C. Chronic lupus vulgaris
    D. All the above

29. **The term universal tumor applies to:**
    A. Papilloma   B. Lipoma
    C. Neurofibroma   D. Hemangioma

30. **Moon's molars are seen in:**
    A. Tuberculosis   B. Leucoplakia
    C. Syphillis   D. Actinomycosis

31. **Cigerette smoking is associated with the following malignancy:**
    A. Carcinoma of stomach
    B. Oropharyngeal carcinoma
    C. Carcinoma bronchus
    D. Carcinoma bladder

32. **Reactionary hemorrhage is seen:**
    A. At the time of surgery
    B. Within 12 hours of surgery
    C. After 7 days
    D. After 14 days

33. **Risus sardonicus is seen in:**
    A. Gas gangrene
    B. Septicemia
    C. Tetanus
    D. Ludwig's angina

34. **Ultra violet radiation leads to:**
    A. Lupus vulgaris
    B. Sarcoidosis
    C. Basal cell carcinoma
    D. All the above

35. **Potts puffy tumor is:**
    A. Osteomyelitis of the skull with subperiosteal swelling
    B. Infected sebaceous cyst
    C. Liposarcoma
    'D. None of the above

36. **Jod Basedow thyrotoxicosis is:**
    A. Iodine induced thyrotoxicosis
    B. Occurs in Reidl's thyroiditis
    C. Common in intrathoracic goiter
    D. All the above

37. **Primary Sjögren's syndrome consists of:**
    A. Xerostomia
    B. Conjunctivitis
    C. No connective tissue disorder
    D. All the above

38. **Ameloblastoma is:**
    A. An epithelial neoplasm
    B. Connective tissue neoplasm
    C. Form of hemangioma
    D. None of the above

39. **Prolonged nasogastric suction leads to:**
    A. Hypokalemia
    B. Metabolic alkalosis
    C. Renal failure
    D. All the above

40. **Causes of delayed healing of an ulcer is:**
    A. Diabetes mellitus
    B. Anemia
    C. Foreign body
    D. All the above

41. **Migrating thrombophlebitis is a sign of:**
    A. Visceral malignancy
    B. Buerger's disease
    C. Varicose veins
    D. Aneurysms

42. **A bluish green discharge from an ulcer is the sign of:**
    A. Healing
    B. Pseudomonas infection
    C. *Staphylococcus aureus*
    D. Gas gangrene

43. **Midline perforation of the palate is due to:**
    A. Tuberculosis
    B. Palatal antrostomy
    C. Gumma
    D. Cleft palate

44. **Preauricular sinus occurs due to:**
    A. Failure of fusion of the six tubercles
    B. Failure of fusion between maxillary process and mandibular process
    C. Persistence of second branchial cleft
    D. Incision and drainage of cold abscess

45. **Macroglossia is caused by:**
    A. Lymphangioma
    B. Hemangioma
    C. Muscular macroglossia
    D. All above

46. **Epulis arises from:**
    A. Inner surface of the cheek
    B. Mucoperiosteum of the gum
    C. In relation to carious teeth
    D. Hard palate

47. Glomus tumor is:

A. Sarcoma

B. Angiomyoneuroma

C. Type of astrocytoma

D. Fibroma

48. Chronic subdural hematoma presents with:

A. Convulsions   B. Headache

C. Hearing Loss   D. Vertigo

49. The common glial tumor is:

A. Ependymoma   B. Meningioma

C. Astrocytoma   D. Tuberculoma

50. The common presentation of berry aneurysm is:

A. Pulsating exophthalmos

B. Cavernous sinus thrombosis

C. Subarachnoid hemorrhage

D. Paralysis of 7th cranial nerve

51. The cause of ptosis is paralysis of:

A. Trochlear nerve

B. Facial nerve

C. Third cranial nerve

D. None of the above

52. Calculi are common in submandibular salivary gland due to:

A. Stasis   B. Thin saliva

C. Viscid secretion D. A and C

53. The treatement of submandibular salivary gland calculus is:

A. Excision of the gland

B. Removal of the stone

C. Irradiation

D. No treatement.

54. Most common cause of delayed hemostasis are:

A. Administration of anticoagulants

B. Administration of vitamin K

C. Thrombocytopenia

D. Jaundice

55. Pendreds' syndrome is characterized by:

A. Thyroglossal cyst with deafness

B. Goiter with deafness

C. Goiter and toxicity

D. None of the above

56. Features of cystic hygroma are:

A. Commonly seen in posterior triangle

B. Cystic

C. Brilliantly translucent

D. All of the above

57. Treatment of division of cervical part of thoracic duct are:

A. Immediate end to end anastomosis

B. Immediate ligation of both ends

C. Pressure bandage

D. Close the wound with drainage

58. Treatment of cervical rib is:

A. Application of local heat.

B. Elevation of forearm

C. Extra periosteal resection of the rib.

D. Division of scalenus meduis muscle.

59. The dreaded complication of Ludwig's Angina is:

A. Rupture into mouth

B. Rupture into larynx

C. edema glottis

D. None of the above

60. Epidural administration of morphine causes:

A. Miosis   B. Pain relief

C. Retention of urine D. All of the above

61. The features of postspinal head ache are:

A. Relieved on lying flat in the bed

B. Frontal head ache

C. Occipital headache

D. Relieved by vomiting

62. Rare sequelae of spinal anaesthesia is:

A. Myelitis

B. Hematorachhis

C. Paraplegia

D. Cauda equina syndrome

63. Stellate ganglion block is characterized by:

A. Ptosis   B. Flushing

C. Miosis   D. All the above.

64. Intracranial pressure is reduced in:

A. Blood loss

B. Dehydration

C. Removal of an intracranial space occupying lesion

D. All the above

65. The cerebral blood flow is increased in:
A. Hemiplegia   B. Hypercarbia
C. Hypoxia   D. All the above

66. The surgical emergency of newborn that requires immediate surgery are:
A. Tracheoesophageal fistula
B. Diaphragmatic hernia
C. Intestinal obstruction
D. All the above

67. Brachial plexus is formed by the following:
A. C5T0T1   B. C4T0T2
C. C5T0T2   D. C4T0T3

68. From the Erb's point the following nerves are given off:
A. Nerve to subclavius
B. Suprascapular nerve
C. Anterior and posterior division of upper trunk
D. All the above

69. Carpopedal spasm is seen in:
A. Hypokalemia
B. Hyperkalemia
C. Hypocalcemia
D. Dehydration.

70. Foramen of Bochdalek is found in:
A. Base of the skull   B. Mandible
C. Heart   D. Diaphragm

71. Blood transfusion is indicated when loss is more than:
A. 10% of blood volume
B. 25% of blood volume
C. 20% of blood volume
D. 15% of blood volume

72. The complications of hypothermia are:
A. Damage to brain
B. Bleeding
C. Ventricular fibrillation
D. All the above

73. Cuffed endotracheal tube anesthesia:
A. Provides airtight seal in trachea
B. Prevents dislocation of the tube
C. Avoids damage to trachea
D. All the above

74. Deep vein thrombosis occurs in the following conditions:
A. Prolonged immobilization
B. Thrombophlebitis
C. Myocardial infarction
D. All the above

75. Common site of multiple myeloma are:
A. Skull   B. Hipbone
C. Vertebrae   D. Ribs

ANSWERS

1 A	2 C	3 C	4 C	5 A	6 D	7 B	8 B
9 A	10 B	11 C	12 C	13 C	14 C	15 C	16 C
17 C	18 B	19 D	20 D	21 C	22 B	23 A	24 C
25 A	26 B	27 A	28 D	29 B	30 C	31 B and C	32 B
33 C	34 C	35 A	36 A	37 D	38 A	39 D	40 D
41 A and B	42 B	43 C	44 A	45 D	46 B	47 B	48 B
49 C	50 C	51 C	52 A and C	53 A	54 C	55 B	56 D
57 B	58 C	59 C	60 D	61 A	62 D	63 D	64 D
65 B	66 D	67 A	68 D	69 C	70 D	71 D	72 D
73 A	74 D	75 C					

Plastic Surgery

1. **In a deep injury over eye-brow you should not:**
   A. Clean the wound
   B. Shave the eyebrow
   C. Suture the muscle
   D. Do all of the above

2. **Eyelid skin sutures following repair for trauma should ideally be removed after about:**
   A. 1 day
   B. 5 days
   C. 10 days
   D. 15 days

3. **A traumatic nasal septal hematoma is best treated by:**
   A. Aspiration of blood by a thick needle
   B. Dependent incision and drainage
   C. Incision, drainage and closure of the incision
   D. All of the above

4. **Traumatic division of facial N should be ideally treated by:**
   A. Primary repair of the nerve
   B. Early secondary repair between 3 and 6 weeks following injury
   C. Exploration and repair after 6 months
   D. None of the above

5. **Following division of parotid duct following trauma the treatment may include:**
   A. Repair of the cut duct around a polythelene tube stent
   B. Suturing the proximal end to oral mucosa
   C. Ligating the proximal end
   D. Any of the above

6. **Waters projection view in radiogram will show fracture of:**
   A. Rim of orbit
   B. Nasal bone
   C. Mandible
   D. All of the above

7. **For fracture of angle of mandible the radiological view suitable is/are:**
   A. Lateral oblique view
   B. Lateral view
   C. Both the above
   D. None of the above

8. **In fracture of the body of mandible inter maxillary fixation can help in:**
   A. Reduction
   B. Immobilisation
   C. Both the above
   D. None of the above

9. **In unilateral subcondylar fracture of the mandible, on opening the mouth the mandible:**
   A. Remains in the center
   B. Deviates to the opposite side
   C. Deviates to the same side
   D. Any of the above

10. **A favorable critical fracture of the angle of mandible runs:**
    A. Anteriorly from the buccal plate going back wards to lingual plate posteriorly
    B. Anteriorly from the lingual plate going backwards to buccal plate posteriorly
    C. From the upper border going downwards and backwards
    D. From the lower border going upwards and backwards

11. **An unfavorable vertical fracture of the angle of mandible runs:**
    A. Anteriorly from the buccal plate going backwards to lingual plate posteriorly
    B. Anteriorly from the lingual plate going backwards to buccal plate posteriorly
    C. From the upper border going downwards and backwards
    D. From the lower border going upwards and backwards

12. **A baby with Robin sequence with airway obstruction may be benefited by lying down in:**
    A. Supine position
    B. Prone position
    C. Right lateral position
    D. Left lateral position

13. **A favorable horizontal fracture of mandible runs:**
    A. Anteriorly from the buccal plate going backward to lingual plate posteriorly
    B. Anteriorly from the lingual plate going backward to buccal plate posteriorly
    C. From the upper border going downwards and backwards
    D. From the lower border going upwards and backwards

14. **A Le Fort I fracture is also known as:**
    A. Guerin fracture
    B. Pyramidal fracture
    C. Craniofacial disjunction
    D. All of the above

15. **A Le Fort II fracture is also knows as:**
    A. Guerin fracture
    B. Pyramidal fracture
    C. Craniofacial disjunction
    D. All of the above

16. **A Le Fort III fracture is also known as:**
    A. Guerin fracture
    B. Pyramidal fracture
    C. Craniofacial disjunction
    D. All of the above

17. **Le Fort I fracture line passes through:**
    A. Alveolar process of maxilla above the level of teeth, walls of maxillary sinus, palatine bone and lower portion of pterygoid process
    B. Nasal bone, frontal process of maxilla, lacrimal bone, inferior rim of orbit, floor of orbit, near or through zygomatico maxillary sutures, lateral wall of maxillary, pterygoid plate to pterygomaxillary, fossa.
    C. Nasofrontal, maxillofrontal, zygomatico frontal sutures, through zygomatic arch, floor of orbit, ethmoid and sphenoid bones
    D. All of the above

18. **Le Fort II fracture line passes through:**
    A. Alveolar process of maxilla above the level of teeth, walls of maxillary sinus, palatine bone and lower portion of pterygoid process
    B. Nasal bone, frontal process of maxilla, lacrimal bone, inferior rims of orbit, floor of orbit, near or through zygomatico maxillary sutures, lateral wall of maxillary, pterygoid plate to pterygomaxillary, fossa.
    C. Nasofrontal, maxillofrontal, zygomaticofrontal sutures, through zygomatic arch, floor of orbit, ethmoid and sphenoid bones
    D. All of the above

19. **Le Fort III fracture line passes through:**
    A. Alveolar process of maxilla above the level of teeth, walls of maxillary sinus, palatine bone and lower portion of pterygoid process
    B. Nasal bone, frontal process of maxilla, lacrimal bone, inferior rims of orbit, floor of orbit, near or through zygomatico maxillary sutures, lateral wall of maxillary, pterygoid plate to pterygomaxillary fossa.
    C. Nasofrontal, maxillofrontal, zygomatico frontal sutures, through zygomatic arch, floor of orbit, ethmoid and sphenoid bones
    D. All of the above

20. **Le Fort I fracture line passes through all of the following *except*:**
    A. Nasal bone
    B. Wall of maxillary sinus
    C. Palatine bone
    D. Pterygoid process

21. **Le Fort II fracture of maxilla passes through all of the following *except*:**
    A. Nasofrontal junction
    B. Nasal bone
    C. Floor of orbit
    D. Lacrimal bone

22. **Le Fort III fracture of maxilla passes through all of the following *except*:**
    A. Zygomatic arch
    B. Zygomatico frontal sutures
    C. Maxillofrontal sutures
    D. Nasal bone

23. **Anosmia following division of olfactory nerve due to fracture of cribriform plate is:**
    A. Temporary
    B. Permanent
    C. Does not occur
    D. Depends on the circumstance

24. **About submentovertical view of skull which statement is wrong?**
    A. Can be used in patients with cervical spine injury
    B. Shows whole skull base
    C. Shows both zygomatic arches
    D. Shows mandibular condylar head

25. **The following structure/structures may give a false appearance of a mandibular fracture in X-ray:**
    A. Air in the orpharynx at the angle of mandible
    B. Calcification or ossification of the stylohyoid ligament projected over or just behind the ascending ramus
    C. The hyoid bone shown over the posterior part of the horizontal ramus
    D. All of the above

26. **A subluxated tooth can be treated by:**
    A. Foil splint   B. Acrylic splint
    C. Arch bar   D. Figure of eight wiring
    E. All of the above

27. **Find one that does not belong to the group:**
    A. Eyelet wiring   B. Gunning splints
    C. Cap splints   D. Arch bar

28. **Arch bars for mandibular and maxillary fractures can be used in all of the following *except:***
    A. Insufficient teeth remaining making eyelet wiring difficult
    B. Simple dento alverlar fracture requiring fixation before inter maxillary fixation
    C. Absence of teeth on both the jaws
    D. Presence of teeth on both tragments but unsatisfactory for intermaxillary fixation

29. **A displaced unstable fracture at angle of tooth bearing mandible with no tooth in posterior segment is ideally treated by:**
    A. Only transosseous wiring
    B. Plate fixation of fracture segments + Intermaxillary fixation
    C. Intermaxillary fixation with eyelet wires
    D. Intermaxillary fixation with arch bars

30. **A unilateral fracture of edentulous mandible capable of being reduced and immobilized by intermaxillary fixation (IMF) can be treated by:**
    A. Gunning splint alone
    B. Gunning splint along with circumalveolar wiring for IMF
    C. Eyelet wiring of mandible, maxilla + IMF
    D. Arch bar for mandible and IMF

31. **Plating of mandibular fractures has the following advantages:**
    A. Intermaxillary fixation usually is brief and hence feeding is easier
    B. Allows early mobilization and prevents stiffuers in condylar fracture
    C. Treatment of badly displaced fractures
    D. All of the above

32. **A baby with Robin sequence with airway obstruction:**
    A. May have chocking and cyanotic attacks
    B. May try to maintain airway by straining and crying
    C. May die of exhaustion while straining to maintain the airway
    D. All of the above

33. **Intermaxillary fixation following eyelet wiring for fracture of body of mandible is kept for about:**
    A. 1 week   B. 2 weeks
    C. 6 weeks   D. 24 weeks

34. **Dislocation of condylar head of mandible can occur in which direction (S):**
    A. Anterior   B. Posterior
    C. Lateral   D. Superior
    E. All of the above

35. **The commonest type of displacement of mandibular condyle is:**
    A. Posterior   B. Lateral
    C. Anterior   D. Superior
    E. Medial

36. **The Robin sequence may be associated with all of the following *except:***
    A. Prognathia
    B. Glossoptosis
    C. Airway obstruction
    D. Cleft palate

37. **In unilateral anterior dislocation of condyle without fracture, the mandible:**
    A. Is deviated to opposite side
    B. Is deviated to same side
    C. Is in the midline
    D. None of the above

38. **In unilateral mandibular condylar fracture with dislocation or significant displacement, the mandible:**
    A. Is deviated to same side
    B. Is deviated to opposite side
    C. Is in the midline
    D. None of the above

39. **Complications of pin fixation in mandibular fracture include:**
    A. Damage to inferior dental nerve
    B. Accidental entry of infection to fracture site
    C. Displacement of lingual plate
    D. Damage to facial nerve
    E. All of the above

40. **Least reactive metallic implant is of:**
    A. Titanium   B. Stainless steel
    C. Chrome   D. Aluminium

41. **Craniosynostosis, low hairline, ptosis, deviated nasal septum and brachydactyly are seen in:**
    A. Crouzon's disease
    B. Saethre-Chotzen syndrome
    C. Apert's syndrome
    D. Carpenter's syndrome

42. **The treatment of acute dislocation of mandibular condyle is:**
    A. Immediate reduction followed by immobilization of jaws by intermaxillary fixation (IMF) for 14 days
    B. Only intermaxillary fixation for 14 days
    C. Reduction and immediate mobilization
    D. Reduction after one week to allow the edema to subside

43. **The treatment of recurrent dislocation of mandibular condyle includes:**
    A. Immobilisation by intermixillary fixation for 4 to 6 weeks
    B. Chemical capsulorrhaphy
    C. Surgical correction
    D. All the above

44. **Surgical treatment of recurrent dislocation of temporomandibular joint includes:**
    A. Restitution of capsule and ligament
    B. Augmentation of articular eminence
    C. Removal of activating muscle
    D. All of the above

45. **Treatment of mandibular condylar fracture includes:**
    A. Conservative nonimmobilization
    B. Immobilization by intermaxillary fixation
    C. Surgical alignment of fractured segments
    D. All of the above

46. **A case of combined unilateral fracture of condyle and body of a mandible with full complement of teeth, can be conservatively managed by:**
    A. Reduction and immobilization of mandible by intermaxillary fixation with eyelet wire for 4 weeks
    B. Conservative nonimobilisation
    C. Restoration of occlusion and intermaxillary fixation by crchbar/cap splint and removal of intermaxillary fixation and arch bars/cap splint after 2 weeks
    D. None of the above

47. **Treatment of fracture of maxilla includes:**
    A. Reduction by intermaxillary fixation and immobilization by fixation to skull
    B. Reduction and immobilization by inter maxillary fixation above
    C. Circum zygomatic wire suspension alone
    D. All of the above

48. **Internal skeletal suspension for treatment of fracture of maxilla may be from:**
    A. Zygomatic arch   B. Frontal bone
    C. infraorbital rim   D. Piriform aperture
    E. Any of the above

49. **In a Le fort III fracture internal skeletal suspension is possible from:**
    A. Zygomatic arch
    B. Infraorbital rim
    C. Frontal bone
    D. All of the above
    E. None of the above

50. In a Le Fort II fracture internal skeletal suspension can be from any of the following *except:*
    A. Piriform aperture
    B. Circum zygomatic
    C. Zygomatic
    D. Central part of frontal bone

51. In a Le Fort II fracture internal skeletal suspension can be any of the following *except:*
    A. Circum zygomatic   B. Zygomatic
    C. Central frontal   D. Lateral frontal
    E. Infra orbital

52. External skeletal fixation for treatment fracture of maxilla can be with:
    A. Halo frame
    B. Plaster of paris headcap with metal frames
    C. Box frame
    D. Levant frame
    E. All of the above

53. In Walsham's forceps rubber padding is provided over:
    A. Longer blade   B. Shorter blade
    C. Both the above D. None of the above

54. In traumatic nasoethmoid injuries the telecanthus may present as:
    A. Increased intercanthal distance
    B. Prominent epicanthal fold
    C. Lax medial canthal ligament
    D. Diplopia
    E. All of the above

55. The approach for treatment of fronto nasoethmoidal fracture may be:
    A. Bicoronal
    B. Open sky (H) – shaped local incision
    C. Bilateral Z local incision
    D. W shaped local incision
    E. Any of the above

56. The treatment of fracture of frontonasoethmoid may include:
    A. Restoration of medial wall of orbit
    B. Restoration of medial canthus to it's original position
    C. Restoration of normal function of nasolacrimal apparatus
    D. Imparting adequate contour to the bridge of the nose
    E. All of the above

57. Most common site for a blowout fracture of orbit is:
    A. Roof
    B. Lateral wall
    C. Posteromedial aspect of orbital floor
    D. Anteromedial aspect of orbital floor
    E. Medial wall

58. Most common muscle to be trapped in blowout fracture of orbit is:
    A. Lateral rectus
    B. Superior oblique
    C. Inferior rectus
    D. Lateral rectus
    E. Superior rectus

59. The sign/signs of blowout fracture of orbit may be:
    A. Diplopia
    B. Enophthalmos
    C. Infraorbital N anesthesia
    D. All of the above

60. In blowout fracture of orbit entrapment of inferior rectus muscle:
    A. Causes diplopia during upward gaze
    B. Causes diplopia during downward gaze
    C. Causes diplopia during lateral gaze
    D. Causes exophthalmus
    E. None of the above

61. In blowout fracture of orbit entrapment of inferior rectus muscle:
    A. Causes diplopia
    B. Occurs more with smaller blowout fractures
    C. Can cause enophthalmos
    D. All of the above

62. In orbital blowout fracture enophthalmos may be due to:
    A. Escape of orbital fat in a large blow out fracture
    B. Trapped inferior recturs muscle
    C. Enlargement of orbital cavity
    D. Atrophy of orbital fat
    E. All of the above

63. Subconjuctival echymosis may be due to:
    A. Fracture zygoma
    B. Fracture floor of orbit
    C. Intracranial haemorrhage
    D. All of the above

64. **Proptosis following zygomatico-orbital trauma may be due to:**
   A. Intraconal hemorrhage
   B. Extraconal hemorrhage
   C. Both
   D. None

65. **Following zygomatic orbital injury the lower eyelid imparted a crackling sensation on palpation. The general condition of the patient was normal. This is most probably due to:**
   A. Surgical emphysema
   B. Gas gangrene
   C. Tetanus
   D. Edema of tarsal plate
   E. Hematoma

66. **Regarding surgical emphysema of eyelid following zygomatico-orbital injury all the following are correct *except:***
   A. Indicates communication between periorbital tissue and paranasal or nasal air cavity
   B. Indicates presence of fracture
   C. Needs antibiotic cover because of the potential for infection
   D. Is self-limiting
   E. Can cause air embolism

67. **In the temporal fossa approach for reduction of zygomatic fracture the elevator passes:**
   A. Above the tempralis fascia
   B. Between two layers of temporalis fascia
   C. Between temporalis fascia and temporalis muscle
   D. Beneath the temporalis muscle
   E. None of the above

68. **In the temporal fascia approach for reduction of fracture of zygoma the direction of elevation is:**
   A. Upward and outward
   B. Outward
   C. Upward and medially
   D. Backward and outwards
   E. None of the above

69. **In the temporal fascia approach for reduction of fracture of zygoma elevation is done with:**
   A. Counterpressure (fulcrum of lever) on one hand with elevation by other hand
   B. Counterpressure (fulcrum of lever) on the temporal bone
   C. Both
   D. None of the above

70. **While approaching orbital floor the periosteum in relation to infracrbital rim should be incised and elevated from:**
   A. 5 mm below the rim
   B. On the rim itself
   C. 5 mm inside the rim
   D. Any of the above

WOUND HEALING

71. **Closing a wound within hours of it's occurrence causes:**
   A. Primary healing
   B. Delayed primary healing
   C. Secondary healing
   D. None of the above

72. **When a full thickness skin loss wound heals with wound contraction and epithelialisation it is called:**
   A. Primary healing B. Secondary healing
   C. Both the above D. None of the above

CLEFT LIP AND PALATE

73. **A unilateral cleft of the lip occurs due to failure of fusion between:**
   A. Medial nasal and maxillary prominence on one side
   B. Medial nasal and maxillary prominence on both sides
   C. Lateral nasal and maxillary prominence on one side
   D. Lateral nasal and maxillary prominence on both sides

74. **An unilateral oblique facial cleft (tessier no.3 cleft) occurs due to failure of fusion between:**
   A. Medial nasal and maxillary prominences on one side
   B. Medial nasal and maxillary prominences on both sides
   C. Lateral Nasal and maxillary prominences on one side
   D. Lateral Nasal and maxillary prominences on both sides

75. **Congenital unilateral macrostomia occurs due to failure of fusion:**
   A. Between maxillary and mandibular prominence on one side
   B. Between maxillary and mandibular prominences on both sides
   C. Lateral nasal and maxillary prominences on one side
   D. Lateral nasal and maxillary prominences on both sides

76. **Bilateral cleft of the lip occurs due to failure of fusion between:**
   A. Medial nasal and maxillary prominence on one side
   B. Medial nasal and maxillary prominence on both sides
   C. Lateral nasal and maxillary prominence on one side
   D. Lateral nasal and maxillary prominence on both sides

77. **Secondary palate develops by fusion of:**
   A. Lateral palatine processes
   B. Medial nasal prominence
   C. Both the above
   D. None of the above

78. **During development of secondary palate the orientation of the lateral palatine process changes from:**
   A. Vertical to horizontal
   B. Horizontal to vertical
   C. Both the above
   D. None of the above

79. **In Millard's rotation advancement method of lip repair the advancement flap from the lateral segment is transferred to the:**
   A. Upper part of medial segment
   B. Middle part of medial segment
   C. Lower part of medial segment
   D. None of the above

80. **The lateral triangular flap in Tennison's repair moves into the medial part at it's:**
   A. Upper 1/3rd
   B. Middle 1/3rd
   C. Lower 1/3rd
   D. Any of the above

81. **In submuous cleft of the palate which of the following statements is false:**
   A. Uvula is usually bifid
   B. There is good muscle union in the center of the soft palate
   C. There is notching of the posterior margin of hard palate
   D. Patient can develop nasal speech

82. **Velopharyngeal incompetence may show:**
   A. Hypernasality
   B. Nasal emission
   C. Imprecise consonant production
   D. All of the above

JAW DEFORMITIES

83. **In Angle's class I occlusion:**
   A. The mesiobuccal cusp of the upper first molar is received in the buccal groove of the lower first molar
   B. Lower first molar is located distal to the upper 1st molar
   C. Any of the above
   D. None of the above

84. **In Angle's class II malocclusion:**
   A. The mesiobuccal cusp of the upper first molar is received in the buccal groove of the lower first molar
   B. Lower first molar is located distal to the upper 1st molar
   C. Lower first molar is located distal to the upper 1st molar
   D. None of the above

85. **In Angles class III malocclusion:**
   A. The mesiobuccal cusp of the upper first molar is received in the buccal groove of the lower first molar
   B. Lower first molar is located distal to the upper 1st molar
   C. Any of the above
   D. None of the above

86. Mandibular prognathia causes:
A. Angle's class I occlusion
B. Angle's class II occlusion
C. Angle's class III occlusion
D. None of the above

87. Maxillary retrusion causes:
A. Angle's class I occlusion
B. Angle's class II occlusion
C. Angle's class III occlusion
D. None of the above

88. Midline clefts of lip and nose are tessier:
A. No to 0 cleft
B. No to 1 cleft
C. No to 3 cleft
D. No to 4 cleft

89. Tessier No.2 cleft:
A. Is in the midline
B. Passes through the ala of the nose
C. Passes lateral to the ala is the nose
D. Passes transversely from angle of month

90. Tessier No.3 cleft:
A. Is in the midline
B. Parts the ala of the nose
C. Lifts the ala and ends medial to the puncturm of the of the lower eye lid
D. Passes transversely from angla of month

91. Tessier No.4 cleft:
A. Is in the midline
B. Parts the ala of the nose
C. Lifts the ala and ends medial to the punctum of the lower eye lid
D. Skirts around the nose and ends medial to the puntum of the lower eyelid

92. Tessier No.5 cleft:
A. Is in the midline
B. Parts the ala of the nose
C. Lifts the ala and ends medial to the puntum of the lower eye lid
D. Starts medial to oral commissure, traverses the cheek and ends in the middle 1/3rd of cover eyelid

93. Hemifacial microsomia comes under Tessier:
A. No 4 cleft
B. No 5 cleft
C. No 6 cleft
D. No 7 cleft

94. A number 8 Tessier cleft extends:
A. From midline of lip to glabella
B. From Cupid's bow to medial canthal area
C. From near angle of month to lower eyelid
D. From lateral canthus to temporal region

95. Crouzon's diseases is characterized by all exept:
A. Craniosynostosis
B. Frog like facies
C. Exorbitism and midface retrusion
D. Symmetrical syndactyly of hand and feet

96. Acrocephallo syndactyly is also known as:
A. Crouzon's disease
B. Apert's syndrome
C. Pfeiffer's syndrome
D. Carpenter's syndrome

97. Craniosynostosis, enlarged thumbs and great toes, exorbitism and midface hypoplasia are seen in:
A. Crouzon's disease
B. Apert's syndrome
C. Pfeiffer's syndrome
D. Carpenter's syndrome

98. Craniosynostosis, polysyndactyly of the foot, short hands and variable soft tissue syndactyly are seen in:
A. Crouzon's disease
B. Apert's syndrome
C. Pfeiffer's syndrome
D. Carpenter's syndrome

ANSWERS

1 B	2 B	3 B	4 A	5 D	6 D	7 A	8 C
9 C	10 A	11 B	12 B	13 D	14 A	15 B	16 C
17 A	18 B	19 C	20 A	21 A	22 D	23 B	24 A
25 D	26 E	27 B	28 C	29 B	30 B	31 D	32 D
33 C	34 E	35 B	36 A	37 A	38 A	39 E	40 A
41 B	42 A	43 D	44 A	45 D	46 D	47 A	48 E
49 C	50 A	51 E	52 E	53 A	54 E	55 E	56 E
57 C	58 C	59 D	60 A	61 D	62 E	63 D	64 C
65 A	66 E	67 C	68 A	69 A	70 A	71 A	72 B
73 A	74 C	75 A	76 B	77 A	78 A	79 A	80 C
81 B	82 D	83 A	84 B	85 C	86 C	87 C	88 A
89 B	90 C	91 D	92 D	93 D	94 D	95 D	96 B
97 C	98 D						

Oral Maxillofacial Surgery

1. Which flap is considered as 'work horse' of reconstructive surgery?

A. Deltopectoral flap
B. Pectoralis major flap
C. Trapezius flap
D. Latissmus dorsi flap

2. Danger space in the head and neck, during spread of odontogenic infections lies between:

A. Space among infrahyoid muscles
B. Between platysma and investing fascia
C. Prevertebral fascia and alar fascia
D. Space within prevertebral fascia

3. Ludwig's angina involves all of the following spaces, *except:*

A. Submandibular space
B. Sublingual space
C. Buccal space
D. Submental space

4. Which is the most common form of oral cancer?

A. Basal cell carcinoma
B. Squamous cell carcinoma
C. Adenoid cystic carcinoma
D. Mucoepidermoid carcinoma

5. Bird face deformity or Andy Gump deformity is seen in:

A. TMJ dislocation   B. TMJ ankylosis
C. Condylar fractures D. Apert's syndrome

6. Sialoliths are commonly formed in which salivary gland?

A. Submandibular salivary gland
B. Sublingual salivary gland
C. Parotid gland
D. Minor salivary glands

7. Campbell's lines are marked on which radiograph:

A. Submentovertex view
B. Paranasal sinus view
C. Skull – PA view
D. CT scan

8. Rule of 10 applies to:

A. Burns
B. Facial asymmetry
C. Cleft lip and cleft palate
D. Corticosteroids

9. Average volume of buccal pad of fat is:

A. 5.2 ml   B. 6.9 ml
C. 9.6 ml   D. 15.2 ml

10. Which of the following are highly aggressive jaw lesions with a high rate of recurrence after enucleation?

A. Ameloblastoma
B. Odontogenic keratocyst
C. Odontogenic myxoma
D. All of the above

11. The radionuclide material used in PET scans:

A. $^{18}F2$ – Fluoro-2- deoxy-D-glucose
B. Technetium – 99 m
C. Caesium
D. F1-Chloro-1-deoxy-D-lactose

12. Nalatan's method is used in the treatment of:

A. TMJ ankylosis
B. TMJ dislocation
C. TMJ internal derangement
D. TMJ arthritis

13. **Trigeminal neuralgia is due to compression caused by:**
    A. Vertebral artery
    B. Superior cerebellar artery
    C. Sigmoid sinus
    D. Superior sagittal sinus

14. **Eagle's syndrome is caused by:**
    A. Elongated styloid process
    B. Fracture of styloid process
    C. Elongated coronoid process
    D. Fracture of coronoid process

15. **Massive osteolysis of the mandible is seen in:**
    A. Treacher Collin's syndrome
    B. Apert's syndrome
    C. Gorham-stout syndrome
    D. Down's syndrome

16. **Sclerotherapy can be done by using which of the following:**
    A. Sodium tetradecyl sulphate
    B. 50% dextrose
    C. Sodium morrhuate
    D. All of the above

17. **Clinical features of silent sinus syndrome includes all, *except*:**
    A. Unilateral enopthalmos
    B. Hypoglobus
    C. Maxillary sinus bone thinning
    D. Ipsilateral large maxillary sinus

18. **Rate of growth of salivary calculi:**
    A. 0.5 mm-year   B. 1-1.5 mm-year
    C. 2 mm-year   D. 5 mm-year

19. **Definitive diagnosis of carotid-cavernous sinus fistula can be obtained by:**
    A. Plain radiographs
    B. CT scan
    C. MRI
    D. Carotid angiography

20. **Complications of Intermaxillary fixation includes all, *except*:**
    A. Respiratory arrest
    B. Weight loss
    C. Decreased pulmonary function
    D. Increased postoperative range of motion of mandible

21. **Ramsay-Hunt syndrome is caused by:**
    A. Reactivation of herpes zoster in geniculate ganglion
    B. Glossophagyngeal nerve
    C. Oculomotor nerve
    D. Paralysis of auriculotemporal nerve

22. **Complications of hyperbaric oxygen treatment includes all, *except*:**
    A. Dysfunction of Eustachian tube
    B. Pneumothorax
    C. Deafness
    D. CSF otorrhoea

23. **Embolization can be done by:**
    A. Autogenous muscle
    B. Gel foam
    C. Lyophilized dura
    D. All of the above

24. **Chylous fistula is a complication during:**
    A. TMJ surgery
    B. Radical neck dissection
    C. Orthognathic surgery
    D. Midface fractures.

25. **Marginal mandibular nerve is damaged during:**
    A. Retro mandibular incision
    B. Submandibular incision
    C. Pre auricular approach
    D. Endaural approach

26. **Central giant cell granuloma – treatment options includes all, *except*:**
    A. Anti angiogenic drugs
    B. Intralesional corticosteroids
    C. Intralesional calcitonin therapy
    D. Placentrix

27. **Antral sign (Holmer Miller) is seen in:**
    A. Mucoepidermoid carcinoma
    B. Angiofibroma
    C. Adenoid cystic carcinoma of maxillary sinus
    D. Lymphangiomas

28. **Beahr's triangle – its clinical significance is to:**
    A. Locate superior laryngeal nerve
    B. Locate recurrent laryngeal nerve
    C. Locate common carotid artery
    D. Locate vagus nerve

29. Griesinger's sign is seen in:

A. Cavernous sinus thrombosis

B. Lateral sinus thrombosis

C. Mastoiditis

D. Basal skull fractures

30. Woodruff's plexus is commonly known as:

A. Nasopharyngeal plexus

B. Cervical plexus

C. Pterygoid plexus

D. None of the above

31. Brachytherapy can be done by using:

A. Radium

B. Caesium^{137}

C. Gold^{198} seeds

D. All of the above

32. Gillette space is also called as:

A. Prevertebral space

B. Retropharyngeal space

C. Reinke's space

D. Space of Burns

33. Which of the bone lesion is most fatal?

A. Fibrous dysplasia

B. Paget's disease

C. Multiple myeloma

D. Osteochondroma.

34. Ameloblastoma is commonly seen in which of the following area?

A. Symphysis region

B. Molar-ramus

C. Maxillary anterior region

D. Maxillary sinus

35. Severe complication of canine space infection is:

A. Blindness

B. Cavernous sinus thrombosis

C. Respiratory paralysis

D. Nasal obstruction

36. The clinical stage grouping of $T_3N_2M_0$:

A. Stage I

B. Stage II

C. Stage III

D. Stage IV.

37. "Cheery blossom appearance" is radio graphically seen in:

A. Adenocystic cell carcinoma

B. Mucoepidermoid carcinoma

C. Clear cell carcinoma

D. Sjögren's Syndrome

38. A traumatic bone cyst is best treated by:

A. Marsupialization

B. Enucleation

C. Opening of the cavity and packing open

D. Opening of the cavity and inducing bleeding

39. Radiographic appearance of osteosarcoma is:

A. Discrete radiolucency with regular borders.

B. Mulicystic radiolucency with a soap bubble appearance

C. Cotton wool appearance with an irregular peripheral border

D. Sunburst pattern with radio–opaque strands extending from the cortical plates.

40. Term metaplasia means:

A. Irregular atypical proliferative changes in epithelial or mesenchymal cell

B. Loss of cell substances producing shrinkage of the cell

C. Replacement of one type of adult cell by another

D. None of the above

41. Coronoid process can be best viewed by:

A. P A View

B. Towne's projection

C. Lateral view of skull

D. Water's view

42. How many weeks of immobilization is required for displaced fracture mandible?

A. 4 to 6 weeks

B. 2 to 4 weeks

C. 6 to 8 weeks

D. 8 to 10 weeks

43. Energy range required to fracture the mandible is:

A. 44.6 Kg/ m to 74.4 kg/m

B. 79.2 kg/m to 98.1 kg/m

C. 30.3. kg/m to 40 kg/m

D. 10.1 kg/m to 28.5kg/m

44. Among the following where one might see bucket handle displacement in a 60 year old patient?

A. Bilateral mandibular fracture

B. Bilateral condylar fracture

C. Bilateral angle fracture

D. None of the above

45. Ecchymosis in the mastoid process is known as:

A. Battle's Sign

B. Guerin's sign

C. Murphy's Sign

D. None of the above

46. **Excessive muscular contraction is one of the frequent cause of:**
    A. Unilateral condylar fracture of mandible
    B. Coronoid fracture of mandible
    C. Fracture of the angle of mandible
    D. Bilateral condylar fracture of mandible

47. **Most common anatomical site of fracture mandible is:**
    A. Angle   B. Coronoid
    C. Condyle   D. Body

48. **Which is the weakest part of the orbit?**
    A. Medial wall   B. Lateral wall
    C. Floor of the orbit D. Roof of the orbit

49. **Posterior displacement of the fractured anterior segment in the bilateral fracture of the mandible in the canine region is due to the action of:**
    A. Thyrohyoid, genioglossus and geniohyoid
    B. Mylohyoid, genioglossus and geniohyoid
    C. Geniohyoid, genioglossus and anterior belly of digastric
    D. Mylohyoid, geniohyoid and anterior belly of digastric

50. **Nasal antrostomy is done through:**
    A. Middle concha   B. Middle meatus
    C. Inferior meatus D. Inferior concha

51. **Lowering the pupillary level of eyeball occurs if:**
    A. The orbit volume increases
    B. Blow out fracture
    C. Detachment of suspensory ligament of lock wood
    D. None of the above

52. **Traumatic telecanthus is seen in:**
    A. Orbital floor fracture
    B. Orbital roof fracture
    C. Fracture of medial wall of orbit
    D. Frontal sinus fracture

53. **Ideal distance in between two bites in sutures is:**
    A. 4 mm   B. 2 mm
    C. 6 mm   D. 1.5 mm

54. **Duration of immobilization for condylar fracture in a 10 yr old patient is:**
    A. 3 weeks   B. 4 weeks
    C. 10 days   D. 20 days

55. **Koleman's sign is seen in:**
    A. Condylar fracture
    B. Angle fractures
    C. Symphysis fracture
    D. Le Fort fracture

56. **Facial paresis is common in:**
    A. Fracture of the condyle
    B. Fracture of the zygomatic arch
    C. Parasymphsysis fracture
    D. None of the above

57. **Direct interdental wiring is also known as:**
    A. Risdon's Wiring
    B. Gilmer's Wiring
    C. Eyelet wiring
    D. Colstout's wiring.

58. **Ptosis of the eye may be caused by a lesion of the:**
    A. Oculomotor nerve
    B. Superior oblique nerve
    C. Optic nerve
    D. Trochlear nerve

59. **Guerin's fracture is also called as:**
    A. Le Fort I fracture
    B. Le Fort II fracture
    C. Le Fort III fracture
    D. Nasal fracture

60. **Trigeminal neuralgia most commonly affects which division of trigeminal nerve:**
    A. Ophthalmic division
    B. Maxillary division
    C. Mandibular division
    D. All the divisions

61. **Blood supply to the palatal flap used to close an oro–antral fistua in the area of upper⑧molar derives from:**
    A. Nasopalatine
    B. Greater Palatine
    C. Posterior superior alveolar
    D. Facial

62. **Ranula is best treated by:**
    A. Electrosurgery
    B. Laser
    C. Excision of sublingual gland
    D. Marsupialization

63. Thiersch's graft is a:
A. Full thickness graft
B. Partial thickness graft
C. Pedicle graft
D. None of the above

64. Bell's palsy affects which nerve:
A. Trigeminal nerve
B. Auriculotemporal nerve
C. Facial nerve
D. Glossophyaryngeal nerve

65. Drug which is diagnostic of trigeminal neuralgia is?
A. Atropine
B. Carbamazepine
C. Lidocaine
D. Morphine

66. CSF Otorrheoa is commonly seen in:
A. Le Fort I fracture
B. Le Fort II fracture
C. Subcondylar fracture
D. Zygomatic complex fracture

67. Trismus is more pronounced in:
A. Sublingual space infection
B. Submasseteric space infection
C. Bucccal space infection
D. Submandibular space infection

68. Name the fissural cyst:
A. Radicular cyst
B. Globulomaxillary cyst
C. Kertocyst
D. Residual cyst.

69. Ostium of the maxillary sinus is present in its:
A. Floor
B. Roof
C. Posterior wall
D. Lateral wall of nose

70. Ohngren's line helps in the assessment of tumor prognosis of:
A. Maxillary sinus
B. Ethmoidal sinus
C. Sphenoidal sinus
D. Frontal sinus

71. CSF leak can be best diagnoed by the estimation of:
A. Glucose
B. Protein
C. Beta-2 transferrin
D. Fat

72. Gillie's temporal approach is used to reduce the fractures of:
A. Temporal bone
B. Zygomatic arch
C. Le Fort III fracture
D. Orbital floor fractures

73. Ectropion of the lower eye lid is commonly seen after using:
A. Subciliary approach
B. Infraorbital approach
C. Transconjunctival approach
D. Crows feet approach

74. Weber's Fergusson approach is used for the exposure of:
A. Zygomatic arch
B. Maxilla
C. Nose
D. Orbit

75. Nerve preserved in modified neck dissection is:
A. Spinal accessory nerve
B. Cranial accessory nerve
C. Transverse cervical nerve
D. Greater auricular nerve

76. Perineural spread is commonly seen in:
A. Mucoepidermoid carcinoma
B. Ameloblastic carcinoma
C. Adenoid cystic carcinoma
D. Giant cell lesion

77. Giant cells are usually seen in all except:
A. Hyperparathyroidism
B. Aneurysmal bone cyst
C. Central giant cell granuloma
D. Fibrous dysplasia

78. Approaches to the TM joint includes:
A. Preauricular approach
B. Alkayat-Bramley approach
C. Endaural approach
D. All of the above

79. Minimal number of lag screws required to fix a symphysis fracture:
A. One
B. Two
C. Four
D. Three

80. **Muscle which is tested in forced adduction test is:**
    A. Superior oblique   B. Lateral rectus
    C. Inferior rectus   D. Medial rectus

81. **Medical line of treatment for retrobulbar hemorrhage includes:**
    A. Mannitol
    B. Mega dose steroid therapy
    C. Acetazolamide
    D. All of the above

82. **Anterior open bite is a classical sign of:**
    A. Bilateral displaced condylar fractures
    B. Symphysis fractures
    C. Angle fractures
    D. All of the above

83. **Trigger zones are seen in:**
    A. Bells palsy
    B. Trigeminal neuralgia
    C. Frey's syndrome
    D. All of the above

84. **Reed Steinberg's cells are kidney shaped cells, histopathologically seen in:**
    A. Paget's disease
    B. Fibrous dysplasia
    C. Hodgkin's disease
    D. Giant cell lesions

85. **Displacement of the fractured condyle usually occurs in which direction:**
    A. Anteromedial
    B. Lateral
    C. Posterior
    D. Superior

86. **Bilateral sagittal split osteotomy is used for correction of:**
    A. Mandibular prognathism
    B. Mandibular retrusion
    C. Anterior open bite
    D. All of the above

87. **Which of the following lesion has no epithelial lining?**
    A. Nasopalatine cyst
    B. Nasolabial cyst
    C. Aneurysmal bone cyst
    D. Dentigerous cyst

88. **Which of the following grafts has the greatest osteogenic potential?**
    A. Autogenous cortical bone
    B. Autogenous cancellous bone
    C. A freeze dried bone
    D. Xenograft

89. **Most common cause of TM joint ankylosis is:**
    A. Osteoarthritis
    B. Trauma
    C. Rheumatoid arthritis
    D. Illness during childhood

90. **Nerve affected in caldwel-luc operation is:**
    A. Facial   B. Lingual
    C. Infraorbital   D. Supraorbital

91. **Tear drop sign is seen in:**
    A. Blow out fractures
    B. Orbital flour fractures
    C. Le fort I fracture
    D. Frontal sinus fractures

92. **Mucoceles are commonly occurs in:**
    A. Floor of the mouth
    B. Tongue
    C. Lower lip
    D. Buccal mucosa

93. **Hyperbaric oxygen is used commonly in the treatment of:**
    A. Osteoradionecrosis   B. Oral cancer
    C. MPDS   D. OSMF

94. **Earliest sign of hemorrhagic shock is:**
    A. Hypotension   B. Vasoconstriction
    C. Tachycardia   D. Dyspnea

95. **The roof of pterygo – mandibular space is formed by:**
    A. Temporalis muscle
    B. Medial pterygoid muscle
    C. Cranial base
    D. Lateral pterygoid

96. **Erb's point is:**
    A. Where the spinal accessory nerve enters the posterior triangle.
    B. Where the common carotid artery bifurcates
    C. Where the spinal accessory nerve enters the sternocleidomastoid muscle
    D. Where the thoracic duct is located

97. Kaban's protocol is used for the treatment of:
A. TMJ ankylosis
B. Osteomyelitits of the jaws
C. Osteoradionecrosis of the jaws
D. All of the above

98. Oroantral fistula is common after extraction of:
A. First maxillary molar
B. Second maxillary molar
C. Third maxillary molar
D. Maxillary canine

99. Antrum of highmore is also called as:
A. Ethmoidal sinus
B. Maxillary sinus
C. Sphenoidal sinus
D. Frontal sinus

100. Anterior epistaxis is commonly due to injury to:
A. Kiesselbach's plexus
B. Pterygoid plexus
C. Pharyngeal plexus
D. All of the above.

ANSWERS

1 B	2 C	3 C	4 B	5 B	6 A	7 B	8 C
9 C	10 D	11 A	12 B	13 B	14 A	15 C	16 D
17 D	18 B	19 D	20 D	21 A	22 D	23 D	24 B
25 B	26 D	27 B	28 B	29 B	30 A	31 D	32 B
33 C	34 B	35 B	36 D	37 D	38 C	39 D	40 C
41 A	42 A	43 A	44 C	45 A	46 B	47 A	48 C
49 C	50 C	51 C	52 C	53 A	54 C	55 C	56 A
57 B	58 A	59 A	60 C	61 B	62 C	63 B	64 C
65 B	66 B	67 B	68 B	69 D	70 A	71 C	72 B
73 A	74 B	75 A	76 C	77 D	78 D	79 B	80 C
81 D	82 A	83 B	84 C	85 A	86 D	87 C	88 B
89 B	90 C	91 B	92 C	93 A	94 C	95 D	96 C
97 A	98 A	99 B	100 A				

Ophthalmology

1. **Characteristic oscillation in pendular nystagmus is:**
   - A. Slow eye movement away from the target
   - B. Rapid eye movement away from the target
   - C. Opposing movement one of equal speed
   - D. Both A and B one correct

2. **The fast component which determines the direction of Jerk nystagmus is:**
   - A. Pursuit
   - B. Saccades
   - C. Opsoclonus
   - D. Flutter

3. **Destructive disorder producing peripheral vestibular nystagmus is usually a jerk nystagmus, having:**
   - A. Slow components towards the affected ear
   - B. Fast component towards the affected ear
   - C. Pendular nystagmus
   - D. All above

4. **Alexander's law in nystagmus comprises:**
   - A. Gaze in the direction of fast components increases the nystagmus intensity
   - B. Gaze in the direction of slow component decreases the intensity of nystagmus
   - C. Gaze in the direction of slow component increases the intensity of nystagmus
   - D. Both A and B are correct

5. **Vogt-Koyanagi-Harada syndrome include:**
   - A. Vitiligo and poliosis
   - B. Chronic granulomatous iritis
   - C. Deafness
   - D. All above

6. **The tumor producing corneal anesthesia is:**
   - A. Pituitary adenoma
   - B. Pineoloma
   - C. Craniopharyngioma
   - D. Acoustic neuroma

7. **Cerebellopontine angle tumors produces:**
   - A. Ipsilateral deafness with vestibular signs
   - B. Hypoesthesia of face and corneal anesthesia
   - C. Ipsilateral paralysis of 6th and 7th cranial nerves
   - D. All above

8. **Which of the following is true about Gradenigo's syndrome?**
   - A. Occurs after middle ear infection
   - B. Produces diplopia
   - C. Ipsilateral facial pain
   - D. All above

9. **Nylen-Barany maneuver induces:**
   - A. Rotatary nystagmus
   - B. Vertical nystagmus
   - C. Jerk nystagmus
   - D. All above

10. **Which statement is true for myasthenia gravis?**
    - A. Never produces nystagmus
    - B. Horizontal or upbeat gaze paretic nystagmus
    - C. Produces congenital nystagmus
    - D. None above

11. **Symmetric gaze paretic nystagmus is produced by:**
    - A. Mental fatique
    - B. Barbiturates
    - C. Anticonvulsants and alcohol
    - D. All above

12. **Up beat nystagmus is caused by lesions that affect:**
    A. Cerebellum and thalamus
    B. Medulla and mid brain
    C. Both A and B
    D. None above

13. **Spasm nutans occurring in a child comprises:**
    A. Pendular nystagmus
    B. Head nodding
    C. Torticollis
    D. All above

14. **Which statement is true about see-saw nystagmus?**
    A. Disconjugate. vertical, pendular nystagmus
    B. Horizontal nystagmus
    C. Right beating nystagmus
    D. Left beating nystagmus

15. **Abducting nystagmus is a feature of:**
    A. Optic nerve glioma
    B. Internuclear ophthalmoplegia
    C. Trochlear nerve paralysis
    D. None above

16. **Horner's syndrome produces:**
    A. Constriction of pupil
    B. Dilatation of pupil
    C. Dilated and fixed pupil
    D. All above

17. **Which statement is true about Argyl Robertson pupil?**
    A. Pupil constricts better to near than to light
    B. Known as light near dissociation
    C. Pupil constricts better to light than to near
    D. Both A and B

18. **Involvement of 3rd cranial nerve is a feature of:**
    A. Common migraine
    B. Migraine with aura
    C. Ophthalmoplegic migraine
    D. None above

19. **Which statement is true about migraine with aura according to classification of international headache society?**
    A. Known as classic migraine
    B. Known as common migraine
    C. Tension type headache
    D. Cluster headache

20. **Scintillating scotoma, multicolored shimmering lights is a feature of:**
    A. Chronic paroxysmal hemicrania
    B. Common migraine
    C. Classic migraine
    D. All above

21. **Sumatriptan, a most effective agent to abort migraine with or without aura is a drug of:**
    A. Parasympathomimetic group
    B. Sympathomimetic group
    C. 5HT, agonist group
    D. None of the above

22. **Which statement is true about temporal arteritis?**
    A. Presence of pain or tenderness around temporal arteries
    B. Produces visual loss as a result of optic nerve or retinal ischemia
    C. 'A' and 'B' correct
    D. None above

23. **Sudden lancinating pain lasting only a few seconds, often recurs is features of:**
    A. Herpes zoster ophthalmicus
    B. Trigeminal neuralgia
    C. Optic neuritis
    D. None above

24. **Visual loss in systemic lupus erythematosus is due to:**
    A. Inflammatory or ischemic optic neuritis
    B. Papilledema
    C. Lens dislocation
    D. Retinal detachment

25. **The target organs commonly affected on sarcoidosis are:**
    A. Eye, lacrimal glands
    B. Lymph nodes, lungs
    C. Salivary glands
    D. All above

26. **Jaw claudication is a feature of:**
    A. Sjogren's syndrome
    B. Behcet's syndrome
    C. Vogt-Koyanagi-Harada syndrome
    D. Giant cell arteritis

27. **Which criteria is helpful for clinical diagnosis of Wegener's granulomatosis?**
    A. Oral ulcers or purulent bloody nasal discharge
    B. Chest radiographs that show nodules, infiltrates or cavities
    C. Microhematuria
    D. All above

28. **Blepharospasm is caused by contraction of:**
    A. Jaw muscles
    B. Levator palpebrae superioris
    C. Orbicularis muscles
    D. Mullers muscle

29. **Which statement is true about Alzheimer's disease?**
    A. Produces progressive neurologic disorder
    B. Produces neural disturbances, defective color vision
    C. Vestibular ocular reflex is normal
    D. All above

30. **Magnetic resonance imaging of brain showing infarction of occipital lobes, cavitary lesion of globus pallidus are seen in poisoning of:**
    A. Carbon monoxide
    B. Carbon dioxide
    C. Digitalis
    D. None above

31. **Pulsating exophthalmos seen occurring within hours is a feature of:**
    A. Pseudotumor of orbit
    B. Cavernous sinus thrombosis
    C. Meningioma of orbital roof
    D. Carotid cavernous fistula

32. **Orbital wall is formed by number of bones:**
    A. Five   B. Six
    C. Seven   D. Eight

33. **Features of orbital blow out fracture comprises:**
    A. Hanging drop appearance of maxillary sinus on radiograph
    B. Infraorbital anesthesia
    C. Restriction of ocular movements
    D. All above

34. **Maxillary antrum growth produces:**
    A. Upward proptosis of eye ball
    B. Downward proptosis of eye ball
    C. Axial proptosis of eye ball
    D. All above

35. **Structures passing through superior orbital fissure:**
    A. 3rd cranial nerve
    B. 6th cranial nerve
    C. 5th cranial nerve
    D. All above

36. **Internal carotid artery is seen:**
    A. Lateral wall of cavernous sinus
    B. Medial wall of cavernous sinus
    C. Floor of cavernous sinus
    D. In the substance of cavernous sinus

37. **The cranial nerves on the lateral wall of cavernous sinus are:**
    A. 3rd cranial nerve
    B. 4th cranial nerve
    C. 1st division of 5th cranial nerve
    D. All above

38. **Thinnest bone of the orbit:**
    A. Nasal bone   B. Lacrimal bone
    C. Lamina papyraceae   D. Palatine bone

39. **The commonest cause for orbital cellulitis in children:**
    A. Ethmoidal sinusitis
    B. Frontal sinusitis
    C. Maxillary sinusitis
    D. Sphenoidal sinusitis

40. **The length of nasolacrimal duct is:**
    A. 4 to 8 mm   B. 8 to 12 mm
    C. 12 to 24 mm   D. 24 to 32 mm

41. **The nerve supply of nasolacrimal duct:**
    A. Supratrochlear nerve
    B. Lacrimal nerve
    C. Infraorbital nerve
    A. Infratrochlear

42. **Optic canal is located between the two roots of:**
    A. Greater wing of sphenoid
    B. Body of sphenoid
    C. Lacrimal bone
    D. Lesser wing of sphenoid

43. **The disease characterized by symmetrical enlargement of lacrimal and salivary gland:**
    A. Harada syndrome
    B. Goldenhar's syndrome
    C. Sjögren's syndrome
    D. Mikulicz's syndrome

44. Epiphora is a symptom of:

A. Acute conjunctivitis
B. Chronic iritis
C. Acute glaucoma
D. Chronic dacryocystitis

45. The length of vertical portion of lacrimal canaliculi is:

A. 1 to 2 mm
B. 2 to 4 mm
C. 4 to 6 mm
D. 6 to 8 mm

46. The surgery for epiphora with canalicular block:

A. Canaliculo dacryocystorhinostomy
B. Conjunctivo dacryocystorhinostomy
C. Any of the above procedure depending the site of obstruction
D. None above

47. Treatment of acute dacryocystitis:

A. Broad spectrum antibiotics
B. Hot fomentation
C. Dacryocystectomy
D. Only a and b are correct

48. How many mm from inner canthus the lacrimal puncta lie on lid margin?

A. 2 mm
B. 6 mm
C. 12 mm
D. 24 mm

49. Normal lacrimal sac when distended is:

A. 15 mm long 5 to 6 mm wide
B. 25 mm long 15 to 20 mm wide
C. 35 mm long 20 to 25 mm wide
D. None above

50. Inflammation of lacrimal gland is known as:

A. Dacryocystitis
B. Lacrimal abscess
C. Mucocoele
D. dacryoadenitis

51. Treatment of congenital dacryocystitis:

A. Hydrostatic pressure
B. Probing of nasolacrimal duct
C. Endoscopic transnasal dacryocystorhinostomy
D. Only A and B are correct

52. Occlusion of the lacrimal puncta and canaliculi:

A. May be congenital
B. May be due to scar or foreign body
C. Less frequenty due to concretions
D. All above

53. The tributaries of the cavernous sinus are all *except:*

A. Superior ophthalmic vein
B. Superior petrosal sinus
C. Inferior ophthalmic vein
D. Angular vein

54. Clinical features of thrombosis of cavernous sinus:

A. Fever, headache and altered sensorium
B. Paralysis of opposite lateral rectus
C. Paresis of ocular motor nerves
D. All above

55. Which of the following is not true about Tolosa Hunt syndrome?

A. Painful ophthalmoplegia
B. Responds promptly to steroid treatment
C. Tolosa described a case in which granulation material was found around carotid artery in the cavernous sinus
D. Infraclinoid aneurysm

56. The orbital space occupying lesion in children:

A. Dermoid cyst
B. Histiocytosis
C. Rhabdo myosarcoma
D. All above

57. Kronlein's operation is:

A. Anterior orbitotomy
B. Transfrontal orbitotomy
C. Medial orbitotomy
D. Lateral orbitotomy

58. Loss of vision in fracture base of skull is due to:

A. Subconjunctival hemorrhage
B. Proptosis
C. Iritis
D. Shearing force injuring the vessels entering the optic nerve on its course in optic canal

59. Quadrantic homonymous hemianopia is produced in lesion of:

A. Optic nerve   B. Temporal lobe
C. Optic chiasma   D. None above

60. **Bitemporal hemianopia is usually caused by:**
   A. Tumors of pituitary
   B. Suprasellor tumors
   C. Lesion of the optic chiasma
   D. All above

61. **The clinical features of vertebrobasilar insufficiency:**
   A. Transient blurred vision
   B. Vertigo, ataxia
   C. Hemiparesis or hemisensory loss
   D. All above

62. **Basilar artery migraine:**
   A. Mimics vertebrobasilar artery insufficiency
   B. Bilateral blurring of vision
   D. All above
   D. None above

63. **In meningitis of middle ear origin, papillitis or papilledema is usually due to:**
   A. Sinus thrombosis   B. Cerebral abscess
   C. All above   D. None above

64. **Which statement is incorrect for multiple sclerosis?**
   A. Occurs in old age
   B. Produces limb weakness and sensory loss
   C. Produces retrobulbar neuritis
   D. Produces internuclear ophthalmoplegia

65. **Which is not true for tumors of parietal lobe?**
   A. Produces upper homonymous quadrantanopia
   B. Auditory hallucination
   C. Abnormal optokinetic response
   D. Upper fibers of optic radiation is involved

66. **Tumors of temporal lobe:**
   A. Produces upper quadrantanopia
   B. Produces visual hallucinations
   C. 3rd nerve may be involved
   D. All above

67. **Which statement is incorrect for Millard Gubler syndrome?**
   A. Lesion in the lower part of pons
   B. Lateral rectus is paralysed
   C. Ipsilateral facial nerve palsy and contralateral hemiplegia
   D. Contralateral facial nerve palsy

68. **Which statement is incorrect with tumors of auditory nerve in cerebellopontine angle?**
   A. Early tinnitus and deafness
   B. Nystagmus
   C. Sixth nerve is usually involved
   D. Corneal anesthesia is never seen

69. **Sunset sign is seen in:**
   A. Hydrocephaly
   B. Occipital lobe lesion
   C. Temporal lobe lesion
   D. None above

70. **Phacomatoses includes:**
   A. Neurofibromatosis
   B. Tuberous sclerosis
   C. von Hippel-Lindau syndrome
   D. All above

71. **Which is not true for Wilson's disease?**
   A. Kayser Fleischer's ring on cornea
   B. High serum caeruloplasmin
   C. Increased concentration of copper in liver biopsy
   D. Excessive copper deposited in brain tissue

72. **The features of Crouzon's disorder:**
   A. Maxillary hypoplasia
   B. Shallow orbits
   C. All above
   D. None above

73. **Facial N block is given by:**
   A. Van lint technique   B. O'brien technique
   C. Nadbath technique   D. All above

74. **Which statement is not true about basal cell carcinoma of lower lid?**
   A. Eearly edged ulcer with central crater that may bleed and crust
   B. May appear as discrete nodule or as a diffuse nodular mass usually on the lid margin
   C. Slow relentless growth over months
   D. Growth may be rapid over few weeks

75. **All of the following structures are located in the lateral wall of cavernous sinus except:**
   A. Optic nerve
   B. Oculomotor nerve
   C. Trochlear nerve
   D. Abducent nerve

76. The average volume of the orbit is:
- A. 6 cc
- B. 12 cc
- C. 30 cc
- D. 40 cc

77. Slow progressive, painless proptosis with downward displacement of globe is seen:
- A. Carcinoma maxillary sinus
- B. Pseudotumor of orbit
- C. Mucocoele of ethmoidal sinus
- D. Mucocoele of frontal sinus

78. Antimongoloid eye position, malformation of external ear and deafness; epibulbar lipodermoid adjacent to limbus are characteristic feature of:
- A. Refsum's syndrome
- B. Usher's syndrome
- C. Goldenhar's syndrome
- D. Greig's syndrome

79. Esinophilic granuloma triad is:
- A. Bony lesion, diabetes mellitus and exophthalmus
- B. Bony lesion, diabetes insipidus and exophtalmus
- C. Bony lesion, diabetes insipidus and ptosis
- D. None above

80. The characteristic location of sphenoidal meningioma in orbital diseases is:
- A. Intraconal
- B. Muscular
- C. Extraconal
- D. All above

81. Café-au-lait spots, optic nerve glioma, sphenoid bone defect causing pulsating proptosis are characteristic of:
- A. Orbital varices
- B. Tuberous sclerosis
- C. Lymphoma of orbit
- D. Neurofibromatosis type 1

82. The upper normal limit of exophthalmometry of the Hertel instrument is:
- A. 10 mm
- B. 18 mm
- C. 28 mm
- D. 30 mm

83. Which wall of the orbit is situated anteroposteriorly in the sagittal plane:
- A. Medial wall
- B. Lateral wall
- C. Floor
- D. Roof

84. Light near dissociation, pinealomas and hydrocephalus absent poor upgaze and convergence retraction nystagmus are feature of:
- A. Parinaud's syndrome
- B. Horner's syndrome
- C. Weber's syndrome
- D. None above

85. Combined horizontal pontine gaze paresis with an internuclear ophthalmoplegia is:
- A. One and a half syndrome
- B. Double syndrome
- C. One-half syndrome
- D. None above

86. Internuclear ophthalmoplegia is due to:
- A. Abducens nuclear lesion
- B. Combined PPRF and MLF lesion
- C. PPRF lesion
- D. MLF lesion

87. Sphenoid ridge meningioma producing ophthalmoplegia due to ocular motor nerves compression is:
- A. Orbital apex syndrome
- B. Eaton lambert syndrome
- C. Superior orbital fissure syndrome
- D. None above

88. Third cranial nerve palsy with contralateral cerebeller ataxia and tremors; involvement of the red nucleus is:
- A. Weber's syndrome
- B. Benedikt's syndrome
- C. Raynaud syndrome
- D. None above

89. Bielschowsky head tilt test is done for:
- A. Oculomotor nerve palsy
- B. Trochlear nerve palsy
- C. Abducent nerve palsy
- D. none above

90. The condition which is first unilateral but becomes bilateral very soon:
- A. Orbital cellulitis
- B. Panopthalmitis
- C. Cavernous sinus thrombosis
- D. All above

91. The features of Usher's syndrome are:
A. Retinitis pigmentosa
B. Sensorineural deafness
C. Both A and B
D. None above

92. Nasolacrimal duct is directed:
A. Downward outward and backward
B. Downward, inward and backward
C. Downward, outward and forward
D. Downward, inward and forward

93. The valve of Hasner in nasolacrimal duct is present at:
A. Upper end   B. Lower end
C. Middle   D. None above

94. Tuberous sclerosis is characterized by:
A. Adenoma sebaceum
B. Mental retardation and seizures
C. Retinal astrocytoma
D. All above

95. Lisch nodules in iris is seen:
A. Medulloepithelioma
B. Granulomatous iritis
C. Keratitis
D. Neurofibromatosis

96. Swelling behind the ear is diagnostic of (mastoid edema):
A. Orbital cellulitis
B. Cavernous sinus thrombosis
C. Bilateral proptosis
D. Pseudotumor of orbit

97. Tears are produced in newborn after:
A. 1 month   B. 2 months
C. 3 months   D. 4 months

98. The most common tumor of lacrimal gland is:
A. Squamous cell carcinoma
B. Basal cell carcinoma
C. Mikulicz syndrome
D. Mixed tumor

99. Synkinetic ptosis is seen in:
A. Myasthenia gravis
B. Marcus gunn phenomenon
C. Bell's palsy
D. All above

100. The feature of pseudotumor cerebri:
A. Headache getting worse during valsalva maneuvre
B. Transient obscuration of vision
C. Occasional diplopia due to 6th nerve palsy
D. All above

101. Ocular involvement of AIDS:
A. Cotton wool spots in retina
B. Cytomegaloretinitis
C. Acute retinal necrosis
D. All above

102. Neurogenic hyposecretin of lacrimal gland is due to lesion of:
A. Frontal nerve
B. Pterygopalatine ganglion
C. Edinger westphal nucleus
D. None above

103. The condition causing congenital hyposecretion of lacrimal gland:
A. Stevens Johnson syndrome
B. Familial dysautonomia (Riley day syndrome)
C. Sjögren's syndrome
D. None above

104. Ishihara test is used to diagnose:
A. Visual acuity
B. Color vision
C. Field of vision
D. All above

105. The retinal sensitivity (threshold) in Auto-perimetry is measured in:
A. Decibel (dB)   B. Diopter
C. Prism diopter   D. All above

ANSWERS

1 C	2 B	3 A	4 D	5 D	6 D	7 D	8 D
9 B	10 B	11 D	12 C	13 D	14 A	15 B	16 A
17 D	18 C	19 A	20 C	21 C	22 C	23 B	24 A
25 D	26 D	27 D	28 C	29 D	30 A	31 D	32 C
33 D	34 A	35 D	36 B	37 D	38 C	39 A	40 C
41 C	42 D	43 D	44 D	45 A	46 C	47 D	48 B
49 A	50 D	51 D	52 D	53 D	54 D	55 D	56 D
57 D	58 D	59 B	60 D	61 D	62 C	63 C	64 D
65 A	66 D	67 D	68 D	69 A	70 D	71 B	72 C
73 D	74 D	75 A	76 C	77 D	78 C	79 D	80 C
81 D	82 B	83 A	84 A	85 A	86 D	87 C	88 B
89 B	90 C	91 C	92 A	93 B	94 D	95 D	96 B
97 A	98 D	99 B	100 D	101 D	102 B	103 B	104 B
105 A							

Neurosurgery

1. **An otolaryngological cause of Gradenigo syndrome is:**
   A. Pontine Glioma
   B. Metastatic tumor from nasopharynx
   C. Petrositis
   D. Fracture base of skull

2. **Anterior cranial fossa fracture commonly associated with:**
   A. Black eye(Raccoon eye)
   B. CSF rhinorrhea
   C. Subconjuctival hemorrhage
   D. Blindness of the eye

3. **CSF Rhinorrhea is confirmed by all *except:***
   A. Halo sign
   B. Glucose content more than 30 mgs/dl
   C. Glucose content less than 10 mgs/dl
   D. Beta -2 transferrin

4. **Transverse fracture of the petrous bone will produce the following *except:***
   A. Otorrhea
   B. Battle sign
   C. Tenderness over temporomandibular joint
   D. Bleeding over the tympanic membrane

5. **Anosmia is produced by a lesion without local abnormality in:**
   A. Fracture anterior cranial fossa through cribriform plate
   B. Olfactory groove meningioma
   C. Allergic rhinitis
   D. To and fro movement of the brain

6. **Intracranial complication of mastoiditis are all *except:***
   A. Lateral sinus thrombosis
   B. Temporal lobe abscess
   C. Gradenigo syndrome
   D. Ninth nerve palsy

7. **Basal meningitis with multiple cranial nerve involvement is produced by all *except:***
   A. Tuberculous meningitis
   B. Carcinomatous meningitis
   C. Maxillary sinusitis
   D. Meningovascular syphilis

8. **Facial pain with impaired sensation and numbness over the face is produced by:**
   A. Trigeminal neuralgia
   B. Atypical facial pain
   C. Intracranial infiltration of nasopharyngeal carcinoma
   D. Temporal arteritis

9. **Otolaryngological cause of vertigo is:**
   A. Acoustic neuroma
   B. Vestibular Neuronitis
   C. Migraine
   D. Complex partial seizures

10. **Paroxysmal pain in the region of the tonsil, posterior pharyngeal wall, back of the tongue and middle ear is commonly produced by:**
    A. Trigeminal neuralgia
    B. Jugular foramen tumor
    C. Glossopharyngeal neuralgia
    D. Ramsay-Hunt syndrome

11. A congenital intracranial tumor which is found in the ear also is:

A. Teretoma
B. Dermoid
C. Epidermoid
D. Chordoma

12. Nine, tenth, eleventh and twelfth cranial nerve palsies with Horner's syndrome is seen in:

A. Vernets syndrome
B. Villarets syndrome
C. Cerebello pontine angle syndrome
D. Collet sicard syndrome

13. Ramsay-Hunt syndrome is caused by:

A. Bacterial infection
B. Parasitic infection
C. Viral infection
D. Tuberculous infection

14. Infection from dangerous area of face commonly spreads to cause:

A. Superior sagittal sinus thrombosis
B. Cavernous sinus thrombosis
C. Lateral sinus thrombosis
D. Middle cerebral vein thrombosis

15. The predisposing diseases to produce Bell's palsy are all *except*:

A. Diabetes insipidus
B. Geniculate herpes
C. CP angle tumor
D. Exposure to cold

16. Tinnitus is caused by all *except*:

A. CP angle acoustic neuroma
B. Repeated exposure to noise
C. Menier's disease
D. Psychomotor epilepsy

17. Gradenigo syndrome is caused by all *except*:

A. Mastoiditis
B. Fracture petrous bone
C. Otitis media
D. Intraorbital cellutis

18. Otitic hydrocephalus is most commonly produced by:

A. Cavernous sinus thrombosis
B. Petrous sinus thrombosis
C. Lateral sinus thrombosis
D. Superior sagittal sinus thrombosis

19. Ramsay-Hunt syndrome is caused by a lesion in the:

A. Sphenopalatine ganglion
B. Gasserian ganglion
C. Geniculate ganglion
D. Pterygopalatine ganglion

20. Temporal lobe abscess caused by otitis media is:

A. *Staphylococcus*
B. Pneumonia
C. Enteric bacteria
D. *Streptococcus*

21. Sensory neural deafness is produced by all *except*:

A. Otitis media
B. Mumps
C. Acoustic neuroma
D. Streptomycin toxicity

22. Tinnitus deafness and vertigo is caused by all *except*:

A. Herpes zoster of ganglia of corti and scarpa
B. Menier's disease
C. Otitis media
D. Acoustic neurinoma

23. Dysphagia is caused by all *except*:

A. Collet-Sicaral syndrome
B. Progressive bulbar palsy of lower motor neuron type
C. Glossitis
D. Myasthenia gravis

24. Ramsay-Hunt syndrome is characterized by:

A. Sixth nerve palsy
B. Third nerve palsy
C. Lower motor neuron type of facial palsy
D. Upper motor neuron type of facial palsy

25. Frontal sinusitis produces:

A. Seasonal headache
B. Perodic headache
C. Tension headache
D. Pressure headache

26. Frontal sinusitis produces:

A. Cerebellar abscess
B. Temporal lobe abscess
C. Frontal lobe abscess
D. Parietal lobe abscess

27. **Neurological complication of mastoidectomy is:**
   A. Fifth cranial nerve palsy
   B. Seventh cranial nerve palsy
   C. Eighth cranial nerve palsy
   D. Nineth, tenth, eleventh cranial nerve palsies

28. **CSF rhinorrhea is produced by fracture of all except:**
   A. Anterior cranial fossa B. Roof of ethmoid
   C. Cribriform plate   D. Zygomatic bone

29. **Inracranial extension of infection to produce brain abscess is all except:**
   A. Metastasis
   B. Trauma
   C. Osteomyelitis of adjacent skull bones
   D. Intracranial surgery

30. **Otorrhea is produced by all except:**
   A. Middle cranial fossa fracture
   B. Petrous bone fracture
   C. Occipital bone fracture
   D. Defect in the external auditory canal wall

31. **The investigation of choice for the diagnosis of acoustic neuroma is:**
   A. X-ray skull
   B. MRI with gadolinium contrast
   C. CT scan brain
   D. Cerebral angiography

32. **Enlargement of the internal auditory meatus in acoustic neuroma can be clearly seen in the following views of X-ray skull except:**
   A. Towne's view
   B. Stenwer's view
   C. Skull PA projection
   D. Tomogram in the coronal plane

33. **Intracanalicular acoustic neuroma with sparing of hearing is excised in collaboration with an otologists through the following approach:**
   A. Suboccipital transmeatal approach
   B. Middle cranial fossa approach
   C. Translabyrinthine approach
   D. Radiosurgery

34. **Acoustic neuroma arises from:**
   A. Laterally near the inner ear
   B. Entirely within the CP angle
   C. Medially at porous acousticus
   D. Schwan cell-glial junction in the vicinity of the vestibular division of the eighth cranial nerve in the internal auditory canal

35. **The growth rate of acoustic neuroma in tumor diameter is:**
   A. 0.5 cm to 0.75 cm per year
   B. 1 cm to 2 cm per year
   C. 0.25 cm to 0.4 cm per year
   D. 2 cm to 4 cm per year

36. **The size of an acoustic neuroma is commonly expressed by the following tumor dimensions except:**
   A. Anteroposterior (parallel to the petrous ridge)
   B. Medial-lateral (perpendicular to petrous ridge)
   C. Irregular in shape
   D. Superior-inferior

37. **The internal auditory canal is traversed by the following structures except:**
   A. Vestibular nerve B. Facial nerve
   C. Abducent nerve   D. Cochlear nerve

38. **The rare stage of acoustic neuroma growth is:**
   A. Canalicular
   B. Cisternal
   C. Brainstem compression
   D. Jugular foramen compression

39. **The size of the canalicular acoustic neuroma is:**
   A. 2 cm to 3 cm   B. 1 cm to 2 cm
   C. 3 cm to 4 cm   D. Exceeding 4 cm

40. **The internal auditory artery which traverses through the internal acoustic meatus along with cranial nerves is a branch of:**
   A. Posterior inferior cerebellar artery
   B. Superior cerebellar artery
   C. Anterior inferior cerebellar artery
   D. Vertebral artery

41. **An audiological test which is abnormal in 100% of cases of acoustic neurinoma is:**
   A. Pure tone audiometry
   B. Caloric tests
   C. Loudness recruitment test
   D. Tuning fork test

42. **Auditory brainstem evoked response is useful in the diagnosis of acoustic neuroma by the presence of changes in:**
   A. Wave one—cochlear nerve
   B. Wave three—superior colliculus
   C. Wave five—inferior colliculus
   D. Absence of all waves after wave one

43. **The common operative approach for the excision of acoustic neuroma are all *except*:**
    A. Sub occipital [retrosigmoid]
    B. Translabrynthine [anterosigmoid]
    C. Middle fossa [subtemporal]
    D. Stereotactic radio surgery

44. **The size of the acoustic neuroma which can be undetected by CT scan even with contrast is:**
    A. 1.5 cm to 2 cm   B. 2 cm to 3 cm
    C. 0.9 cm to 1 cm   D. 3 cm to 4 cm

45. **During acoustic neuroma surgery, preservation of facial nerve function is related to all *except*:**
    A. Tumor size
    B. Anatomic integrity of the nerve
    C. Biological behavior of the tumor [adherent or easily dissectable]
    D. Surgical technique

46. **The common sites of fracture to produce CSF rhinorrhea are all *except*:**
    A. Fracture of ethmoid bone
    B. Fracture of cribriform plate
    C. Fracture of orbital plate of frontal bone
    D. Fracture of Tegman tympani

47. **The investigation of choice in identifying the site of CSF leak is:**
    A. X-ray skull with loss or deformity of normal bone laminae
    B. Insufflation of air into the subdural space
    C. Iohexol-enhanced computed tomography
    D. Radioisotope cisternography

48. **Otorrhea is commonly produced by:**
    A. Middle cranial fossa fracture
    B. Longitudinal fracture of petrous bone
    C. Fracture Tegmen tympani
    D. Rupture of tympanic membrane

49. **The common intracranial tumor which protrudes through the external auditory meatus is:**
    A. Acoustic neuroma
    B. Cholesteatoma
    C. Meningioma
    D. Glomus jugulare tumor

50. **Nonoperative treatment of cerebrospinal fluid fistula are all *except*:**
    A. Head elevation to thirty degree to forty degree
    B. Continuous lumbar drainage
    C. Diamox, gardinal and lasix
    D. Antibiotics

51. **Operative procedure of choice for cerebrospinal fluid fistula are all *except*:**
    A. Ventriculo peritoneal shunt
    B. Lumboperitoneal shunt
    C. Direct repair through extradural approach
    D. Endoscopic repair

52. **Indication for operative management of cerebrospinal fistulae are all *except*:**
    A. Failure of conservative management
    B. Persistent and copious CSF leakage or very large fistula site
    C. Recurring meningitis
    D. Epilepsy

53. **The common substances used for sealing the CSF fistulae are all *except*:**
    A. Cyanoacrylate monomer
    B. Fascia lata femoris
    C. Temporalis fascia
    D. Muscle or fat

54. **The commonest complications of untreated CSF fistulae are all *except*:**
    A. Recurring meningitis
    B. Low pressure headache
    C. Anosmia
    D. Pneumocephalus

55. **The glomus jugulare tumor is:**
    A. Carotid body like tumor
    B. Glomus tympanicus tumor
    C. Chemodectoma
    D. Pheochromocytoma

56. **The investigation of choice in the diagnosis of the glomus jugulare tumor is:**
    A. X-ray skull
    B. Computed tomography of brain
    C. Jugulare phlebography
    D. Magnetic resonance imaging of brains and neck with angiography

57. The best operative approach to remove a large glomus jugulare tumor is:
A. Lateral skull base approach
B. Infratemporal fossa approach
C. Medial lateral skull base approach
D. Suboccipital approach

58. Chronic otitis media causing brain abscess is in:
A. Frontal lobe
B. Temporal lobe
C. Parietal lobe
D. Occipital lobe

59. Mastoiditis causes brain abscess in:
A. Parietal lobe
B. Frontal lobe
C. Cerebellum
D. Temporal lobe

60. Temporal bone fracture producing CSF oto-rhinorrhea through:
A. Frontal sinus through nasofrontal duct
B. Ethmoidal sinus through ethmoid roof
C. Mastoid air cells through Eustachian tube
D. Sphenoid sinus

61. The investigation of choice in localization of even inactive sites of CSF leakage is:
A. High resolution thin section contrast enhancing computed tomography
B. X-ray skull or polytomography
C. Radioisotope scanning
D. MRI cisternography

62. Bleeding from ear due to temporal bone fracture can be confirmed by all except:
A. Facial nerve palsy
B. Conductive hearing loss
C. Tenderness over temporomandibular joint
D. Battle's sign [retroauricular ecchymosis]

63. Vestibular dysfunction, acute vertigo, sensory neuronal hearing loss and seventh nerve palsy is caused by:
A. Middle cranial fossa fracture
B. Otic capsule-sparing fractures
C. Occipital bone fracture
D. Otic capsule disrupting fractures

64. Timing of surgery for cerebrospinal fluid leak is:
A. Within 24 hours   B. Within 5 to 7 days
C. Within 10 to 13 days   D. Within 2 to 4 days

ANSWERS

1 B	2 D	3 C	4 C	5 D	6 D	7 C	8 C
9 B	10 C	11 C	12 B	13 C	14 B	15 A	16 D
17 D	18 C	19 C	20 C	21 A	22 C	23 C	24 C
25 B	26 C	27 B	28 D	29 D	30 C	31 B	32 C
33 A	34 C	35 C	36 C	37 C	38 D	39 B	40 C
41 A	42 D	43 D	44 C	45 B	46 D	47 C	48 B
49 B	50 D	51 C	52 D	53 A	54 C	55 C	56 D
57 B	58 B	59 C	60 C	61 D	62 C	63 D	64 C

Miscellaneous-I

1. **The most common cause of acquired postlingual deafness in children is:**
   A. ASOM
   B. Secretory otitis media
   C. Meningitis
   D. Ototoxicity

2. **The most common cause of mucoepidermoid carcinoma is:**
   A. Parotid gland
   B. Submandibular gland
   C. Sublingual gland
   D. Minor salivary gland

3. **Most common cause of acute simultaneous bilateral facial palsy is:**
   A. Bells palsy
   B. Guillain-Barré syndrome
   C. Melkerson-Rosenthal syndrome
   D. Ramsay-Hunt syndrome

4. **The length of fallopian canal is:**
   A. 5 mm
   B. 10 mm
   C. 20 mm
   D. 30 mm

5. **The most common childhood malignancy in head and neck is:**
   A. Rhabdomyosarcoma
   B. Osteosarcoma
   C. Chondrosarcoma
   D. Lymphosarcoma

6. **The type of Hodgkin's lymphoma having best prognosis is in:**
   A. Lymphocytic predominant
   B. Lymphocytic depleted
   C. Nodular sclerosis
   D. Mixed cellularity

7. **Carhart's notch in otosclerosis is most commonly seen at:**
   A. 1 KHZ
   B. 2 KHZ
   C. 3 KHZ
   D. 4 KHZ

8. **The least common complication of CSOM is:**
   A. Lateral sinus thrombosis
   B. Otitic hydrocephalus
   C. Labrynthitis
   D. Brain abscess

9. **The most severe type of congenital dysplasia of labyrinth is:**
   A. Michele dysplasia
   B. Mondini dysplasia
   C. Bing-siebenmann dysplasia
   D. Scheibe dysplasia

10. **The most common virus causing sensorineural deafness is:**
    A. Rubella
    B. Rhino virus
    C. Para influenza virus
    D. Cytomegalovirus

11. **The first nerve to be myelinated in CNS is:**
    A. Facial nerve
    B. Cochlear nerve
    C. Vestibular nerve
    D. Olfactory nerve

12. **The commonest craniofacial syndrome is:**
    A. Down's syndrome
    B. Edwards syndrome
    C. Treacher-Collins syndrome
    D. Crouzan's syndrome

13. **The most effective way of testing nonorganic hearing loss is:**
    A. Pure tone audiometry
    B. Impedance audiometry
    C. BERA
    D. Speech audiometry

14. **External frontoethmoidectomy is otherwise known as:**
    A. Lynch-Howarth operation
    B. Jansen-Horgan operation
    C. McBeth's operation
    D. Denker's operation

15. **The most common benign neoplasm of nose and PNS is:**
    A. Angioma
    B. Osteoma
    C. Inverted papilloma
    D. Fibroma

16. **The commonest isolated single cranial nerves to be involved in nasopharyngeal cancer are:**
    A. V and VI
    B. VII and VIII
    C. IX and X
    D. XI and XII

17. **The diagnostic titer of viral capsid antigen to TgA in nasopharyngeal cancer is:**
    A. 1/10
    B. 1/20
    C. 1/30
    D. 1/40

18. **Michulitz cells in rhinoscleroma are to be demonstrated for:**
    A. Stage 1
    B. Stage 2
    C. Stage 3
    D. Stage 4

19. **Coffin's corners is related to:**
    A. Base of tongue
    B. Pyriform fossa
    C. Ventricle of larynx
    D. Retromolar trigone

20. **Klebs-Loeffler bacillus is otherwise known as:**
    A. Corynebacterium diphtheria
    B. Frisch's bacillus
    C. Mycobacterium tuberculosis
    D. Friedlander's bacillus

21. **Verrucae body is found in:**
    A. Glommus tumor
    B. Schwanomas
    C. Sarcoidosis
    D. Rhinoscleroma

22. **Meckels cave is related to:**
    A. Otic ganglion
    B. Geniculate ganglion
    C. Spiral ganglion
    D. Gasserian ganglion

23. **Cartilage of santorini is otherwise known as:**
    A. Corniculate cartilage
    B. Cuneiform cartilage
    C. Aryterial cartilage
    D. Cricoid cartilage

24. **All the following reticulo-endothelial diseases are components of histocytosis-x *except*:**
    A. Eosinohillic granuloma
    B. Wegners granuloma
    C. Hand-schuller-christian disease
    D. Letterer-sieve disease

25. **All the following hereditary syndromal disease usually cause sensoneural deafness *except*:**
    A. Wardenberg syndrome
    B. Alports syndrome
    C. Treacher Collins syndrome
    D. Ushers syndrome

26. **All the following classification are used for non-Hodgkin's lymphoma *except*:**
    A. Kiel's classification
    B. Luke-Collin classification
    C. Ruppaport classification
    D. Rye classification

27. **The classification used for craniofacial defects is:**
    A. Sunderland's classification
    B. Ohngren's classification
    C. Ledermann's classification
    D. Tessier's classification

28. **All the following statements regarding Lymes disease are true *except*:**
    A. Its otherwise known as Bannwarth's syndrome
    B. It's a viral disease
    C. It causes facial palsy
    D. Its characterized by erythema chronicum migrans

29. **All the following foramens are related to CSF circulation *except*:**
    A. Foramen of Luschka
    B. Foramen of magendi
    C. Foramen of monro
    D. Foramen of morgagni

30. **All the following statements are true regarding fossa of Rosenmuller *except*:**
   A. It's otherwise known as pharyngeal recess
   B. Its present behind the posterior margins of torustubaris
   C. It's a common site for nasopharyngeal cancer
   D. It opens above the foramen lacerum

31. **Birbeks granules are found in:**
   A. Langerhans cells
   B. Plasma cells
   C. Myoepithelial cells
   D. Acinar cells

32. **Loop of Galen is related to:**
   A. Trigeminal nerve
   B. Facial nerve
   C. Vagus nerve
   D. Hypoglossal nerve

33. **All the following surgical procedures are indicated for zenkers diverticulum *except*:**
   A. Frenkner's operation
   B. Dohlman's operation
   C. Glasscock's operation
   D. Goldman's operation

34. **Phelp's sign on lateral tomography is seen on:**
   A. Vestibular schwanoma
   B. Glomus jugulare
   C. Nasopharyngeal angiofibroma
   D. Parapharyngeal tumors

35. **Thumb sign is the radiological picture seen in:**
   A. Acute epiglottitis
   B. Acute laryngitis
   C. Tuberculosis laryngitis
   D. Quinsy

36. **Cozzolino's zone is related to:**
   A. Meniere's disease
   B. Meniere's syndrome
   C. Otosclerosis
   D. None of the above

37. **The most suitable approach for small intracanalicular acoustic neuroma:**
   A. Translabrynthine approach
   B. Retrosigmoid approach
   C. Suboccipital approach
   D. Middle cranial fossa approach

38. **Petrous apex cholesterol granulomas exhibit which of the following characteristics?**
   A. The substrate is isodense with CSF
   B. They have a non-enhancing rim
   C. They occur in poorly pneumatised petrous apex
   D. The substrate is isodense with brain

39. **All the following statements about glommus tumor is true *except*:**
   A. Its otherwise known as paraganglioma
   B. 10% of them are with synchronous lesions
   C. 3% of them metastatize
   D. 20% of them produce catacholamines

40. **The most accurate test in diagnosis of acoustic neuroma is:**
   A. Auditory brainstem response (ABR)
   B. CT with contrast
   C. MRI with gadolinium
   D. Bekesy's audiometry

41. **Ground glass appearance in CT is seen in:**
   A. Stewart granuloma
   B. Fibrous dysplasia
   C. Wegner's granuloma
   D. Benign giantcell repairative granuloma

42. **The salivary gland cell most frequently affected by radiotherapy is:**
   A. Acinar cells   B. Myoepithelial cells
   C. Intercalated cells   D. Duct cells

43. **In salivary gland malignancy, facial paralysis is more common in:**
   A. Adenocystic carcinoma
   B. Mucoepidermoid cancer
   C. Oncocytic cancer
   D. Squamous cell cancer

44. **All the following drugs can cause sialomegaly *except*:**
   A. Thiouracil   B. Phenyl butazone
   C. Iodide   D. Biguanides

45. **All the following are present in Sjogren's syndrome *except*:**
   A. Kerato conjunctivitis
   B. Sarcoidosis
   C. Xerostomia
   D. Rheumatoid arthritis

46. Swiss cheese appearance on histopathological examination is found in:
  A. Adenocarcinoma
  B. Oncocytic carcinoma
  C. Adenocystic carcinoma
  D. Mucoepidermoid carcinoma

47. The LASER used in photodynamic therapy is:
  A. Tunable dye laser   B. CO_2 laser
  C. Krypton laser   D. Nd:Yag laser

48. The gas used in cryo unit is:
  A. Carbon dioxide   B. Nitrous oxide
  C. Nitrogen   D. Carbon monoxide

49. Which of the following cells is more radiosensitive?
  A. Muscle cells
  B. Bone cells
  C. Lymph nodes
  D. Connective tissue cells

50. TiS lesion over vocal cords should be best treated with:
  A. Radiotherapy
  B. Chemotherapy
  C. Total laryngetomy
  D. Stripping of cord

ANSWERS

1 C	2 A	3 B	4 D	5 A	6 A	7 B	8 B
9 A	10 D	11 C	12 D	13 C	14 A	15 C	16 A
17 A	18 C	19 D	20 A	21 B	22 D	23 A	24 B
25 C	26 D	27 D	28 B	29 D	30 D	31 A	32 C
33 A	34 B	35 A	36 C	37 D	38 D	39 D	40 C
41 B	42 A	43 A	44 D	45 B	46 C	47 A	48 B
49 C	50 D						

Miscellaneous-II

1. **"Steeple sign" appearance of airway in X-ray neck-A P view is diagnostic of:**
   - A. ALTBS
   - B. Acute epiglottitis
   - C. Subglottic edema
   - D. Laringismus stridulus

2. **Collagen disease most commonly affecting esophagus is:**
   - A. Scleroderma
   - B. SLE
   - C. Poly arteritis nodosa
   - D. Wegner's disease

3. **Common site of unknown primary in secondaries neck are all *except*:**
   - A. Pyriform fossa
   - B. Posterior third tongue growth
   - C. Nasopharynx
   - D. Glottis

4. **Maximum stridor occurs in which type of the vocal cord palsy:**
   - A. Unilateral complete paralysis
   - B. Unilateral incomplete paralysis
   - C. Bilateral complete paralysis
   - D. Bilateral incomplete paralysis

5. **Signet shaped cartilage in larynx is:**
   - A. Thyroid
   - B. Cricoid
   - C. Cuneiform
   - D. Corneculate

6. **Lateralization of vocal cord is done for:**
   - A. Bilateral abductor palsy
   - B. Bilateral adductor palsy
   - C. Unilateral abductor palsy
   - D. Unilateral adductor palsy

7. **Blackish nasal discharge in an elderly diabetic is due to:**
   - A. Mucormycosis
   - B. Candidiasis
   - C. Histoplasmosis
   - D. Aspergilosis

8. **Earliest symptom of acoustic neuroma is:**
   - A. Deafness
   - B. Tinnitus
   - C. Vertigo
   - D. Facial weakness

9. **Genetic disorder of deafness after birth are all *except:***
   - A. Alport syndrome
   - B. Cogan syndrome
   - C. Usher's syndrome
   - D. Refsum's disease

10. **Battle's sign is seen in:**
    - A. Middle cranial fossa fracture
    - B. Anterior cranial fossa fracture
    - C. Posterior cranial fossa fracture
    - D. All of the above

11. **Ramadier's operation is done in:**
    - A. Meniere's diseases
    - B. Bell's palsy
    - C. Petrositis
    - D. None of the above

12. **Cochlear implant is introduced in:**
    - A. Oval window
    - B. Round window
    - C. Internal auditory meatus
    - D. Lateral semicircular canal

13. **Angular movements are tracked by:**
    - A. Utricle
    - B. Saccule
    - C. Semicircular canal
    - D. All of the above

14. "Drop attacks" are characteristic of:
    A. Otosclerosis
    B. Meniere's disease
    C. Vestibular neuronitis
    D. Acoustic neuroma

15. The chromosome associated with Meniere's disease is:
    A. Chromosome 7   B. Chromosome 14
    C. Chromosome 18   D. Chromosome 11

16. Otoacoustic emissions are sound arising from:
    A. Inner hair cells
    B. Outer hair cells
    C. Both inner and outer haircells
    D. None of the above

17. Valvasori criteria is useful in the diagnosis of:
    A. Acoustic neuroma
    B. Otosclerosis
    C. Meniere's disease
    D. None of the above

18. Trautman's triangle is formed by all except:
    A. Superior petrosal sinus
    B. Sigmoid sinus
    C. Lateral semicircular canal
    D. Bony labyrinth

19. Middle ear ossicles are fully developed at the fetal age:
    A. 8 weeks   B. 12 weeks
    C. 16 weeks   D. 20 weeks

20. The sinus not present at birth is:
    A. Maxillary   B. Frontal
    C. Ethmoid   D. Sphenoid

21. The first step in FESS is:
    A. Ethmoidectomy
    B. Uncinectomy
    C. Bullectomy
    D. Middle meatal antrostomy

22. The commonest site of osteoma of PNS is:
    A. Maxillary   B. Frontal
    C. Ethmoid   D. Sphenoid

23. T_{is} lesion over vocal cord is best treated by:
    A. Radiotherapy
    B. Chemotherapy
    C. Stripping of cord
    D. Total laryngectomy

24. Which of the following is used in photodynamic therapy?
    A. Tunable dye laser
    B. CO_2 laser
    C. Nd. YAG laser
    D. Krypton laser

25. Which of the following is most radiosensitive?
    A. Lymphocytes
    B. Muscle cells
    C. Bone cells
    D. Connective tissue cells

26. The commonest childhood soft tissue tumor in head and neck is:
    A. Chondrosarcoma
    B. Osteosarcoma
    C. Rhabdomyosarcoma
    D. Lymphosarcoma

27. Synchronous lesions in paraganglioma is found in:
    A. 2%   B. 5%
    C. 10%   D. 20%

28. Ground glass appearance on CT scan is found in:
    A. Fibrous dysplasia
    B. Osteoma
    C. Angiofibroma
    D. Cystic hygroma

29. The most accurate test in the diagnosis of acoustic neuroma is:
    A. ABR   B. MRI
    C. CT scan   D. MRI with gadolinium

30. Incidence of catecholamine secreting glomus tumor is:
    A. 1%   B. 3%
    C. 8%   D. 10%

31. Histiocytosis 'X' does not include:
    A. Eosinophillic granuloma
    B. Wegner's granuloma
    C. Hand schuller christian complex
    D. Letter-swierer disease

32. **Birbek granules on electron microscopy is found in:**
    A. Glomous tumor
    B. Cholesterol granuloma
    C. Steward granuloma
    D. Langerhan cell histiocytosis

33. **Verrucay bodies are found in:**
    A. Facial neuroma
    B. Vestibular schwanoma
    C. Cholesterol granuloma
    D. None of the above

34. **The most suitable approach for small intracanalicular vestibular neuroma is:**
    A. Middle cranial fossa
    B. Translabyrnthine
    C. Retrosigmoid
    D. None of the above

35. **The salivary gland cells most affected by radiotherapy is:**
    A. Myoepithelial cells
    B. Intercalated cells
    C. Duet cells
    D. Acinar cells

36. **The swiss cheese appearance in histopathological examination found in:**
    A. Adenocystic cancer
    B. Mucoepidermoid tumor
    C. Warthins tumor
    D. Mixed parotidtumor

37. **The histogenesis of oncocytoma is from:**
    A. Acinar cells
    B. Striated duct cells
    C. Excretory duct cells
    D. Myoepithelial cells

38. **The length of fallopian canal:**
    A. 5 mm
    B. 10 mm
    C. 20 mm
    D. 30 mm

39. **Beverly-Douglas procedure is done for:**
    A. Wardenberg syndrome
    B. Treacher Collin syndrome
    C. Pierre Robin syndrome
    D. Cruzon syndrome

40. **All the following surgeries are indicated for zenkers diverticulum *except:***
    A. Glosscock's operation
    B. Goldman's operation
    C. Dohlman's operation
    D. Denker's operation

41. **External frontoethmoidectomy is otherwise know us:**
    A. Lynch-Howarth's operation
    B. Patterson's operation
    C. Jansen-Horgan operation
    D. McBeth's operation

42. **Meckel's cave is related to:**
    A. Otic ganglion
    B. Gasserian ganglion
    C. Spiral ganglion
    D. Scarpas ganglion

43. **The diagnostic titer for viral capsid antigen to IgA in nasopharyngeal cancer is:**
    A. 1/10   B. 1/20
    C. 1/30   D. 1/40

44. **The cranial nerve not involved in Hugling-Jackson's syndrome is:**
    A. CN IX   B. CN X
    C. CN XI   D. CN XII

45. **The best prognosis in Hodgkins lymphoma is in:**
    A. Lymphocytic predominant type
    B. Lymphocytic depletion type
    C. Nodular sclerosis type
    D. Mixed cellularity type

46. **Cuzzolino's zone is related to:**
    A. Acoustic neuroma
    B. Menier's disease
    C. Otosclerosis
    D. None of the above

47. **Coffin corner is related to:**
    A. Pyriform fossa   B. Retromolar trigone
    C. Base of tongue   D. Ventricle of larynx

48. **Most common cause of acquired postlingual deafness is:**
    A. Mumps   B. Rubella
    C. Toxoplasmosis   D. Meningitis

49. Most common cause of acute simultaneous bilateral facial palsy is:

A. Bell's palsy

B. Ramsay-Hunt syndrome

C. Guillain-Barré-syndrome

D. Melkerson-Rosenthal syndrome

50. The most common neurological lesion in sarcoidosis is:

A. 5th cranial nerve

B. 7th cranial nerve

C. 8th cranial nerve

D. 10th cranial nerve

51. The most common virus causing sensorineural deafness in children is:

A. Mumps virus

B. Parainfluenza virus

C. ECHO virus

D. Cytomegalovirus

ANSWERS

1 A	2 A	3 D	4 D	5 B	6 A	7 A	8 A
9 C	10 A	11 C	12 A	13 C	14 B	15 A	16 B
17 A	18 C	19 D	20 B	21 B	22 B	23 C	24 A
25 A	26 C	27 C	28 A	29 D	30 B	31 B	32 D
33 B	34 A	35 D	36 A	37 B	38 D	39 C	40 D
41 A	42 B	43 A	44 A	45 A	46 C	47 B	48 D
49 C	50 B	51 D					

Miscellaneous-III

1. **Branchogenic carcinoma occurs in:**
   A. Apical segment lung
   B. Pancoast tumor
   C. Branchial cyst wall
   D. Horner's syndrome

2. **Pharyngeal ears are:**
   A. Accessory auricles seen in upper part of neck
   B. Dog ear in sutured pharyngeal wound
   C. Type of congenital ear
   D. Contrast picture of elderly showing normal bulges from tonsillar and pyriform fossa

3. **Neoglottis construction was designed by:**
   A. Asai
   B. Staffieri
   C. Billroth
   D. Schobinger

4. **Lyre sign may be detected in contrast pictures of:**
   A. Glomus tumor
   B. Warthin's tumor
   C. Verrucous tumor
   D. Carotid body tumor

5. **Oort's anastomosis is:**
   A. Vestibulocochlear nerve anastomosis
   B. Vestibulocochlear artery anastomosis
   C. Arteriovenous anastomosis in internal acoustic meatus
   D. Anastomosis of internal and recurrent laryngeal nerve

6. **Morgagni-Stewart-Morel syndrome consists of the following *except*:**
   A. Hyperostosis frontalis interna
   B. Obesity and dizziness
   C. Psychological disturbance and inverted sleep rhythm
   D. Menarche

7. **Gallen's loop is formed by nerve fibers that pass between:**
   A. Anteromedial branch of recurrent laryngeal and external laryngeal nerve
   B. Posteromedial branch of recurrent laryngeal and internal branch of superior laryngeal nerve
   C. External and internal branch of superior laryngeal nerve
   D. None of the above

8. **Prominent Passavant's ridge is seen in:**
   A. Oropharyngeal growth
   B. Berry's syndrome
   C. Cleft palate
   D. Steven Johnson's syndrome

9. **Meige's syndrome is:**
   A. A type of jugular foramen syndrome
   B. An oromandibular syndrome
   C. A chorieform syndrome
   D. None of the above

10. **Vestibular neuronitis is characterized by the following *except*:**
    A. Episode of URI
    B. Nystagmus
    C. SNHL
    D. Vertigo

11. **Myringoplasty is the choice of treatment in:**
    A. Inactive CSOM with perforation and 70db PTA
    B. Active CSOM with perforation and 45db PTA
    C. Inactive CSOM with perforation and 30db PTA
    D. Quiescent CSOM with perforation and 55db PTA

12. **Nasal cholesteatoma is:**
    - A. Rhinophyma
    - B. Rhinitis cascosa
    - C. Rhinitis sicca
    - D. Crusting ozaena

13. **Perforation of bony nasal septum is mostly due to:**
    - A. Pick ulcer
    - B. Over use of snuff
    - C. AFRS
    - D. Syphilis

14. **Quincke's disease is:**
    - A. Peritonsillar abscess
    - B. Lateral sinus thrombosis
    - C. Acute uvular edema
    - D. Acute epiglottitis

15. **Steeple's sign is seen radiologically in:**
    - A. Acute epiglottitis
    - B. Acute laryngotracheobronchitis
    - C. Subglottic stenosis
    - D. Esophageal malignancy

16. **The commonest site of perforation of esophagus is:**
    - A. Narrow area of esophagus at aorta crossing
    - B. Near upper esophageal sphincter
    - C. Near the indentation in esophagus caused by Lt main bronchus
    - D. Near lower esophageal sphincter

17. **Heller's operation is done in:**
    - A. esophageal stricture
    - B. Lieomyoma of esophagus
    - C. Schatzki's ring
    - D. esophagectasia

18. **Laimer-Hackerman's point is the weak area between:**
    - A. Superior and middle constrictors
    - B. Middle and inferior constrictors
    - C. Longitudinal muscles of esophagus
    - D. Thyro and crico pharyngeus

19. **Rhinitis sicca has the following features *except*:**
    - A. Common in dusty surroundings
    - B. Crusting present
    - C. Leads to septal perforation
    - D. Affects posterior part

20. **Mike's dot is a cribriform area in:**
    - A. Lamina cribrosa ethmoidalis
    - B. Macula cribrosa medialis vestibuli
    - C. Macula cribrosa superioris vestibuli
    - D. Cribriform area over fovea mastoideum

21. **Stereotactic radiosurgery of the acoustic neuroma can be deleterious in:**
    - A. Solid tumors
    - B. Peritumoural edema
    - C. Hemorrhagic tumors
    - D. Cysts with acoustic neuroma

22. **Particle repositioning maneuver may obviate surgery in:**
    - A. Endolymphatic hydrops
    - B. Canalolithiasis
    - C. Iatrogenic vertigo
    - D. Post concussional syndrome

23. **Marble bone disease is:**
    - A. Sclerosteosis
    - B. Osteoectasia
    - C. Osteitis deformans
    - D. Osteopetrosis

24. **Evoked otoacoustic emissions are released from:**
    - A. Inner hair cells
    - B. Outer hair cells
    - C. Spiral ganglia
    - D. Organ of corti

25. **Open-roof deformity is a complication seen in:**
    - A. Laryngeal stenosis
    - B. Reduction rhinoplasty
    - C. CSF fistula repair
    - D. Cochlear implant surgery

26. **Goldman's technique improvises:**
    - A. Ossiculoplasty with gold prosthesis
    - B. Tippoplasty
    - C. Mentoplasty
    - D. Dohlmann's operation

27. **Brun's nystagmus is:**
    - A. An optokinetic railway nystagmus
    - B. A direction changing nystamus seen in acoustic neurofibroma
    - C. A benign positional nystagmus seen in vestibular neuronitis
    - D. A type of congenital nystagmus

28. **Anemometry refers to:**
    - A. Embryonic inner ear fluid analysis
    - B. Assessment of middle ear fluid in barotraumas
    - C. Study of pressure changes in dysbarism
    - D. Measure of nasal air flow to assess velopharyngeal insufficiency

29. **Collaural fistula is due to:**
   A. 1st branchial cleft anomaly
   B. 2nd branchial cleft anomaly
   C. 3rd branchial cleft anomaly
   D. Measure of nasal air flow to assess velopharyngeal insufficiency

30. **Cookie bite audiometric air conduction curve suggests:**
   A. Acoustic neuroma
   B. Acoustic trauma
   C. Cochlear otosclerosis
   D. Early Meniere's disease

31. **The most common symptom of glomus tumor is:**
   A. Tinnitus   B. Vertigo
   C. HOH   D. Diplopia

32. **Neurovascular conflict is detected in Obersteiner-Redlich zone in cases of:**
   A. Tinnitus
   B. Trigeminal neuralgia
   C. Hemifacial spasm
   D. Disabling positional vertigo

33. **The landmarks encountered in endolymphatic sac surgery are the following except:**
   A. Donaldson's line B. Irv's ridge
   C. Bill's island   D. Mike's dot

34. **Fluctuating sensorineural hearing loss may be associated with the following except:**
   A. Meniere's disease
   B. Perilymph fistula
   C. Cogan's disease
   D. Multiple sclerosis

35. **Diagnosis of silent otitis media does not include:**
   A. HOH
   B. Vertigo
   C. Pressure or pain
   D. Dry perforation of pars tensa

36. **Mogiphonia is:**
   A. Hesitation of conversation
   B. Stammering
   C. Defective articulation
   D. Phonic spasm during professional speech

37. **Visual aphasia is:**
   A. Word deafness   B. Word blindness
   C. Congenital alexia D. Hemianopia

38. **PRM is not indicated in:**
   A. Cupulolithiasis   B. Canalolithiasis
   C. BPPV   D. VBI

39. **Botulism toxin is successfully used in the following ENT problems except:**
   A. Spasmodic dysphonia
   B. Hemifacial spasm
   C. Spastic deaf mutes
   D. Torticollis

40. **Leptothrix are associated with:**
   A. Leptospirosis with aphthous ulcers
   B. Tophi
   C. Keratosis pharyngis
   D. Leptomeningitis

41. **'Dish-face' deformity is seen in:**
   A. JNA
   B. Aprosexia
   C. Guerin's fracture
   D. Complication of rhinoplasty

42. **Prelaryngeal node is also known as:**
   A. Henle's node
   B. Rouviere's node
   C. Delphian node
   D. Wood's node

43. **The nerve of 3rd pharyngeal arch is:**
   A. Trigeminal
   B. Vagus
   C. Facial
   D. Glossopharyngeal

44. **'Reversed ear' is seen in:**
   A. Congenital anomaly
   B. Sonoinversion
   C. Complication of otoplasty
   D. Barotrauma of external ear canal

45. **One of the components of Beahr's triangle is:**
   A. Superior semicircular canal
   B. Facial nerve
   C. Recurrent laryngeal nerve
   D. Middle fossa dura

46. **In laryngeal verrucous carcinoma:**
   A. Warty papillomatous appearance is uncommon
   B. Supraglottic site is more than glottic
   C. Lymphatic spread is common
   D. Radiotherapy is not better than surgery

47. Functional laryngeal dyskinesia requires:
- A. Tracheostomy
- B. Assertiveness training
- C. Distraction technique
- D. Invasive investigations

48. Palatal nystagmus may be consequent to:
- A. Laryngeal vertigo
- B. Torticollis
- C. Multiple sclerosis
- D. Velopharyngeal insufficiency

49. Endonasal DCR was first described by:
- A. Rebiz
- B. Caldwell
- C. Bowlds
- D. Pankrator

50. Choanal adenoidectomy is relatively safer and incomplete with:
- A. Microdebrider
- B. Transnasal Weil's forceps removal
- C. Adenotome curettage
- D. Endoscopic suction diathermy curettage

51. Who introduced cartilage in reconstructive middle ear surgery?
- A. Utech
- B. Sheehy
- C. Hildman
- D. Helms

52. Stennert's protocol is followed in:
- A. Taking Stenver's view X-ray
- B. Preparation for endolymphatic sac decompression
- C. Treatment of Bell's palsy
- D. Diagnosis of dysbarism

53. Cartilage palisading in tympanoplasty is done primarily to prevent:
- A. PORP dislocation
- B. Atelectasis
- C. Warping
- D. TORP dislocation

54. "Anatomy of the nasal cavity and its pneumatic appendices" was published by:
- A. Messerklinger
- B. von Graefe
- C. Emil zuckercandl
- D. Draf

55. In a month old total facial paralysis the EDT that determines status of nerve is:
- A. Nerve excitability test
- B. Electroneuronography
- C. Electromyography
- D. None of the above

56. Griesel's syndrome is a complication of:
- A. Lateral sinus thrombosis
- B. Dorello's canal suppuration
- C. Adenoidectomy
- D. Petrosectomy

57. Cochlear implants:
- A. Provide normal hearing
- B. Note done below 10 years
- C. Enables sound detection but hearing is not normal
- D. Done for anyone with SNHL

58. Treatment of glomus jugulare does not include:
- A. Radiotherapy
- B. Surgical excision
- C. Internal jugular vein ligation
- D. Vascular embolisation

59. Bone conductor hearing aid should not be used in:
- A. CSOM with persistently wet ear causing deafness
- B. Bilateral meatal atresia
- C. Intractable ext otitis
- D. Presbyacusis

60. Congenital SNHL can be caused by:
- A. Treacher Collins syndrome
- B. Wardenburg's syndrome
- C. Down's syndrome
- D. None of the above

61. Nonperipheral vestibular disorder is:
- A. ANF
- B. BPPV
- C. Iatrogenic dizziness
- D. Meniere's disease

62. A patient with anosmia should respond to inhalation of:
- A. Oil of lemon
- B. Coffee
- C. Ammonia
- D. None of the above

63. Olfactory sensibility:
- A. Provides flavor component to taste
- B. Is unaffected by total laryngectomy
- C. May be lost after of cribrifrom plate
- D. Fatigues quickly

64. Radiological diagnosis of adenoid hypertrophy is possible in:
- A. Hypogammaglobulinaemia
- B. Wiskott-Aldrich syndrome
- C. Griesel's syndrome
- D. Guy's aprosexia

65. Nasal congestion in women is uncommon in:
- A. Pregnancy
- B. Myxoedema
- C. Progesterone contraceptive pill intake
- D. None of the above

66. Rodent ulcer does not cause:
- A. Pain
- B. Non metastasizing ulcers
- C. Non healing ulcerations
- D. None of the above

67. Functional voice disorders exist when:
- A. Abnormal laryngeal functions are present
- B. No abnormality is seen
- C. Cough is abnormal and voice is normal
- D. Swallowing is abnormal but cough and voice are normal

68. Intraoperative audiometry during stapedectomy is:
- A. Contraindicated
- B. Impossible
- C. In determining best prosthesis and its placement for optimum hearing
- D. Unreliable

69. Laser STAMP surgery is done in:
- A. Locus valsalvae micro angiomas
- B. Berry aneurysms
- C. Localised fissula antefenestral otosclerosis
- D. CSF fistulas

70. Abnormally patulous Eustachian tube is not diagnosed by:
- A. Autophony
- B. Elevated oestrogen levels
- C. Weight loss
- D. Absolutely normal hearing

71. Fungus cerebri is:
- A. Fungal infection of the brain
- B. Endaural encephalocele
- C. Variant of malignant otitis externa
- D. None of the above

72. Grolin's syndrome does not include:
- A. Frontal bossing
- B. Pigmented basal cell carcinoma
- C. Hypoplastic mandible
- D. Hyperpteliorism

73. CSF leak encountered in middle ear is usually through:
- A. Glasserian fissure
- B. Santorini's fissure
- C. Korner's fissure
- D. Hyrtl's fissure

74. Salicylism is:
- A. Sialadenitis
- B. Hypersalivation
- C. NSAID toxicity
- D. Rhinophonia

75. The importance of Chassaignac's triangle identification and dissection is in clearing:
- A. Henle's node
- B. Wood's node
- C. Scalene node
- D. Delphian node

76. Phonomicrosurgical management of vocal cord polyp is done by:
- A. Cold knife resection
- B. Laser resection
- C. Epithelial cordotomy and subepithelial resection
- D. Micro shaver resection

77. Pseudotumor of orbit does not cause:
- A. Immune based inflammation
- B. Complicate Tolosa-Hunt syndrome
- C. Low sedimentation rate
- D. Proptosis

78. The maximum incidence of mucoceles is seen in:
- A. Posterior ethmoid
- B. Sphenoid
- C. Maxillary
- D. Frontoethmoid

79. Fungal balls are diagnosed by the presence of:
- A. Allergic mucin
- B. Tissue invasion detected on histopathology
- C. Mass of fungal hyphe in the lumen of sinus
- D. Immunodeficiency

80. The gold standard investigation in laryngo-pharyngeal reflux is:
- A. Endoscopy
- B. Pharyngeal pH monitoring
- C. Barium esophagogram
- D. Radionuclide scintigraphy

81. **Bull's eye lense was devised by:**
    - A. Bull
    - B. Morrel mackinze
    - C. Van troltsche
    - D. Kramer

82. **CSOM is not characterized by:**
    - A. Otorrhoea
    - B. Hearing impairment
    - C. Pain
    - D. Dry spells

83. **Cavum minor is created in:**
    - A. Cavity obliteration
    - B. Blind sac closure
    - C. Type IV tympanoplasty
    - D. Skin grafting after maxillectomy

84. **Shian-Lee technique is attempted in:**
    - A. Laryngeal stenosis
    - B. Dysphagia
    - C. Drooling of saliva
    - D. Meatoplasty

85. **In a normal ear:**
    - A. Tensor tympani and stapedius muscles are not innervated by the motor branch of maxillary nerve
    - B. Stapedius doesn't contract to alter stapes movement in response to loud sound
    - C. Levels of discomfort and sound intolerance occurs at 60 db
    - D. Action of stapedius may not be detected by tympanometry

86. **Deafness in a 2 yr old child is commonly due to:**
    - A. Neonatal jaundice
    - B. Cholesteatoma
    - C. Glue ear
    - D. Wax

87. **Primary mastoid exploration is not warranted in CSOM with:**
    - A. Onset of facial paralysis
    - B. +ve fistula sign
    - C. Ipsilateral headache
    - D. Onset of vertigo

88. **Laser STAMP surgery requires:**
    - A. Schucknecht wire prosthesis
    - B. Teflon piston
    - C. No prosthesis
    - D. Laser fenestration of LSC

89. **REZ (root entry zone) in vascular compression in cases of hemifacial spasm lie at Magnan's division of:**
    - A. Superior level
    - B. Intermediate level
    - C. Inferior level
    - D. None of the above

90. **Adenoids:**
    - A. Secrete mucus
    - B. Cause snoring as they move
    - C. Involved in immune reactions
    - D. Source of chronic sepsis

91. **Nasal swab in an asymptomatic patient may reveal:**
    - A. *Staphylococcus aureus*
    - B. *Streptococcus β hemolytic type*
    - C. Haemophilus influenza
    - D. *Coagulase positive streptococcus*

92. **Symptoms of septal perforation may not include:**
    - A. Whistiling
    - B. Crusting
    - C. Nasal discharge
    - D. Obstruction

93. **Autoimmune inner ear disease:**
    - A. Presents with normal hearing
    - B. May be picked up by Western blot assays
    - C. Does not improve with steroid therapy
    - D. Is never associated with systemic autoimmune disease

94. **Gold standard treatment of esthesio-olfactory neuroblastoma is:**
    - A. Radiotherapy
    - B. Endoscopic excision
    - C. Lateral rhinotomy excision and adjunct radiotherapy
    - D. Radiotherapy and chemotherapy

95. **Branchial cysts are common in:**
    - A. Anomalous 1st branchial cleft
    - B. Anomalous 2nd branchial cleft
    - C. Anomalous 3rd branchial cleft
    - D. Anomalous 4th branchial cleft

96. **Specific infectious causes of hoarseness include the following *except*:**
    - A. Tuberculosis
    - B. Candida
    - C. Sarcoidosis
    - D. Syphilis

97. Gastroesophageal reflux in children:

A. Is uncommon in the newborn
B. Is not associated with sliding hernia
C. May be associated with recurrent respiratory tract infections in older children
D. Does not require usually endoscopy

98. Important symptom for esophageal disease includes:

A. Sensation of lump in the throat
B. Pain on swallowing
C. Difficulty in swallowing
D. All of the above

99. Pleomorphic adenoma of the parotid is not:

A. A benign tumor
B. Surrounded by pseudocapsule
C. Excised with a wide margin
D. Operable when recurrent

100. Congenital choanal atresia:

A. Is diagnosed early if unilateral
B. Usually has membranous defect
C. Does not require surgical management if bilateral
D. May be associated with other congenital defects

ANSWERS

1 C	2 D	3 B	4 D	5 A	6 D	7 B	8 C
9 B	10 C	11 C	12 B	13 D	14 C	15 B	16 C
17 D	18 C	19 D	20 C	21 D	22 B	23 D	24 B
25 B	26 B	27 B	28 D	29 A	30 C	31 C	32 C
33 D	34 C	35 D	36 D	37 B	38 D	39 C	40 C
41 C	42 C	43 D	44 D	45 C	46 D	47 B	48 C
49 B	50 B	51 A	52 C	53 C	54 C	55 C	56 C
57 C	58 C	59 D	60 B	61 C	62 C	63 B	64 D
65 C	66 A	67 B	68 C	69 C	70 D	71 B	72 C
73 D	74 C	75 C	76 C	77 C	78 D	79 C	80 B
81 B	82 C	83 C	84 A	85 A	86 C	87 C	88 C
89 B	90 C	91 A	92 C	93 B	94 C	95 B	96 C
97 C	98 C	99 D	100 D				

Miscellaneous-IV

1. **Otogenic retropharyngeal abscess is caused by:**
   - A. Lateral sinus phlebits
   - B. Extradural perisinus abscess
   - C. Otic cholesteatoma
   - D. Petrositis

2. **The commonest symptom of foreign body in a child is:**
   - A. Cough
   - B. Wheezing
   - C. Vomiting
   - D. Dyspnea

3. **Which of the following is not a complication of tracheostomy?**
   - A. Subglottic stenosis
   - B. Subcutaneous emphysema
   - C. Rupture of internal jugular vein
   - D. Infection

4. **Which of the following is a characteristic sign of oesophageal atresia in child?**
   - A. Dribbling of saliva
   - B. Dyspnea
   - C. Cyanosis
   - D. Distension of abdomen

5. **The following are recognized complications of diptheria except:**
   - A. Myocarditis
   - B. Periuvular abscess
   - C. Polyneuritis
   - D. Nephritis

6. **White striae presenting a lace pattern on the buccal mucosa with possible skinlesions:**
   - A. Leukoplakia
   - B. Fordyces spots
   - C. Lichen planus
   - D. None of the above

7. **What is the most possible diagnosis— Necrotising gingivitis and oropharyngeal ulcerations in a patient with severe halitosis?**
   - A. Infectious mononucleosis
   - B. Oropharyngeal candidiasis
   - C. Vincents' angina
   - D. None of the above

8. **Riolan's bouquet is:**
   - A. Styloid process
   - B. Stylomandibular ligament
   - C. Stylohyoid
   - D. Styloid apparatus

9. **Lancinating pain around the tonsils during eating is indicative of:**
   - A. Trigeminal neuralgia
   - B. Glossopharyngeal neuralgia
   - C. Facial neuralgia
   - D. None of the above

10. **The cause of white patch in mouth is all except:**
    - A. Candida
    - B. Aphthous ulcer
    - C. Leukoplakia
    - D. Lichen planus

11. **The most common danger of fiberoptic bronchoscopy is:**
    - A. Hypoxemia
    - B. Hypercapnia
    - C. Respiratory acidosis
    - D. Low arteriolar CO_2

12. **Lump in the throat not interfering with swallowing is:**
    - A. Globus hystericus
    - B. Cervical spondylosis
    - C. Pharyngeal diverticulum
    - D. Carcinoma esophagus

13. **Key hole appearance of glottis is seen on laryngoscopy in:**
    A. Functional aphonia
    B. Bilateral complete paralysis of vocal cords
    C. Bilateral imcomplete paralysis of vocal cords
    D. Phonasthenia

14. **All are related to OSAS except:**
    A. Respiratory effort
    B. Snoring
    C. Periodic breathing
    D. Cardiac complications

15. **Total length of fallopian canal is:**
    A. 20 to 25 mm   B. 25 to 29 mm
    C. 28 to 33 mm   D. 33 to 38 mm

16. **Rearding tuning fork tests all are possible in conductive deafness except:**
    A. Positive rinne
    B. Negative rinne
    C. Lateralised weber
    D. Reduced ABC

17. **Boiler marker's notch in pure tone audiogram is:**
    A. Dip at 2000 Hz in bone conduction audiogram
    B. Dip at 4000 Hz in bone conduction audiogram
    C. DIP at 3000 Hz in bone conduction audiogram
    D. None of the above

18. **SP/AP widening in electrocochleogram is a feature of:**
    A. Otosclerosis
    B. Acoustic neuroma
    C. Meniere's disease
    D. Vestibular neuronitis

19. **All are true regarding nystagmus except:**
    A. Presence of nystagmus indicates vestibular pathology
    B. Severest form of nystagmus is the third degree nystagmus
    C. Peripheral nystagmus is suppressed by fixation
    D. Irritative lesions of labyrinth produces nystagmus to opposite side while paralytic to same side

20. **All are tests in vertiginous patients except:**
    A. Fistula test   B. Corneal reflex
    C. Romberg's tests   D. Caloric test
    E. Patch test

21. **Match the following type of deafness with features:**

Table A		Table B
A. Conductive deafness	i.	Meniere's disease
B. Sudden sensorineural hearing loss	ii.	Presbyacusis
C. Fluctuant sensorineural hearing loss	iii.	Alzhiemer's disease
D. Reversible sensorineural hearing loss	iv.	Viral
E. Central deafness	v.	Pathology upto foot plate of stapes
F. Bilateral symetric sensorineural hearing loss	vi.	Ototoxicity
	vii	Cochlear otosclerosis

22. **All are true regarding malignant external otitis except:**
    A. Invasive/necrotising otitis
    B. Causative organism-Pseudomonas
    C. Immunocompromised patients
    D. Skull base osteomyelitis
    E. Commonest cranial nerve involved is VII nerve

23. **Fill in the blanks:**
    A. Commonest tympanic meembrane finding in eustachian tube dysfucntion is ....
    B. Commonest cause of conductive deafness in a child is ....
    C. Adult male with unilareal OME, rule out ....
    D. Commonest cause of bilateral OME in a child ....
    E. Severe ear ache and blocked sensation in a perosn immediately after air travel ....

24. **Where do you see the following otoscopic findings on the tympanic membrane?**
    A. Cart wheel appearance
    B. Hair line with air bubbles
    C. Blue drum
    D. Chalky patches
    E. Rising sun sign
    F. Irregular perforation
    G. Multiple perforations

25. **Regarding CSOM the true statement is:**
    A. Central perforations means tubotympanic disease and are never associated with cholesteatoma
    B. Anterior perforations cause more hearing loss than posterior perforations
    C. Reniform perforations are comparatively rare
    D. Most common ossicle to be affected by cholesteatoma is long process of incus

26. All of the following are related to glomus tumors *except:*
    A. Non chromaffin paraganglioma
    B. Ascending pharyngeal artery
    C. Sensory neural deafness
    D. Bleeding aural polyp

27. Earliest sensory modality to be impaired in acoustic neuroma ....

28. Impairment of sensation of posterior meatal wal of EAM is known as ....

29. Investigation of choice in acoustic neuroma is ....

30. Uveoparotitis with bilateral pacial palsy is a feature of:
    A. Ramsay-Hunt syndrome
    B. Melkerson-Rosenthal syndrome
    C. Heerfordts syndrome
    D. Moebius syndrome

31. Rehabilitation option following bilateral acoustic neuroma surgery is ....

32. An instrument used to confim velopharyngeal incompetence and quantify is ....

33. The rarest type of tracheoesophageal fistula is:
    A. Esophageal atresia with distal tracheo esophageal fistula
    B. Esophagal atresia with proximal and distal tracheo esophageal fistula
    C. Esophageal atresia without tracheo esophageal fistula
    D. Esophageal atresia with proximal tracheo esophageal fistula

34. CHARGE association in choanal atresia includes all *except:*
    A. Ear deformities
    B. Genital hypopalsia
    C. Colobomatous blindness
    D. Radial dysplasia
    E. Retarded growth and development

35. All are anatomical structures related to paranasal sinuses *except:*
    A. Accessory ostium   B. 1st molar
    C. Internal carotid artery D. Lamina papyracea
    E. Crest of maxilla

36. Space between superior constrictor and base of skull is:
    A. Killian's Dehiscence
    B. Sinus of morgagni
    C. Sinus of His
    D. Space of Boyers

37. Lupus perino in a patient with multisystem involvement is a feature of:
    A. Tertiary syphilis
    B. Tuberculosis
    C. Midline nonhealing granulomas
    D. Sarcoidosis
    E. None of the above

38. Potts puffy tumor is feature of:
    A. Osteomyelitis of maxilla
    B. Mucocoele
    C. Intracerebral abscess
    D. Osteomyelitis of frontal bone

39. Diplopia, enophthalmos, difficulty in elevating, the globe with infraorbital anesthesia constitute:
    A. Tripod fracture of zygoma
    B. Jarjauay fracture
    C. Blow out fracture of orbit
    D. Lefort's fracture

40. Clown's cap deformity is a feature of:
    A. Pfeiffers syndrome
    B. Aperts syndrome
    C. Crouzon's syndrome
    D. Treacher Collin syndrome

41. A facet between the columella and lateral rim of the nostrial is referred to as:
    A. Nasolabial angle B. Dome
    C. Soft triangle   D. All of the above

42. Palatal palsy, retro-orbital pain and conductive deafness are components of:
    A. Gradenigo's syndrome
    B. Trotter's triad
    C. Avelli's syndrome
    D. Samter's triad

43. The surface area of nasopharynx in an adult is:
    A. 60 cm^2
    B. 55 cm^2
    C. 50 cm^2
    D. 65 cm^2

44. Pendred syndrome is_____with nerve deafness:
   A. Meniere's syndrome
   B. Thyroid swelling
   C. Cardiac defect
   D. Renal defect

45. Ramadier's operation is done in:
   A. Bells palsy
   B. Meniere's disease
   C. CSOM
   D. Petrositis

46. Stapedius reflex is mediated by:
   A. V and VI nerves
   B. V and VII nerves
   C. VII and VI nerves
   D. VII and VIII nerves

47. The volume of mastoid antrum in adult is_____.
   A. 2.5 ml
   B. 7.0 ml
   C. 1 ml
   D. 15 ml

48. Albright's syndrome consists of all of the following *except*:
   A. Polyostotic fibrous dysplasia
   B. Pigmented skin lesion
   C. Precocious puberty
   D. Endocrine abnormalities
   E. Epistaxis

49. The primary etiological factor in contact ulcer of the larynx is:
   A. Syphilis
   B. Tuberculosis
   C. Viral
   D. Vocal abuse

50. Mogiphonia means:
   A. Hesitation in starting conversation
   B. Frequent interruptions during speech
   C. Sudden glottic spasm during ordinary conversation
   D. Sudden glottic spasm at the start of professional speech

ANSWERS

1 D   2 B   3 C   4 A   5 B   6 B   7 C   8 D
9 B   10 D   11 A   12 A   13 D   14 C   15 C   16 D
17 B   18 C   19 D   20 F   21 A–v, B – iv, C – i, D – vi, E – iii, F – ii   22 E

23 A – RETRACTED TYMPANIC MEMBRANE
   B – SEROUS OTITIS MEDIA
   C – NASOPHARYNGEAL CARCINOMA
   D – ADENOIDS
   E – OTITIC BAROTRAUMA

24 A – ASOMCACUTE SUPPURATIVE OTITIS MEDIA
   B – SEROUS OTITIS MEDIA
   C – HAEMOTYMPANUM
   D – TYMPANOSCLEROSIS
   E – GLOMUS TUMOUR
   F – TRAUMATIC PERFORATION
   G – TUBERCULOSIS   25 D   26 C

27 CORNEAL REFLEX
28 HITSELBERGER'S SIGN
29 MRI WITH GADOLINIUM ENHANCEMENT   30 C
31 AUDITORY BRAIN STEM IMPLANT
32 PERCI (PALATAL EFFICIENCY RATING COMPUTED INSTANTANEOUSLY)
33 B   34 D   35 E   36 B   37 D   38 D   39 C   40 C
41 C   42 B   43 C   44 B   45 D   46 D   47 C   48 E
49 B   50 D

44. Pendred syndrome is _____ with nerve deafness.

A. Morizzo's syndrome
B. Thyroid swelling
C. Goitre nodal
D. Renal distal cysts

45. Ramadier's operation is done in:

A. Bell's palsy
B. Meniere's disease
C. CSOM
D. Tinnitus

46. Stapedius relex is mediated by:

A. V and VI nerves
B. V and VII nerves
C. VI and VII nerves
D. VII and VIII nerves

47. The volume of mastoid antrum in adult is _____

A. 2 ml
B. 12 ml
C. 6 ml
D. 15 ml

48. Albright's syndrome consists of all of the following except:

A. Polyostotic fibrous-dysplasia
B. Pigmented skin lesion
C. Precocious puberty
D. Endocrine abnormalities
E. Epistaxis

49. The primary etiological factor in contact ulcer of the larynx is:

A. Syphilis
B. Tuberculosis
C. Viral
D. Vocal abuse

50. Mophonia means:

A. Healthcare in single conversation
B. Frequent alteration during speech
C. Sudden glottic basm during ordinary conversation
D. Sudden shift in pitch ahead of professional speech

ANSWERS

1. C	2. B	3. C	4. A	5. B	6. B	7. A	8. D
9. B	10. D	11. A	12. A	13. D	14. C	15. C	16. D
17. D	18. C	19. D	20. T	21. A	22. B—W, C—I, D—V, E—III, F—II	22. E

23. A – RETRACTED TYMPANIC MEMBRANE
B – SEROUS OTITIS MEDIA
C – NASOPHARYNGEAL CARCINOMA
D – ADENOIDS
E – OTITIC BAROTRAUMA

24. A – ACUTE SUPPURATIVE OTITIS MEDIA
B – SEROUS OTITIS MEDIA
C – HAEMOTYMPANUM
D – TYMPANOSCLEROSIS
E – GLOMUS TUMOUR
F – TRAUMATIC PERFORATION
G – TUBERCULOSIS

27. CORNEAL REFLEX
28. LITTLE.BERGER'S SIGN
29. MRI WITH GADOLINIUM ENHANCEMENT   30. C
31. AUDITORY BRAIN STEM IMPLANT

32. FERDI (FAL ATAE EFFRIGENCY RATING COMPUTED INSTANT AND DUST V)

33. E	34. D	35. E	36. C	37. D	38. D	39. C	40. C
41. C	42. E	43. C	44. B	45. D	46. D	47. C	48. E
49. B	50. D

Bibliography

1. Stell and Maran's Head and Neck Surgery, Fourth Edition, 2000 by Reed Educational and Professional Publishing Ltd.
2. A Synopsis of Otolaryngology by John C Ballantyne and John Grones, 5th Edition.
3. Essential Otolaryngology and Head and Neck Surgery by KJ.
4. Lee, 8th Edition, McGraw-Hill Medical Publishing Division, 2003.
5. Textbook of Pathology, 2nd Edition by Harsh Mohan
6. Grant's Method of Anatomy (A Clinical Problem Solving Approach), 71th Edition by Basmajan, Slonecker, Williams and Wilkins International Edition Textbook of Head and Neck Anatomy of James L Hiatt, LP Gartner.
7. Plastic and Reconstructive surgery of Head and Neck (Vol. 1) Proceedings on 40th International Symposium on Asthetic Surgery.
8. An Introduction to Neurotology by Anirban Biswas, Second Edition.
9. Pye's Surgical Handicraft, 21st Edition, Edited by James Kyle (Centenary edition).
10. The Otolaryngologic Clinics of North America, April 2003, Edited by Aristides Sismanis (WB Saunders Company).
11. Maxillofacial Injuries by NL Rowe and Williams (Vol. 1) Published by Churchill Livingstone, 1985.
12. Harper's Biochemistry, Twenty fifth edition, 2002.
13. Nelson Textbook of Paediatrics, 17th edition, 2004.
14. Harrison's Principles of Internal Medicine, 15th Edition, 2001.
15. Goodman and Gillman's. The Pharmacological Basis of Therapeutics, 11th Edition, 2006.
16. Robbin's Pathologic Basis of Disease, 6th Edition, 2000.
17. Guyton and Hall, Textbook of Medical Physiology, 10th edition, 2000.
18. Bailey and Love's, Short Practise of Surgery, 23rd edition, 2000.
19. Bailey and Scott's Diagnostic Microbiology, 11th edition, 2002.
20. Comprehensive Textbook of Psychiatry, HI Kaplan and BJ Sadock, 7th edition, 2005, Williams and Wilkins Company, Philadelphia.
21. Essentials of Psychiatry, V Eapen, P Kulhara, R Raguram, 1st edition 2005, Paras Medical Publisher Hyderabad.
22. Year Book of Psychiatry, JA Talbotl et at. 2006, Mosby Elsveir, Philadelphia.
23. Uncommon psychiatric syndromes, David Enoch and Hadrian Ball. 4th edition, 2004, Viva Book Pvt Ltd.
24. Short Textbook of Psychiatry, Niraj Ahuja, 6th edition, 2006, Jaypee Brothers Medical Publishers, New Delhi.
25. Scott-Brown's Otolaryngology, 6th edition. Volume 1-Vol.6 Edited by David A, Adams and Micheel J Cinnmod.
26. Cancer of the Head & Neck, Stephan and Ariyan, MD Published by CV Mosby Company.
27. Operative Otorhinolaryngology. Edited by Nigel Bleach. Chris Mitford. Andrew Van Hasselt.
28. Glasscock and Shambaugh-Surgery of the ear Fifth Edition.
29. Ballenger's Otorhinolaryngology Head and Neck Surgery. Sixteenth Edition James B Snow Jr, MD John Jacob Ballenger, MD.
30. Cummings Otolaryngology, Head and Neck Surgery Fourth Edition, Volumes 1-Volume 4.
31. Byron J. Bailey, Head and Neck Surgery Otolaryngology. Third Edition Volume One and Two.

32. Radiation Oncology Management Decisions KS Cufford Chao MD, Carlos - A - Perez MD, Luther W. Bready MD - 2002. St Louis, Missouri and Philadelphia.

33. Textbook of Radiotherapy Gilbert H Fletcher MD; MD Anderson Hospital Texas, 1980.

34. Technological Basic of Radiation Therapy Pratical and Clinical Applications. Levitt and Tapley's Seymour H, Levitt MD. Paiz M Khan PhD, Roger A, Potish MD, 2nd edition, 1992.

35. Principles and Practice of Radiotherapy Charier M Wastington-Texas Dennis Leaver-Portland, Edition - 2004.

36. Neurological Differential Diagnosis John Patten, 2nd edition, 2001 Springer.

37. Principles of Neurology. Raymond D Adam Maurice Victor, Fourth edition, 1989 McGraw Hill International Edition.

38. Neurological Surgery Julian. R. Youmans Fourth Edition, 1996 WB Saunders Company.

39. Merritts Textbook of Neurology, Edited by Lewis R Rowland 9th Edition, 1995 William and Wilkins

40. Operative Neurosurgical Techniques. Schmidek and Sweet 4th Edition, 2000 WB Saunders Company.

41. Parson's Diseases of the Eye, Edited by Ramanjit Sihota, Radhika Tandon, 20th Edition, Elsevier Publications.

42. Textbook of Ophthalmology. Yanoff. 1st Edition Mosby Publications.

43. Essentials of Ophthalmology. Pradeep Sharma, 1st Edition, Modern Publishers.

44. Basic Ophthalmology, Renu Jogi, 3rd Edition Jaypee Brothers Medical Publishers New Delhi.

45. A Synopsis of Anaesthesia by Atkinson, RS, Rushman, GB, Lee AJ, 10th Edition, 1987.

46. A Practise of Anaesthesia, 5th Edition by Churchill Davidson HC, Year Book, Medical Publishers, Chicago 1984.

47. Anaesthesia, A Comprehensive Review, 3rd edition Mosby Publications.

48. A Textbook of Anaesthesia, 2nd Edition Aitkenhead AR and Smith G, Churchill Living Stone, Edinburgh.

49. GoodMan and Gillman's pharmacological basis of therapeutics, 8th edition, Pergamon Press, Oxford.

50. Textbook of Medical Physiology by Guyton AC, 7th Edition 1986.

51. Gray's Anatomy, 37th Edition, Churchill Livingstone, Edinburgh.

52. Anaesthesia by Miller RD, 3rd Edition, Churchill Livingstone, Edinburgh.

53. Bailey and Love's, Short Practice of Surgery, 24th Edition, 2004, RCG Russell, Norman S William Christopher JK Bulstrode.

54. Oxford Textbook of Surgery, 2nd Edition, 2000, Peter J Morris William C Wood.

55. Schwartz's Principles of surgery, 18th Edition, 2005. F Charles Brunicardi.

56. Sabiston Textbook of Surgery 17th Edition, 2004 Courtney M Townsend, Jr MD.

57. Textbook of surgery, The Association of Surgeons of India, 1st Edition, 2003, Dr Ahmad A Hai Dr Rabindra B Shrivastava.

58. Textbook of Biochemistry DM Vasudevan 4th Edition, 2005.

59. Textbook of Medical Biochemistry MN Chatterjee Rana Shinde 5th Edition, 2002.